biostatistics

an applied introduction for the public health practitioner

PUBLIC HEALTH PROFESSIONAL

biostatistics

an applied introduction for the public health practitioner

first edition

heather m. bush

series editor f. douglas scutchfield

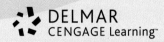
DELMAR
CENGAGE Learning™

Australia • Brazil • Japan • Korea • Mexico • Singapore • Spain • United Kingdom • United States

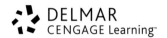

Biostatistics: An Applied Introduction for the Public Health Practitioner, First Edition
Heather M. Bush

Vice President, Editorial: Dave Garza

Director of Learning Solutions: Matthew Kane

Senior Acquisitions Editor: Tari Broderick

Managing Editor: Marah Bellegarde

Associate Product Manager: Meghan E. Orvis

Editorial Assistant: Nicole Manikas

Vice President, Marketing: Jennifer Ann Baker

Senior Marketing Manager: Michele McTighe

Marketing Coordinator: Scott A. Chrysler

Production Manager: Andrew Crouth

Senior Content Project Manager:
    Kathryn B. Kucharek

Senior Art Director: Jack Pendleton

For product information and technology assistance, contact us at
Cengage Learning Customer & Sales Support, 1-800-354-9706
For permission to use material from this text or product,
submit all requests online at **cengage.com/permissions**
Further permissions questions can be emailed to
permissionrequest@cengage.com

Library of Congress Control Number: 2011925054

ISBN-13: 978-1-1110-3514-3

ISBN-10: 1-1110-3514-8

Delmar
5 Maxwell Drive
Clifton Park, NY 12065-2919
USA

Cengage Learning is a leading provider of customized learning solutions with office locations around the globe, including Singapore, the United Kingdom, Australia, Mexico, Brazil, and Japan. Locate your local office at:
international.cengage.com/region

Cengage Learning products are represented in Canada by Nelson Education, Ltd.

To learn more about Delmar, visit **www.cengage.com/delmar**

Purchase any of our products at your local college store or at our preferred online store **www.cengagebrain.com**

Notice to the Reader
Publisher does not warrant or guarantee any of the products described herein or perform any independent analysis in connection with any of the product information contained herein. Publisher does not assume, and expressly disclaims, any obligation to obtain and include information other than that provided to it by the manufacturer. The reader is expressly warned to consider and adopt all safety precautions that might be indicated by the activities described herein and to avoid all potential hazards. By following the instructions contained herein, the reader willingly assumes all risks in connection with such instructions. The publisher makes no representations or warranties of any kind, including but not limited to, the warranties of fitness for particular purpose or merchantability, nor are any such representations implied with respect to the material set forth herein, and the publisher takes no responsibility with respect to such material. The publisher shall not be liable for any special, consequential, or exemplary damages resulting, in whole or part, from the readers' use of, or reliance upon, this material.

Printed in the United States of America
1 2 3 4 5 6 7 15 14 13 12 11

This book is dedicated
with love to
Josh and Beatrix.
SDG

CONTENTS

LIST OF TABLES

CHAPTER 7

APPENDIX A

APPENDIX B

USING THIS TEXT TO IMPLEMENT DATA ANALYSIS IN PUBLIC HEALTH

There are many textbooks on biostatistics. Some are conceptual and some are heavily based on formulas and mathematics. Very few textbooks offer readers a conceptual explanation of statistical concepts and examples of how to implement methods. The purpose of this textbook is to provide a guide to using statistics for the public health practitioner. It is written with the expectation that the reader needs to conduct some straightforward statistical analysis and/or to read papers using statistical analyses.

AUTHOR'S VISION

Whenever I tell people that I teach biostatistics, I get one of two responses:

1. "Oh, I had a statistics course, I got a bad grade. It was useless."
2. "Oh, I had a statistics course, I got an A, but it was useless and I didn't learn anything."

Not everyone will love or appreciate the study of statistics, but the troubling part of these statements is that students (current and past) find the course useless and are not retaining the material. It is difficult to find an area of study with more applications and pertinence than the field of statistics, suggesting that these comments do not stem from the lack of relevance of statistics but in the way statistical methods are presented to this audience.

Public health students enter introductory graduate biostatistics courses with the primary goal of learning a skill: the application of statistical methods. They become easily frustrated in the presence of "too much mathematics" and often become disinterested in the topic if they cannot see the direct implications to their individual research or work. Furthermore, these students find it difficult to understand the practicality of learning how to do it "by hand" if ultimately a computer is used. In an effort to meet the needs of my students, the introductory courses I teach are designed to emphasize the application of statistical methods through the use of data analysis projects and assigned readings of articles that make use of the methods discussed in lecture. Unfortunately, it has been difficult to find a text that provides a wide breadth of statistical methods common to public health *and* emphasizes concepts over computations.

The content and layout of the text were motivated by requests from students, researchers, and practitioners, who often approach me for help with the design of a research study and/or the analysis of data. Investigators rarely come to my office knowing what statistical issues to consider or the appropriate methods to use. Instead, they approach me with a description of the study, a research question, and/or a particular outcome. Most biostatistics texts are organized by method. Given the many statistical methods to choose from, it can be baffling to try to match up the research question to the appropriate statistical method. Hence, to make the text easier to navigate, the chapters of the text are organized not by method but by type of outcome and motivating research question.

The first chapter provides a general overview of statistical concepts discussed throughout the text. Although this text is not intended as a reader's first exposure to statistics, this first chapter provides a survey of the concepts taught in elementary statistics courses. Even the practitioner with a good deal of statistical experience may find this first chapter helpful because it provides conceptual insights to describing data, making inferences, and planning studies. The ensuing chapters provide a discussion of the statistical methods that are common in public health research studies for continuous, categorical, dichotomous, count, and time to event outcomes.

Chapters 2 and 3 address research questions where the outcomes are continuous. Research questions for comparing a continuous outcome between groups are discussed in Chapter 2, and the methods for research questions involving associations and relationships between a continuous variable and other variables are described in Chapter 3. Methods for categorical outcomes are provided in Chapter 4, and a more detailed look at dichotomous outcomes is given in Chapter 5. Common methods for handling count data are discussed in Chapter 6, and the text ends by discussing methods for time to event data in Chapter 7.

For the interested reader, the text can be read from Chapter 1 to Chapter 7, providing a complete overview of the statistical concepts most often used in public health applications. For the more focused investigator, this text may be used as a reference, using only the chapters applicable to the research question and outcome of interest.

For the student, this text provides a conceptual treatment of topics appropriate for a two-course series in biostatistics. Initial chapters provide an introduction to describing data and simple statistical tests, and later chapters introduce multiple variable relationships or more sophisticated methods. Specifically, Chapters 1, 2, and 4 provide an introduction to statistical methods with straightforward comparisons and relationships, while Chapters 3, 5, 6, and 7 discuss topics that may be more appropriate for a second course in biostatistics.

CHAPTER FEATURES

Public Health Applications: These Methods Really Are Used

Each chapter has a similar layout and begins with a **Public Health Application**. These applications provide a current example of research studies in public health that give rise to a particular type of outcome. Using the Public Health Application as a starting point, the chapter proceeds with a sample study that could be used to help answer the research question. Data from this sample study are used in introducing topics and in demonstrating the implementation of a statistical analysis. Essentially, the public health application serves as a foundation for each chapter and motivates the theories and formulas of biostatistics in an understandable, real-world example. Using a real-life research study also allows readers to identify with the Public Health Application as an example of a study they themselves may participate in as public health professionals and how they would be able to utilize their knowledge of biostatistics in a professional arena.

Research Questions

Just as the public health applications motivate the methods presented in each chapter, potential research questions are posed to frame different statistical methods. **Research Questions** are provided as examples of the types of questions an investigator may have. Data are analyzed using the methods of each section to demonstrate how biostatistics can help address public health research questions. Although these research questions may not be the same for every investigator, they can be used to help identify the appropriate statistical method for similar research questions. Research questions are highlighted to remind the reader that the discussion of every statistical method or test originated from a public health research question.

Hypotheses and Conclusions

Regardless of whether this text is to be used for a first graduate course in biostatistics or as a refresher, the one thing all practitioners, researchers, or students seem to know is that they need biostatistics in order to get a p-value. Fewer users of biostatistics fully understand what a p-value is, and even fewer understand the mathematical mechanics to calculate this value. It is a challenge to make this famous little value less mysterious while keeping the discussion at a conceptual level. A common problem is that p-values are easily obtainable but less easily interpreted. They result from hypothesis tests, and one way to make sure that they are used correctly is to remember what hypothesis is being tested. Therefore, for each statistical test, the **hypotheses** being tested are provided. Making **conclusions** and interpretations from the statistical test is much more straightforward if the hypothesis being tested is clear. Thus, after each statistical test, the p-value and a conclusion relating to the hypothesis being tested is provided.

Application of Formulas

One of the most common complaints about statistical texts from public health practitioners is that there are too many formulas and that the formulas are used to explain topics. The emphasis of this text is not on formulas, symbols, or mathematical calculations. Most readers of this text would not be expected to utilize formulas to perform pencil-and-paper or calculator calculations in order to analyze data; they would simply implement the appropriate analysis with statistical software. However, formulas can be instructive. Understanding how the statistical software comes up with the results is helpful in determining the appropriate method as well as better understanding the concepts. Therefore, formulas are presented when needed.

The **Application of Formula** feature is a mathematical presentation of the statistical formula (with mathematical notations and symbols) followed by a step-by-step explanation using the data motivated by the public health application. When appropriate, this feature is then followed by the results from a statistical software package so that the reader can confirm the results. Hence, the formulas serve as a behind-the-scenes look at what is being done by software programs. Consequently, corresponding SAS, R, and STATA codes are provided for the application of formulas, tables, and figures for each chapter in the Premium Web site. Thus, the formulas presented in this text are not meant to be the focus, but rather simply an additional tool for understanding concepts.

Statistical Software Help

Generally datasets are too large or statistical problems are too complicated to perform analyses without using statistical software. To implement an analysis, some software packages offer options for simply pointing and clicking, while others require statistical programming. In public health research, the most commonly used programmatic software packages are SAS, STATA, and R. The Internet provides a variety of resources, from introductory to sophisticated instructions, on using these packages.

However, seeing a full example with an interpretation of the results is often helpful. Although SAS was used as the statistical software package for implementing the analyses in the text, any statistical software package can be used with the data to recreate the results. Therefore, in addition to providing the data used for the text, codes for using SAS, STATA, and R are also provided electronically on the Premium Web site.

Practice with Data and Concepts

Problems are provided at the end of each chapter to give the student an opportunity for additional practice with the concepts and methods presented. These problems involve additional practice with the data presented in each chapter as well as problems on statistical concepts.

Practice with Data questions range from describing the data to making statistical inferences. Using the same data used in the chapter, questions are posed that require the use of statistical software to perform different aspects of data analysis. As the name of these questions suggests, the purpose of these questions is to provide additional practice with data analysis. Therefore, answers to these questions, along with statistical programming help, can be found in the Premium Web site.

Practice with Concepts questions provide students with additional examples of the uses of statistical methods in other public health applications. Additional public health examples from published works are presented, and questions about statistical concepts are provided. These questions are intended to provide readers with additional practice and to show further evidence of the use of statistical principles in practice. Additionally, because one of the challenges of biostatistics is determining the correct statistical methods, examples of public health research questions are provided, and students are asked to identify the most appropriate method for each scenario. Again, since these are practice problems, example responses are provided in the Premium Web site.

Points to Ponder: An Exercise in Critical Thinking

Most biostatistics graduate courses require a lot of information to be provided very fast. Students often do not have the time to think through the concepts. The study of statistics might actually be simpler and make more sense for the student if there were an opportunity to take a breath and really think about what is being said. Throughout the chapters, **Points to Ponder** provide students with a pause to think about what is being presented. Points to Ponder may be in the form of open-ended questions or just comments on the concepts. They are positioned in places where it might be helpful to take a pause and think about the concepts being presented. In a classroom setting, these points may also provide an opportunity for class discussion.

Summary of Chapter Concepts

Each chapter concludes with a **Summary of Chapter Concepts**. The summary is provided to remind students how the methods were used to answer research questions motivated from the Public Health Application. Moreover, Chapters 2–7 also conclude with a table of methods so that investigators can quickly match up research questions with the most appropriate methods for describing data and testing hypotheses.

A TEMPLATE FOR EXTENSIONS TO OTHER PUBLIC HEALTH APPLICATIONS

The public health applications presented in each of the chapters are not the only possibilities for public health research questions or public health data. Many other examples of public health problems could have easily been chosen as example applications. Although other texts provide many different examples of public health applications for the methods presented, I find that investigators are often in search of a road map to statistical analysis. Therefore, each chapter starts with the description of data, based on the Public Health Application, and progresses to estimation and statistical testing (inference). Using a single set of data throughout the chapter, readers have an example of a complete data analysis.

Even if an investigator understands the statistical concepts, however, writing up the interpretation for a paper or a presentation can be somewhat difficult. Many of my consultations involve helping students, researchers, and practitioners construct appropriate figures, tables, and summary statements of methods and results. Therefore, the results of the analyses are presented as a guide to summarizing the results of an analysis. Tables and figures are presented in ways that are common to public health research. Analyses in this text are accompanied with a conclusion, a paragraph or two, describing the results. These descriptions are similar to what can be found in published public health papers. Therefore, the analyses described in the chapters provide readers with a template for executing their own analyses and an outline for providing interpretations of the results.

SUMMARY

The purpose of this text is to try to bring relevance and application to the study and use of biostatistics. Most readers of this text have a practical need for using biostatistics, whether in a course or for public health research or practice. The content and design of this text were created with this audience in mind. The features of this text were intended to help support a public health investigator in understanding the concepts and the issues for utilizing statistical methods in public health research.

As our nation grapples with rising health care costs, there is an understanding that only through prevention will we be able to effectively reverse the trend of rising expenses related to heath care. With this recognition, more individuals are seeking the knowledge and skills to allow them to practice population health, whether in a health department, insurance company, hospital or other health care organization. Led by Dr. F. Douglas Scutchfield, the *Public Health Professional* series, emphasizes the competencies needed to practice population health and spans the gamut of contemporary public health and preventive medicine practice. Drawing on his vast experience and expertise in public health, Scutchfield has crafted a series to help the modern student of public health and prevention to develop the capacity to make a difference in the health of populations they serve.

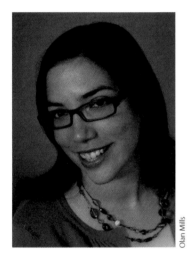

Olan Mills

Heather M. Bush, PhD, is an assistant professor in the Department of Biostatistics at the University of Kentucky College of Public Health. In addition to teaching in the MPH, DrPH, and PhD programs, Dr. Bush provides guest lectures in introductory biostatistics and collaborates on a variety of projects in the Colleges of Medicine, Dentistry, Public Health, Behavioral Sciences, and Health Sciences. She also has a successful track record of collaborating with, advising, and teaching researchers and other established professionals. Dr. Bush received the Golden Apple Award for teaching in the College of Public Health in 2008 and the Provost's Outstanding Teaching Award in 2009. Before joining the University of Kentucky faculty, she served as a senior biostatistician for disease and product registries in the pharmaceutical industry.

ACKNOWLEDGMENTS

I am very thankful for the teaching and research opportunities I have had at the University of Kentucky. The idea for this text originated from many conversations with practitioners, researchers, and students while at the university. I would especially like to thank the College of Public Health and the students in the Biostatistics II courses who have provided motivation, encouragement, and suggestions for this text. Also, I would like to thank my research assistants, Hsin-Fang Li and Catherine Starnes, for helping with statistical software aids, supplemental materials, and all the many other things they do so well.

I would also like to thank the reviewers, whose feedback was invaluable to the revision process and who contributed to the success of this textbook:

Martha M. Perryman, PhD, MBA, MT (ASCP)
Associate Professor
Florida A&M University, Tallahassee, FL

Amy M. Cantrell, PhD
Clinical Assistant Professor
University of Florida, Gainesville, FL

Yuequin Zhao, PhD
Assistant Professor
Eastern Virginia Medical School, Norfolk, VA

Heather M Bush, PhD
Assistant Professor
University of Kentucky, Lexington, Kentucky

Delmar/Cengage Learning
Executive Woods
5 Maxwell Dr.
Clifton Park, NY 12065 - 2919
Phone: 1-800-648-7450

Heather M. Bush, PhD
heather.bush@uky.edu
University of Kentucky
College of Public Health
Department of Biostatistics
Lexington, KY

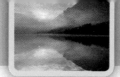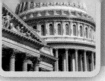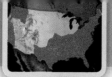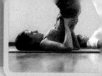

CHAPTER 1

an overview of statistical concepts

Public health is a multidisciplinary field involving stakeholders from politics, advocacy groups, and scientific disciplines coming together to address complex research questions.

- Why are some children obese?
- Does contaminated groundwater adversely affect pregnancies?
- Why do some households neglect to use insecticide-treated nets to prevent malaria?
- What factors are related to new fractures in osteoporotic women?
- What impacts the time it takes a student athlete to return to play after an injury?

Public health researchers and practitioners, (investigators) seek answers to these and other research questions by designing studies, collecting evidence, and interpreting the results.

Research questions are somewhat general; so hypotheses are constructed to make a research question testable. *Hypotheses* are statements that describe an expected result and can be thought of as proposed explanations or claims regarding the research question. They are precisely defined statements that can be tested with data. In biostatistics, *data* are pieces of information that result when measurements are obtained from subjects of interest. The principles of biostatistics can help investigators choose the appropriate items (the *variables*) to measure and to create informative summaries of the data so that conclusions can be made about whether the proposed explanation (hypothesis) is valid. Using the data to make conclusions about a research question or hypothesis is referred to as *statistical inference*.

This text describes the methods needed to accurately describe (graphically and numerically) data and explains how to use statistical evidence to make conclusions. One challenge of biostatistics is that many different methods are available for describing, summarizing, estimating, and testing. However, identifying appropriate statistical methods can be simplified by focusing on the research question. The research question drives the design of the study, including the choice of variables to be measured. Different variables result in different types of information or data. Statistical methods transform data into evidence. So certain types of data correspond to certain statistical methods. Therefore, choosing between statistical methods is made easier because the type of data (outcome) and the statistical method just need to be matched.

This chapter provides an overview of the statistical issues associated with investigating research questions and is organized according to the issues a researcher might face when conducting a study: determining whom to study, how to study them, and what to measure. Once data are obtained, the researcher must then make decisions about what summaries to use, what estimates to provide, and how to test hypotheses. The concepts presented in this first chapter lay a foundation for the chapters that follow; which provide specific information for summarizing data, estimating, and testing hypotheses for the different types of data that result from studies in public health.

LEARNING OBJECTIVES

How do I get the subjects?
Understand the differences between populations and samples.
Understand issues associated with sample selection.

What variables do I measure?
Understand that different types of variables provide different types of information.
Be able to distinguish between the different types of variables.

How do I describe the data?
Identify strategies for describing data graphically and numerically.
Use proper notation for parameters and statistics.

How do I estimate the parameter?
Understand the concept of sampling variability and how it is involved with the creation of interval estimates.
Be able to articulate how the use of interval estimates can aid in estimation and making inferences.

How do I test the hypothesis?
Understand the concept of sampling variability and how it is involved with hypothesis testing.
Be able to articulate how the use of statistical tests can aid in testing and making inferences.
Identify the issues involved with testing a hypothesis.

What do I need to consider to plan a study?
Distinguish the issues for planning a study for estimation or for testing.
Understand the roles that power, effect size, and sample size play in designing a study.

Public Health Application

Sedentary behavior is associated with obesity, and the risk factors for obesity appear to have origins in childhood and adolescence (Freedman et al. 1987). Efforts to develop an active lifestyle early in children may be a successful strategy to increase physical activity among adults (Taylor et al. 1999) and therefore diminish the incidence of overweight and obesity. It has been recommended that children accumulate 1–2 hours of physical activity each day to receive health benefits (Corbin & Pangrazi 1998). However, increasingly, leisure time activities are becoming more sedentary, with television watching, video games, and personal computing among the most popular pastimes (Andersen et al. 1998). [Heelan, K.A., Donnelly, J.E., Jacobsen, D.J., Mayo, M.S., Washburn, R., Greene, L. (2005). Active commuting to and from school and BMI in elementary school children—preliminary data. *Child: Care, Health and Development, 31,* 341–349.]

Data Description

Suppose a study is conducted to better understand childhood obesity. Children between the ages of 6 and 10 who attend public schools are given questionnaires involving lifestyle. The questionnaire includes items such as whether they participate in school lunch programs, their activity level, and the amount of television watched and video games played. In addition, clinical assessments of height and weight are obtained for calculating body mass index (BMI). A total of 610 children participate in the study.

RESEARCH QUESTION:
What factors are associated with obesity?

Defining the Subjects and Population

One of the key steps to clearly defining the research question is to state clearly who or what needs to be studied, the *subjects* to study. Although many studies in public health involve human beings as subjects, this is not a requirement. The subjects can be anything. Examples are children, extracted teeth, pregnant women, water sources exposed to bacteria, cell cultures, households in the tropics, muscle tissues, women with osteoporosis, different geographic regions, student athletes, or homeless teenagers. The subjects (human or not, living or not) in a study are the sources of information or data. Data are obtained by measuring the characteristics of the subjects.

Defining who or what is going to be studied means defining the **population**, which consists of all possible subjects of interest. In some studies the population is defined in general: all children. In other studies, the population is defined in more detail: children ages 6–10 who attend public school. When the population is specifically defined, the subjects are more similar to one another than the subjects of a population that is more loosely defined. Subjects with characteristics in common are less complicated to describe, and answers to research questions are easier to identify when there are fewer differences among subjects. However, the more specific the population, the harder it is to generalize the findings to groups outside the specific population. Therefore, defining the population is a critical first step because it defines the subjects to be studied and the subjects to whom the conclusions will be applicable.

In this example, the population consists of children between the ages of 6 and 10 who attend public schools. The goal is to collect information from these children to investigate the research question. How will this information be obtained? One strategy is to offer the clinical exam and questionnaire to every child between the ages of 6 and 10 attending public school. This strategy is called a census of the children. A **census** is the collection of information on all members of the population. Although taking a census would provide information about the lifestyle characteristics and body mass index for this population, the approach may not be practical. Consider the number of surveys that would have to be collected, the time needed to get the responses, and the efforts needed to reach every child. The endeavor would be very costly, if not impossible.

Samples: A Subset of the Population

An alternative to a census, in which data are obtained on every member of the population, is to obtain data only on some of the subjects, that is, to take a sample from the population. A **sample** is a smaller set (or a subset) of the population; a representative sample is a subset that provides an accurate picture of the whole population. The data obtained from a sample of subjects may not be exactly the same as data collected on the whole population. However, when the sample is representative, the sample data should be very similar to what would be found in the whole population.

To better understand how a representative sample relates to the population, consider an analogy: a landscape and a photograph. A person who sees a landscape in person has access to every color, shape, and aspect of the view. In contrast, someone who views a photograph of the landscape may not be able to fully experience this same level of detail. However, the person who views the photograph has a fairly good depiction of what the landscape looked like in person without having to physically go there. Suppose, however, that, instead of the photograph, someone was given a picture of only the grass, or only the sky, or only the things that were green in the landscape. That picture would not provide an accurate representation of the landscape, and the viewer may not get an accurate depiction of it. Similarly, a representative sample provides an accurate picture of the population but an unrepresentative sample may be misleading.

If only certain members of the population are chosen so that the sample systematically misrepresents the population, the sample is a **biased sample** and may not be effective for investigating the research question. Biased samples can occur because of how the subjects

Point to Ponder

Ideally, a population will be chosen based on who (or what) is impacted by the public health problem. However, the population does not always match up with the subjects that are actually studied. Why might this be a problem?

are selected. Allowing subjects to select themselves for the sample (voluntary response) or selecting subjects that are convenient to the investigator (convenience sample) are ways the sample can become biased. One way to obtain a representative sample and avoid bias is to allow random chance to choose the subset of subjects from the population, that is, to conduct a **random sample**. Random samples can be implemented with a variety of methods. Random number generators (online or through software) are a common method and provide an easy option for incorporating randomness into sample selection.

Strategies for Obtaining a Random Sample of the Population

The strategies for choosing a random sample depend on the research question and how feasible it is to implement the randomization. When selecting a random sample, the role randomness plays in selection can vary. There are three primary types of random samples: simple, stratified, and systematic. Each type of random sample requires a list of the population, known as the **sampling frame**. Usually the sampling frame is ordered, and every subject in the sampling frame is assigned a unique number. From these unique identifiers, a random number generator can be used to randomly select the sample.

In a *simple random sample*, each subject in the population has the same chance of being selected. The random number generator randomly selects numbers from the range of unique identifiers in the sampling frame. The selected identifiers are then matched with the subjects to select the sample. For example, suppose an investigator wants a simple random sample of 610 children from the population of children between the ages of 6 and 10 enrolled in public schools. The sampling frame is a list of all these children. If each child is assigned a unique number, a random list of 610 numbers can be generated from all possible numbers (children) in the sampling frame. Children whose numbers appear in the random list are selected as the sample.

Simple random samples, however, are not without problems. On average, they are representative, but a single simple random sample may not reflect the true population. Furthermore, for large populations, a simple random sample may not be feasible. In this example, there are approximately 30 million public school children between the ages of 6 and 10; a simple random sample in this setting would be quite cumbersome.

An alternative to a simple random sample is *stratified random sampling*. In a stratified random sample, the sampling frame is divided into subgroups or strata and simple random samples are conducted within the strata. For example, children between the ages of 6 and 10 attending public schools may be stratified by location. Suppose the sampling frame were divided into five regions: Northeast, Southeast, Midwest, Southwest, and Northwest. Simple random samples conducted within each of these regions would make the sampling frames more manageable and would ensure that students from each region were represented in the sample. The total sample for the study consists of all the subjects selected from each region. The total sample will be representative as long as the number of subjects sampled in each region is proportional to the population size of the region.

Systematic random sampling provides an additional option for choosing a sample. In a systematic random sample, the sampling frame is ordered, and a number s is selected so that every s^{th} subject is selected to be in the sample; this is the systematic part. The selection process is still random because the starting point for choosing the sample is based on random chance. For example, suppose that an investigator was interested in a school district with 2000 students aged 6–10. The sampling frame would consist of all these students. For a sample of 200 students, the investigator may decide to enroll every tenth student in the study: $s = 10$. Using a random number generator, 3 is selected as the starting point. The sample consists of the students numbered 3, 13, 23, 33, etc. Although systematic random samples are a strategy for choosing subjects at random, the systematic component can lead to bias. If the sampling frame is ordered so that a characteristic of the population repeats for every s subjects, choosing every sth subject could result in a sample with or without the characteristic, depending on the starting point.

Regardless of the random sampling strategy (simple, stratified, systematic, or some combination), the sampling frame provides the foundation for choosing the sample. Consequently, a representative sample depends on having a complete sampling frame. Unfortunately, a list of the whole population may not be feasible for the sampling frame. For example, in a study where physicians are the subjects, investigators may solicit a roster from a professional organization as the sampling frame. This sampling frame, however, is incomplete because it would only include the physicians who were members of the organization. As another example, investigators may use ZIP codes or phone numbers as a sampling frame. National studies, like the Behavioral Risk Factor Surveillance System (BRFSS) conducted by the Centers for Disease Control and Prevention, use lists of telephone numbers as the sampling frame. Subjects are selected by randomly selecting digits of the phone numbers. In the past, this was a reasonable approach because almost all households had a land-line phone. However, the strategy has become less effective as increased cell phone use has led many households to discontinue their land-line phone. Any time a sampling frame systematically excludes a portion of the population, there is the potential for a biased sample. If the sampling frame is grossly incomplete, investigators may be forced to redefine the population of interest.

Ideally, samples are chosen from complete sampling frames using an element of random chance. When a sample systematically misses a group of subjects in a population, the sample suffers from selection bias. Bias can occur when the sampling frame omits a particular group of subjects, when subjects are either self-selected or investigator-selected. Although eliminating all sources of bias from the sample selection process may not be possible, selecting a sample requires careful consideration and procedures should be carefully planned so that potential biases are minimized.

HOW TO STUDY THE SUBJECTS: STUDY DESIGNS

The *study design* is how information (data) on the subjects will be collected. In public health research, prospective, retrospective, and cross-sectional are common study designs.

In a *prospective study*, subjects are identified and followed for a specific period of time. Data collection starts at the beginning of the study and continues as subjects are followed during the study. The investigator controls what variables are measured and how they are measured. In public health, prospective studies are often conducted when the goal is to compare groups. Groups with particular characteristics are identified at the start of the study and then followed to determine whether a particular outcome occurs. A difference in outcomes suggests that group membership is related to the outcome.

In public health, these groups are called *cohorts*, and a prospective study involving the comparison of cohorts is called a *cohort-study*. An example of a cohort-study might involve following two groups of children: those that participated in a school lunch program and those who did not. Suppose a sample of nonobese, healthy-weight children are recruited and followed over a 5-year period to investigate the relationship of participating in school lunch programs and obesity. Children in this study are randomly assigned to either participate or not in the school lunch program. After 5 years, obesity in the two groups is compared. This is an example of a prospective cohort study.

In a *retrospective study*, an outcome is identified, after the data have already been collected. Previously collected data are reviewed to determine whether any characteristics impacted the outcome. Retrospective studies are often conducted when the outcome is not very common and when it would require a long time to follow subjects prospectively. By identifying subjects with a particular outcome and looking backward for factors that might be related to the outcome, the investigators can be sure to obtain enough cases (subjects with the outcome). Because data collection occurs prior to the start of the study, the groups are defined based on data that have already been collected. This means investigators do not have control over the variables collected or how they were collected.

In public health, retrospective studies are usually conducted as case-control studies. In a *case-control study*, case subjects (those having the outcome) and control subjects (those not having the outcome) are identified. Existing data are then obtained to determine what factors were related to subjects becoming either a case or a control. Suppose, for example, an investigator selects obese (cases) and nonobese (control) children to examine the relationship between school lunches and obesity. School records are accessed to determine whether each child participated in the school lunch program. Because the outcome has already occurred and past factors are investigated to distinguish between children with and without the outcome, this represents an example of a case-control study where data are collected retrospectively.

In a *cross-sectional study*, data are collected at a particular time point and represent a *cross-section* of time. The outcome and the variables of interest are all measured at the same time. Surveys that measure the responses of subjects at a particular point in time are typically conducted as part of a cross-sectional study. The study description that opened this chapter is an example of a cross-sectional study because surveys measuring lifestyle characteristics and clinical exams measuring obesity are given to students at one point in time. This is an example of a cross-sectional study because the outcome and the factors of interest are obtained at the same time. Many times, cross-sectional studies are limited in their conclusions because the data are only collected at a single point in time.

WHAT TO MEASURE ON THE SUBJECTS: VARIABLE TYPES

To address a research question, studies are conducted with the goal of collecting data on subjects, that is, obtaining measurements of certain characteristics on each subject. The collection of data means that a set of *variables* is measured on each subject. In this example, the research question involves the relationship between obesity (measured by BMI) and the lifestyle characteristics of children (between 6 and 10 years old) who attend public school. The body mass index is used to determine whether a child is obese. Therefore, it represents the outcome of interest, or the *primary endpoint*, for the study. However, lifestyle characteristics are also important variables because differences in a child's BMI might be related to differences in these characteristics. Therefore, the following variables are measured on each child: BMI, activity level, consumption of fruits and vegetables, and time spent watching television or playing video games. Multiple variables are often measured on a subject because different types of variables measure different things and can take many different forms.

The research question drives the type of variables to collect in the study. Different types of research questions call for different types of information. Variables can be broadly grouped into two types:

- *Categorical:* Variables whose measurements represent a limited set of possible values, such as the child being defined as obese or nonobese.
- *Continuous:* Variables whose measurements represent an unlimited set of possible values, such as the child's BMI measured in kg/m².

Categorical variables can be further subdivided into:

- Ordinal
- Nominal
- Dichotomous

Each type of variable gives a different amount of information about the subject. In this example, the BMI measured in kg/m² (continuous variable) gives more information than the weight or obesity classifications (categorical variables). The research question motivates the level of information measured and the type of variable to be collected: continuous, ordinal, nominal, or dichotomous (Figure 1-1).

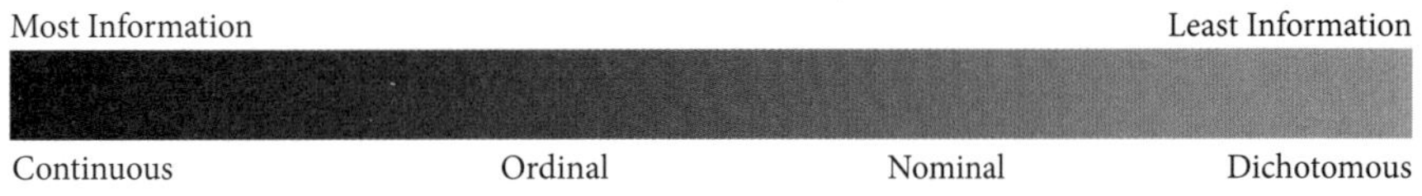

Figure 1-1 Variable types.
© *Cengage Learning, 2012.*

Most Information			Least Information
Continuous	Ordinal	Nominal	Dichotomous

Categorical Variables

Categorical variables are variables whose potential measurements for each subject are limited to a certain set of values. Because only a limited set of values are possible, categorical variables are known as *discrete* variables. These values represent different groups, different classifications, different categories, and/or different levels. The set of values can be expressed in either numbers or in characters and words. Because the values represent different categories or levels, multiplying, dividing, adding, or subtracting the values does not make sense. Categorical variables are best analyzed using procedures that try to count the number of subjects with a particular category or level. Ordinal, nominal, and dichotomous variables are specific types of categorical variables with varying amounts and types of information.

Ordinal Variables

Ordinal variables are categorical variables with different levels or categories whose order matters. From the variables measured in this study, the child's activity levels is an example of an ordinal variable. Students who are very active are more active than those who are moderately active, who are in turn more active than those who are somewhat sedentary, who are more active than those who are very sedentary. Because these categories can naturally be ordered, activity level is an ordinal variable. Other examples of ordinal variables in public health include pain scores (rating pain on a scale of 0–5), stages of cancer, and educational attainment.

Nominal Variables

Nominal variables are categorical variables with different levels or categories whose order does *not* matter. From the variables measured in this study, the color of the student's favorite fruit or vegetable is an example of a nominal variable because colors have no predefined order. Whereas ordering an ordinal variable like activity levels (sedentary, somewhat sedentary, moderately active, very active) makes sense, ordering a nominal variable like fruit/vegetable color (white/yellow, red, orange, green, blue/purple) does not. Examples of nominal variables in public health include tooth color, race, marital status, and political affiliation.

Dichotomous Variables

Dichotomous variables are a very special kind of categorical variable that can have *only two levels*. Because many public health questions involve outcomes with only two levels, these variables are used often in public health research. Examples include yes/no variables, gender (M/F), and so on.

Continuous Variables

Continuous variables can have only numeric values. They are called continuous because there are no natural *gaps* between the numbers. Unlike discrete variables, all "in-between" values are possible (17.56 kg/m^2, 17.561 kg/m^2, 17.5611 kg/m^2 . . . are all valid), and the level of detail measured by a continuous variable is limited only by the level of detail of the measuring instrument. Examples of continuous variables found in public health research include BMI, Viral Load, average probing depths, and so on. Continuous variables are different from categorical because the values no longer represent a limited set of levels or categories. Therefore, procedures that try to count the number of responses in a continuous variable are not useful. Instead, continuous data are best analyzed by procedures that allow for multiplying, dividing, adding, or subtracting the values.

Count Variables

Count variables are variables that can take on only positive, whole number values (0, 1, 2, . . .). Count variables are considered discrete because values in-between whole number counts do not occur. Examples of count variables in public health research include the number of cavities in a mouth, the number of side effects, the number of sexual partners, and the number of cigarettes.

Simple descriptions of count variables depend on how varied the counts are. For example: When counting the number of fruits and vegetables a child eats per day, the possible counts are 0, 1, 2, 3, 4, and 5. Most children do not eat more than five fruits or vegetables per day; so using the same summaries as in *categorical* data may be helpful. If, however, the number of steps taken per day is counted, many different values are possible for the counts and methods for describing *continuous* data may be more appropriate. Although count variables can be analyzed as categorical variables and as continuous variables, they are different and research questions resulting in count outcomes require a special set of statistical methods.

HOW TO DESCRIBE THE SUBJECTS: NUMERICAL SUMMARIES

Categorical Variables

For categorical variables or for variables with a limited number of possible values, numerical summaries include:

- *Counts:* For each level or category, a subject either belongs in the category or not. The total number of subjects with a particular category or level is a count.
- *Proportions:* The proportion is simply the count for a category divided by the total number of subjects.
- *Percentages:* The percentage is the proportion times 100.

Continuous Variables

For continuous variables, there are many options for summarizing the responses numerically. Typically, numerical summaries of continuous variables are the mean, standard deviation, median, first and third quartiles, and minimum and maximum. Some of these numerical summaries describe the *center* of the distribution, and some describe the *spread* (Table 1-1).

A measure of center provides a description of the "average" response. A measure of spread provides a description of how varied the responses are. A measure of how spread out the responses are tells the investigator whether the responses are clustered close to the center or dispersed farther away from the center.

TABLE 1-1 **POSSIBLE NUMERICAL SUMMARIES FOR DESCRIBING CONTINUOUS VARIABLES**

Numerical Summary	Measures	How to Find It
Mode	Center	Most common response
Mean	Center	Sum of responses divided by number of responses
Variance	Spread	Mean squared distance of responses from the mean
Standard deviation	Spread	Square root of the variance
Median	Center	Middle value of the responses
First quartile	Spread	Middle value of the first half of the responses
Third quartile	Spread	Middle value of the last half of the responses
Interquartile range	Spread	Third quartile minus First quartile
Minimum	Spread	Lowest value
Maximum	Spread	Highest value
Range	Spread	Maximum minus Minimum

© Cengage Learning, 2012.

Because continuous variables can take on any value, describing *both* the center and the spread of a variable is critical. For example, stating that the mean weight of children is 50 lb is not a sufficient summary. A standard deviation of 0.5 lb would suggest that all of the weight observations were very close together—that there was little deviation from the mean of 50 lb. On the other hand, a standard deviation of 15 lb would suggest that the responses were much more variable and spread out.

Ideally, all of the numerical summaries in Table 1-1 would be used to give a clear and complete description of the continuous variables. However, because space may be limited or a simpler description may be desired, presenting all of these summaries might not be practical. Therefore, investigators often choose one measure of center and one measure of spread to describe continuous outcomes.

The mean is commonly used to describe the center of the responses. However, when extremely large or small values are present, the mean is no longer a good measure of the center. In this case, the median, which is the middle of the responses, is a better measure of the center. The choice for the measure of spread depends on the measure of center. Mixing and matching measures of center and spread is not appropriate. If the mean is chosen as the measure of center, then an appropriate measure of spread is the standard deviation. If the median is chosen to summarize the center of the data, then an appropriate measure of spread is the range. The range can be presented either as the difference between the maximum and the minimum or as the interval of values (minimum, maximum).

Notations for Parameters and Statistics

Because it is rarely feasible to investigate a research question by obtaining data from the entire population, variables are measured on the sample. The very same numerical summaries that are of interest for a population are the numerical summaries used to describe the data collected on the sample. Numerical summaries that describe the population are called **parameters**, while numerical summaries that describe the sample are called **statistics**. If the sample is representative of the population, then the numerical summaries obtained from the sample (statistics) will provide a good approximation or estimate for the numerical summaries of the population (parameters). If a sample is a poor representation of the population, then the statistics will not do a good job of estimating the population parameters.

Parameters are generally represented in a special way so that it is clear that the summaries refer to the population. Likewise, statistics are presented in a special way so that it is clear that the sample is being summarized. Although parameters and statistics represent the same numerical summary, they describe different sets of subjects. Therefore, parameters are different from statistics. Parameters are the numerical summaries that an investigator wants but can not obtain directly because collecting data on the entire population is not feasible.

- *Parameters* are actual numerical summaries that exist, the specific value is just not known (which is why a study was conducted in the first place).
- A *statistic* is the same numerical summary as the parameter but provides a summary of the sample.

Use the following statement to remember these definitions: "**S**tatistics describe the **s**ample, and **p**arameters describe the **p**opulation."

To see the similarities between statistics and parameters, consider examples of potential summaries for this study (Table 1-2). Notice that the names of the numerical summaries of the sample are the same as the numerical summaries of the population. However, the notations for the parameters and statistics are different because the parameters describe the population, whereas statistics can be calculated from the data. To avoid confusion, statistics need to be presented (have notations) so that they are clearly different from parameters.

TABLE 1-2 **EXAMPLES OF NOTATIONS FOR STATISTICS AND PARAMETERS**

Example Questions	Example Numerical Summaries	Example Notation for a	
		Population (Parameter)	Sample (Statistic)
What do the children weigh?	The mean (and standard deviation) weight	mean (μ) standard deviation (σ)	mean ($\bar{x}$) standard deviation (s)
Are they participating in school lunch programs?	The proportion participating in school lunch programs	proportion (p)	proportion ($\hat{p}$)
What color is their favorite fruit or vegetable?	The proportion whose favorite fruit/vegetable is green, yellow/white, orange, red, blue/purple.	green (p_g), yellow/white (p_{yw}), orange (p_o), red (p_r), or blue/purple (p_{bp})	green ($\hat{p}_g$), yellow/white ($\hat{p}_{yw}$), orange ($\hat{p}_o$), red ($\hat{p}_r$), or blue/purple ($\hat{p}_{bp}$)
What is the activity level?	The proportion who are very sedentary, somewhat sedentary, moderately active, or very active	very sedentary (p_1), somewhat sedentary (p_2), moderately active (p_3), or very active (p_4)	very sedentary ($\hat{p}_1$), somewhat sedentary ($\hat{p}_2$), moderately active ($\hat{p}_3$), or very active ($\hat{p}_4$)
How many hours are spent watching television or playing video games?	The median (and range) number of hours	median (M) range (R)	median ($\bar{m}$) range ($\bar{R}$)

© Cengage Learning, 2012.

One of the reasons statistical formulas can be intimidating is that the symbols for statistics and parameters are not always presented in a standard way. Different texts and publications use different conventions to represent statistics and parameters. So deciding which symbol to use can be confusing. However, two rules are always true:

1. Although Greek letters can be used to represent parameters, they are *never* used alone to represent statistics.
2. Often, a statistic is presented as a letter with a bar ($^-$) or hat ($^\wedge$) on top, but a parameter *never* has a bar or hat.

For presenting hypotheses and results, be very clear about which numerical summaries refer to the population (parameters) and which refer to the sample (statistics).

HOW TO DESCRIBE THE SUBJECTS: GRAPHICAL SUMMARIES

Each type of variable has its own special properties, and the distribution of each type of variable has a particular shape and characteristics. The **distribution** of a variable consists of a summary of the possible values the variable can have and the number of subjects with each of these values. A distribution that uses counts to describe the number of subjects with a particular value is called a *frequency distribution*. A distribution that uses proportions to describe the number of subjects with a particular value is called a *probability distribution*. Understanding the shape and characteristics of a distribution will provide an investigator with greater insights and can help in answering research questions.

Categorical Variables

Because categorical variables have only a limited number of possible values (discrete), the distribution can be displayed with either a table or a picture (graph). In this example, a child's activity level is a categorical variable where each child provides a response for one (and only one) category: Very Sedentary, Somewhat Sedentary, Moderately Active, or Very Active. A child could not provide a response between, say, Somewhat Sedentary and Moderately Active. Only these four categories are observed; these are the only values the activity level variable can have.

The distribution of the activity level consists of the possible values of the categories and the number of subjects (children) in each category or value (Table 1-3). The table represents a distribution of the activity level variable because it provides a listing of all

TABLE 1-3 DISTRIBUTION OF ACTIVITY LEVELS

Activity Level Categories	Count of Participants	Proportion
Very Active	78	0.13
Moderately Active	101	0.17
Somewhat Sedentary	252	0.41
Very Sedentary	179	0.29

© Cengage Learning, 2012.

the possible values (activity level categories) and the number of times these values were observed in the study. This table can be converted to a picture, which often is more meaningful than a table of values. Pictures (graphs and charts) enable an investigator to better understand the shape and characteristics of the distribution.

Two types of graphs are used to summarize categorical variables: pie charts and bar graphs. A *pie chart*, as the name suggests, looks like a pie. Each level of a categorical variable is a slice of pie, and the size of the slice represents the number of subjects in that category. Pie charts can be presented using frequencies (counts of the number of subjects) or proportions. A pie chart describes how the pieces relate to the whole. So the counts for all the slices (categories) must add up to the total number of subjects, and/or the proportions for all the slices (categories) must add up to 1 (or 100% if percentages are used). Therefore, pie charts are generally used when trying to demonstrate how the categories within a variable relate to each other.

A *bar graph* is a graph whose vertical axis represents the number of times a value occurs and whose horizontal axis represents the possible values of the categorical variable. Typically, a bar graph is used to describe the distributions of categorical variables. For each value or category, a bar is drawn. The heights of the bars indicate how many subjects were in each value or category. The height of the bar (vertical axis) can represent either the number of subjects (frequency) or the proportion (probability) of subjects in a particular category (Figures 1-2a and b). Because the shape of the graph does not change when using the count or proportion of participants, many times the proportion of participants is preferred because it takes the total number of subjects into account. Because the heights of the bars can easily be compared, these graphs are particularly useful when the research question involves comparisons.

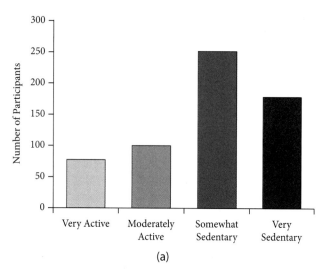
(a)

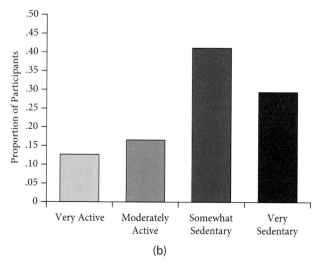
(b)

Figure 1-2 (a) Frequency distribution of activity level; (b) probability distribution of activity level. © *Cengage Learning, 2012.*

Notice that in these bar graphs, fewer children (bars with the lower heights) rate themselves as very and moderately active as compared to those who rate themselves as very or somewhat sedentary. The somewhat sedentary category is the most common (bar with the highest height) observed response in this study. In this example, the activity levels have an order to them and could be treated as ordinal variables. Therefore, the bars are ordered in a predefined way, and the shape or trend moving across the horizontal axis (moving from the very active category to the very sedentary category) can be described.

In this study, the children were also asked about the color of their favorite fruit/vegetable. Diets that include a variety of fruits and vegetables have been found to help in weight control. The children were asked to think of their favorite fruit or vegetable and were asked which of the following food color groups it belonged to: green, yellow/white, orange, red, blue/purple. The color of the fruit and vegetable food group is a nominal variable because the color of foods does not have a natural order; any arrangement of the categories could make sense. In a bar graph, the shape of the distribution depends on the ordering of the categories (food color groups) (Figures 1-3a and b). Because the ordering of the groups changes the shape, the shape of the distribution cannot really be discussed. However, the bar graph makes it easy to see that more participants in the study prefer foods in the yellow/white category (highest bar) above all others. When dealing with nominal variables, the categories are generally provided in descending order by the number of times a value is observed (Figure 1-3b).

When children in the study were also asked whether they partake in the school lunch program, the response has only two values: yes or no. This is a dichotomous variable (Figure 1-4).

The distribution of a dichotomous variable is not very interesting because only two values are possible. Given only two options, the ordering of the variables does not matter. The bar graph in Figure 1-4 shows that the children in this study are not likely to be participating in the school lunch program (bar with the lowest height). Further, once the percentage of those who do participate in a school lunch program (20%) is known, the percentage of those who do not (80%) can be easily found by subtracting the participating percentage from 100%. Because variables with only two levels are very common and have nice properties, the probability distribution that occurs when dichotomous variables are measured on subjects in a sample, is given a particular name: the *binomial distribution*.

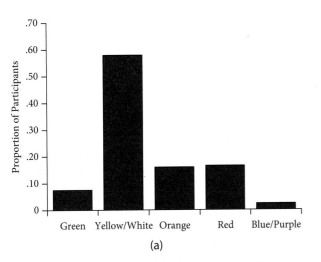 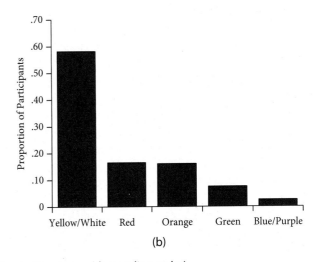

Figure 1-3 (a) Distribution of food color groups; (b) distribution of food color groups (descending order).
© Cengage Learning, 2012.

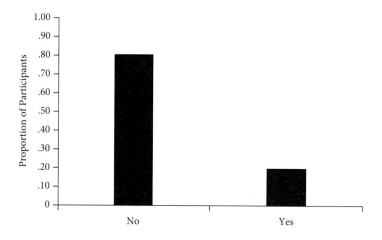

Figure 1-4 Distribution of participating in the school lunch program.
© *Cengage Learning, 2012.*

Bernoulli and Binomial Distributions

When the categorical variable is dichotomous, each subject has only two possibilities: have the characteristic or do not have the characteristic. Often these two options are measured by a variable where subjects are assigned a 0 for not having the characteristic and a 1 for having it.

When a variable has only two possible outcomes, the data for each subject come from a *Bernoulli distribution*, which has only two possible outcomes. However, research questions are investigated by obtaining information on a sample of subjects, not just one subject. When a sample of *n* subjects are measured and the variable has only two options, the data come from a binomial distribution. Therefore, the probability distribution of binomial data has the two possible values on the horizontal axis and the proportion (probabilities) of subjects with those values on the vertical axis (Figure 1-4).

Because of the gap between the two possible values, binomial variables are said to be *discrete.*

- The *mean* of the binomial distribution is simply the number of subjects with the characteristic or the proportion multiplied by the sample size.
- The *variance* of the binomial distribution is a little more complicated. It is the proportion of the sample with the characteristic multiplied by the proportion without it, all divided by the sample size.

Continuous Variables

Suppose the actual weight (in pounds) is measured for each child. A variable, such as the child's weight, is not discrete like a categorical variable; 50 lb and 51 lb are possible values, as well as 50.1 lb, 50.11 lb, 50.112 lb, and so on. The only limit to the in-between values is how precisely the scale measures the weight. So there are really infinite possibilities for the weight of the child, making weight a continuous variable. For continuous variables (e.g., weight measured in pounds), many different values (weights of all the children) are possible. Perhaps only one or two children will have exactly the same weight. Therefore, listing all the possible values of weight and counting the number of children with each weight, as was done with categorical values, does little to summarize children's weight; this summary is little more than a list of all the possible values.

Because of the potential for an infinite number of possible values, a histogram is the best way to describe the distribution of a continuous variable. A histogram is a graphical representation of a variable in which the observed values are categorized, a bar is drawn for each category, and the number of participants in each category is represented by the height of the bar.

The histogram of the weight variable (Figures 1-5a and b) offers a range of the possible weight values and the number of participants in each range, Like the graphs of the discrete variable, a histogram provides a quick picture of the distribution of a variable, and it can be presented with counts or proportions of participants (Figures 1-5a and b). Also like discrete variables, when counts are used on the vertical axis, the distribution is referred to as a *frequency distribution*. Likewise, the histogram is called a *probability distribution* when the vertical axis consists of proportions. Unlike the distribution of the discrete variable, however, there are no gaps between the bars of the histogram; all of the bars are touching. The touching bars demonstrate that all in-between values are possible.

For example, for each weight category that is created, the number of participants is counted, providing the frequency distribution (Figure 1-5a). Because proportions take the total sample size into account, a more useful summary may be the probability distribution, where the count is replaced by the proportion (Figure 1-5b). The horizontal axes in Figures 1-5a and b represent the midpoints for each range; this is typical for histograms.

In this example, seven categories were created, resulting in seven bars. However, there is no hard rule on the number of bars that should appear in a histogram. Although statistical software often has a default method of determining the number of categories to create, the investigator can also control the number of categories (or bars). The number of categories to create depends on the data, but as a general rule the chart must have

Figure 1-5 (a) Frequency distribution of weight (lb); (b) probability distribution of weight (lb).
© *Cengage Learning, 2012.*

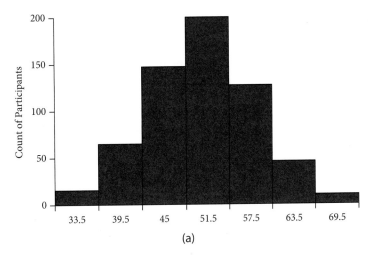

(a)

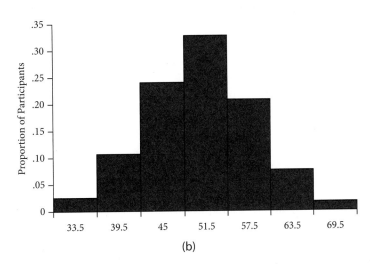

(b)

Application of Formula: HISTOGRAM

Histograms are obtained by taking the range of values and dividing the values evenly into groups.
   What you need to construct a histogram:

1. *The range of values:* In this example, the weight of the children ranged from 30.5 lb to 72.5 lb. The range of the weight is $72.5 - 30.5 = 42$.
2. *The number of bars:* In this example, there are seven bars.
3. *The width of bars:* Divide the range into equal parts, (1)/(2). So $42/7 = 6$. There are 6 pounds for each bar.
4. *Ranges of the bars:* Starting with the lowest possible value, the number found in (3) is added to make the range of each bar. The lowest weight is (30.5). So the first bar is $30.5 - 36.5$, the second bar is $36.5 - 42.5$, and so on.
5. *The height of the bars:* This comes from the number of subjects in each category:
   a. Count the number of subjects in each bar range for a frequency histogram.
   b. Divide the counts (5) by the total number of subjects for a probability histogram.

DISTRIBUTION FOR WEIGHT (lb)

Weight Ranges	30.5–36.5	36.5–42.5	42.5–47.5	48.5–54.5	54.5–60.5	60.5–66.5	66.5–72.5	Total
Number of Participants	15	65	147	200	127	46	10	610
Proportion	0.02	0.11	0.24	0.33	0.21	0.08	0.02	1.0

enough bars to present a good picture of the distribution results. Too few or too many categories (bars) hide interesting trends in the data. Obtaining an accurate representation of the data may require trying different numbers of categories (bars) and creating multiple histograms.

Histograms provide information about how spread out the responses are, which responses are the most common, which responses are in the center, and the overall shape of the distribution. Especially in the case of continuous variables, with so many possible values, histograms are particularly helpful for providing a summary. For example, Figure 1-5b represents a probability distribution that is symmetric and unimodal. **Symmetric** distributions can be folded in half so that each half is close to a mirror image of the other. The *mode* of the distribution represents the most common response. A *unimodal* distribution has one mode or one most common value. It is represented by the peak in the histogram. A distribution with two peaks is called *bimodal*.

In Figure 1-5b, the value at the peak (48.5–54.5 lb) represents the mode or most common observed weights for this study. This peak also provides the point at which the data can be folded in half. Hence, this value also represents the middle of the distribution—where 50% of the observations are larger and 50% of the observations are smaller. This value also represents the mean and median weight for the children. Probability distributions with this bell-shaped, unimodal, symmetric shape occur often and are called *normal distributions*. In the normal distribution, the most common value, the middle of the distribution, and the mean are all the same.

The Normal Distribution

When the histogram is bell-shaped, unimodal, and symmetric, with the mean, median, and most common value at the center at the peak, the data come from a normal distribution (Figure 1-6). Because there are no gaps between possible values, normally distributed variables are continuous variables. Normally distributed variables are characterized by two values: the mean and the standard deviation (or variance). Therefore, normally distributed variables have the same overall shape but may have

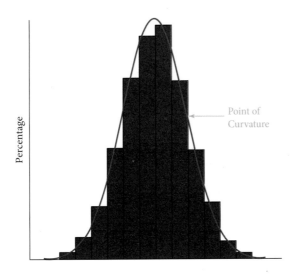

Figure 1-6 The normal distribution.
© Cengage Learning, 2012.

Point of Curvature

Percentage

different centers and/or different spreads (e.g., be skinny or fat), depending on the mean and the standard deviation (or variance). In the normal distribution, knowing the mean indicates nothing about the spread, and knowing the standard deviation (or variance) indicates nothing about the center.

A normal curve, like the one in Figure 1-6, can be thought of as having two shapes: concave up and concave down. A concave down curve looks like an upside down U or a cup that is dumping its contents. A concave up curve looks like a U or a cup that could hold its contents. At the peak of the normal curve, the curve is concave down (the shape of an upside down cup). By moving away from the mean in either direction, the curve starts to become concave up (the shape of a cup that can hold its contents). The **point of curvature** (the point at which the curve goes from concave up to concave down) occurs one standard deviation from the mean or center of the distribution.

Using the standard deviation as a unit of distance, 68% of all subjects are within one standard deviation of the mean, 95.4% are within two standard deviations of the mean, and 99.7% are within three standard deviations of the mean. This rule, known as the *empirical rule,* can be applied to any normal distribution. (Recall that different normal distributions result from different means and standard deviations.) The empirical rule can be used to determine if observations are common or extreme. Observations in the middle of the distribution are considered common and those more than three standard deviations from the mean are considered to be very rare.

Skewed Distributions

Continuous distributions are not always normal or even symmetric. Suppose that, instead of the bell-shaped distribution presented in Figure 1-6, there were more subjects with smaller weight values. In the example shown in Figure 1-7, the distribution with more children with smaller weights has a tail that extends to the left.

Figure 1-7 Left-skewed distribution of weights (lb).
© Cengage Learning, 2012.

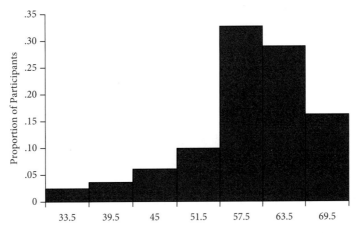

The data diverge in Figure 1-7 from the symmetric pattern of Figure 1-6. Because the left side has a longer tail than the symmetric distribution, this histogram cannot be folded in half to get a mirror image on either side. These data are **skewed** to the left. In this case, the peak still represents the most common value (weights in the range of 54.5–60.5 lb) observed in the sample, but it no longer represents the mean of the data. The mean is pulled away from the peak out toward the tail to account for the observations that are more extreme.

- The distribution is *left skewed* when the distribution has a tail that extends longer to the left, that is, there is a set of observations with lower values than those of the majority of the observed responses.
- Similarly, a distribution is *right skewed* when the distribution has a tail that extends longer to the right, that is, there is a set of observations with higher values than those of the majority of the observed responses.

Count Variables

Sometimes discrete variables may be summarized as a continuous variable, not because all in-between values are possible, but because so many values are possible. This is often the case when participants are asked to provide a count. Count data are discrete because only positive, whole numbers (0, 1, 2, . . .) are allowed as possible values; fractional counts are not possible. Unlike the discrete categorical variables, where only a few categories are possible, count variables can take on many more values. When a large number of counts are possible, a histogram may be a better choice than a bar graph for describing count variables. For example, suppose the children were asked to recall the number of days they exercised for at least 30 minutes in the last 30 days (Figure 1-8).

Because counts increase by whole numbers, there are natural gaps between the possible values. The picture of the probability distribution of count data has the possible counts on the horizontal axis, and the proportion of subjects with those values on the vertical axis (Figure 1-8).

This discrete probability distribution, whose possible values are whole numbers from 0 to infinity, is called the *Poisson distribution* (pronounced PWAH-SAUN), which is not necessarily symmetric like the normal distribution. When the mean is small, the distribution is somewhat skewed. However, as the mean increases, the distribution

Point to Ponder

Histograms also show where natural breaks occur and can help define cutoffs for creating categorical variables. What categories should be created here?

Figure 1-8 Distribution of number of days exercised more than 30 minutes. © *Cengage Learning, 2012.*

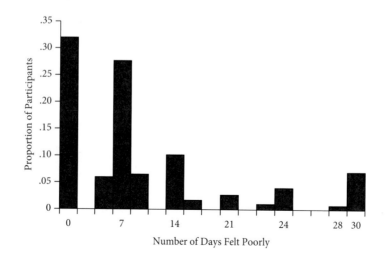

becomes more symmetric. Also unlike the normal distribution, one of the assumptions of the Poisson distribution is that the mean and the variance are the same. In the normal distribution, *both* the mean and the variance are required to describe the distribution. However, because the mean and the variance of a Poisson distribution are the same, only the mean is needed.

An added advantage of the Poisson distribution is that, when the mean is very small, the distribution is similar to the binomial distribution. In fact, when the mean is very small, it is so similar to the binomial distribution that it can be used as an approximation of it. Therefore, depending on the size of the mean, the Poisson distribution can become like the binomial (very small mean) or the normal (large mean) distributions.

Percentiles

Probability distributions (from continuous or discrete variables) can also be used to determine whether values are common or rare. Consider the distribution of the heights (in inches) of children (Figure 1-9). The heights come from a normal distribution where the average heights (those in the middle of the distribution) occur most often and are considered common. On the other hand, the values at the far ends of the distribution are heights that rarely occur (very small and very large). Using the distribution of possible heights (Figure 1-9), an investigator can determine whether a height of 45 in., for example, is common or rare. To determine whether a particular value is common or rare, an investigator can use **percentiles**, which are percentages of all the observations that are less than the value of interest.

Based on Figure 1-9, a child with a height of 47 in. would be in the 99th percentile; that is, 99% of children are shorter or have a height less than this particular height. Because so many children have a shorter height, this child's height would be considered rare; she is quite tall. Similarly, a child with a height of 43 in. would belong to the 4th percentile; 4% of children have heights shorter than 43 in. She is quite short. On the other hand, a child with a height of 45 in. would correspond to a percentile of 53rd. Because only 53% of children are shorter than this child, this height would be considered common, or average.

Percentiles are easily obtained using statistical tables or on-line calculators. Statistical tables are tables that provide the percentiles for all possible values for a standard distribution, for example, a normal distribution with a mean of 0 and a standard deviation of 1. To use these tables the data has to be converted to a standardized distribution. Data from any normal distribution can be converted to a standard normal distribution by subtracting off the mean and dividing by the standard deviation. In fact, heights and weights are often compared using these standardized values, known as z-scores. Percentiles can also be obtained from online distribution calculators that compute the percentage (or proportion) of subjects that would be smaller than the value observed if the variable came from a particular distribution.

Figure 1-9 Probability distribution of heights (in.). *© Cengage Learning, 2012.*

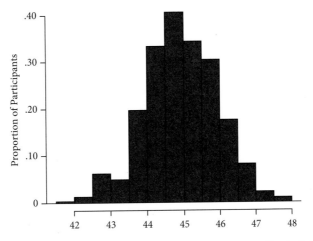

Graphical and numerical summaries provide a strategy for taking all the responses and organizing them in a meaningful way. Numerical and graphical summaries are necessary because variability in responses exists: Not all subjects respond to the same questions or conditions in exactly the same way. If all subjects were exactly the same, with the same characteristics and with the same reaction to treatments or interventions, then statistical methods would not be helpful or necessary. Practicing in public health or in any field would be uninteresting and very simple. Public health practitioners would need to figure out how to help just one person, and the solution could be applied to everyone else. Just as the variability in populations makes practicing public health interesting, variability within and between samples make using statistical methods essential for answering research questions.

Variability Within and Between Subjects

Variability can be defined and described in many ways. *Variability* in measurements occurs when multiple measurements are taken on a subject. If there is little measurement variability, the measurement has **reliability**. For example, if a child's weight was measured at a physician's office three times within an hour, very little to no change would be expected because a scale that measures weight is fairly reliable. On the other hand, if a child is asked what her favorite food is multiple times, the responses are likely to be more inconsistent than when weights were measured. This variable may not be reliable because children have a tendency to change their minds often, and their responses could be very different depending on when the question is asked.

Variability also exists between subjects. In any study, the subjects are generally not the same. Subject-to-subject variability is one of the primary reasons numerical summaries (especially measures of spread) are necessary. Because not every subject is the same, researchers need a systematic approach to describing average measurements on subjects as well as how similar these measurements are. For example, children are not expected to watch the same amount of television. Even though the mean amount of television viewing is 2.1 hours, not every child watches 2.1 hours of television, which is why the standard deviation is 0.5 hours and not 0 hours.

Variability Between Samples

Variability, however, is not limited to differences within subjects (reliability) or between them (spread). It also includes differences between samples. Suppose another sample of 610 children between the ages of 6 and 10 attending public school was selected. Would the same rate of sedentary lifestyle be observed? Would the same number of children be participating in school lunch programs? Would the same average weight or the same number of obese children be observed? It would be very unlikely that any two samples would have exactly the same characteristics; when different samples of subjects are chosen, the sample characteristics will not be exactly the same. The idea that samples may be different is called **sampling variability**.

Because samples are different, the numerical summaries from these samples are expected to be different. Therefore, it is important not to overinterpret the results (numerical and graphical summaries) obtained from a single sample. Although it may seem troubling that different samples could result in different summaries, the study of statistics, in particular *statistical inference*, provides some reassurance.

Ideally, samples chosen from a population should be representative of that population. If each sample represents the population, then the samples should not be wildly different from each other because representative samples are expected to have similar characteristics. If the samples are representative of the population, then their statistics (the numerical summaries of the samples) should be relatively good estimates of the true parameter (the numerical summary of the population). If the statistics (sample summaries) are good estimates of the true parameter (the population summary), then all of the statistics should be relatively close together and "pile up" at the true parameter.

Suppose that all possible random samples (n = 610) are drawn from the population of children (ages 6–10) who attend public school and that, for each sample, the mean weight is calculated. If all the sample mean weights were to be graphed in a histogram, the picture of the probability distribution would reveal that most of the statistics pile up at the center. The center of the pile represents the parameter, the true mean weight of children ages 6–10 who attend public school (Figure 1-10). Only a few of the samples would result in sample means (statistics) that were far from the center of the distribution. The value of the statistics and the number of times the statistics occur from all the possible samples is known as the *distribution of samples*, or the **sampling distribution**.

Just as the distribution provides a description of all possible values obtained from a variable, the sampling distribution provides a description of all possible statistics obtained from samples. In fact, the "average" statistic of all the samples can be described as well as how spread out these statistics are from the "average" statistic. In other words, just as summaries are used to describe the average characteristics of individuals in one sample, summaries can be used to describe the average statistic obtained from a group of samples.

The shape of the sampling distribution in Figure 1-10 is unimodal and symmetric, and it resembles a normal distribution. The value where most of the statistics pile up is the mean of the sampling distribution. This point of the pile-up is also where the true parameter (the true mean weight of children with ages 6–10 attending public school) should be. If the histogram is outlined with a curve (Figure 1-10), the shape of the curve would resemble a bell, the normal curve.

The Central Limit Theorem

If the means obtained from all possible samples are summarized in a histogram:

- The shape will be unimodal and symmetric or normally distributed, as in Figure 1-10.
- The center of the sampling distribution will be the true population mean.
- The distance between the center and the point of curvature will represent one standard deviation, which is equal to the standard error of the mean.

This characterization of all sample means is known as the *central limit theorem (CLT)*.

According to the central limit theorem, the distribution of the means obtained from all possible samples (the sampling distribution of the mean) will result in a normally shaped distribution, in which the center of the distribution is the true parameter (the true population mean) and one standard deviation of the sampling distribution is the standard error of the mean.

The distribution of the sample statistics (the sampling distribution) is different from the other two distributions discussed in this chapter: the distribution of the population and the distribution of data from the sample. If a variable is measured on every

Figure 1-10 Sampling distribution of the mean. © *Cengage Learning, 2012.*

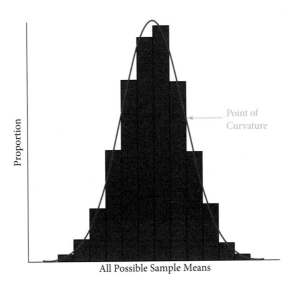

Point of Curvature

Proportion

All Possible Sample Means

subject in the population, the summary of all the possible values of the variable and the number of times the values occurred represents how that variable is distributed in the population. Likewise, when the variable is measured on the subjects in a sample, the summary of all the observed values and how many times they occur provides a distribution of data from the sample. The distribution of the variable measured on a representative sample should resemble the distribution if the variable had been measured on all the subjects in the population. The sampling distribution, however, is different from these two distributions of a variable. A value in a sampling distribution is a statistic. The central limit theorem ensures that, when the statistic is a mean obtained from a reasonably large sample, regardless of the distribution that results from a variable being measured in the population (or sample), the sampling distribution of the mean will always be unimodal, symmetric, and bell-shaped (i.e., normally distributed).

The central limit theorem holds true for large sample sizes. When larger samples (increased sample sizes) are taken, they are more representative of the population and provide an even better estimate of the true parameter. On the other hand, if the sample size is small, then it may not be as representative and the estimates of the parameter may not be as good. When the sample sizes are small, the statistics from these samples are still expected to pile up near the true parameter, but the statistics will have more variability. The greater variability in the statistics results in a distribution that is more spread out and that may not be bell-shaped. However, even with smaller sample sizes the sampling distribution approaches a fairly normal shape rather quickly (Figures 1-11a–f).

Figure 1-11 Changes to sampling distribution of the mean as sample size increases. © *Cengage Learning, 2012.*

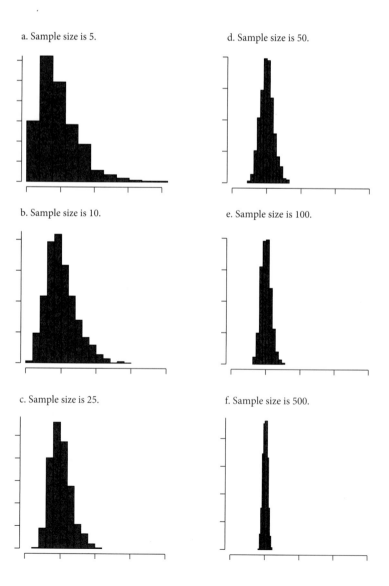

a. Sample size is 5.

b. Sample size is 10.

c. Sample size is 25.

d. Sample size is 50.

e. Sample size is 100.

f. Sample size is 500.

The parameter of interest is not always the mean. When the mean is not of interest, the sampling distribution of all possible statistics may not be normally distributed. Luckily, the sampling distributions of many of these statistics follow distributions that are common and that have well-defined properties. For example, variances have a sampling distribution that follow a chi-square distribution and the ratio of two variances have a sampling distribution that follows an F-distribution. In fact, statistical testing involves transforming numerical summaries obtained from a sample into a value that belongs to one of these commonly used distributions. Numerical summaries (statistics) that are standardized or transformed so that common, known sampling distributions can be used are referred to as **test statistics**. Test statistics with sampling distributions that follow a normal, t-, F-, or chi-square distribution can be used to test a hypothesis while accounting for the fact that different samples may result in different statistics.

CONCEPTS FOR STATISTICAL INFERENCE

A great deal of care (and expense) is taken to conduct a study, so the idea that different samples result in different numerical summaries or statistics can be a little unsettling. Since the results may not be the same from one study to another, it is not wise to use the summaries from a single sample to make conclusions about the population or research question. Luckily, sampling variability (described by sampling distributions) has a predictable pattern, and methods have been developed so that the numerical summaries obtained from a single sample can be used to make conclusions or inferences about the population of interest. These statistical methods are referred to as *methods for statistical inference*. Statistical inference refers to using sample data to estimate a parameter (confidence intervals) or to test a hypothesis (p-values).

Estimation (Confidence Intervals)

Some studies are conducted because an investigator wants to estimate a summary of the population (defined as a parameter). For example, parameters to estimate in this study are the proportion suffering from obesity, the average number of hours spent watching television/playing video games, and the proportion participating in school lunch programs.

Research questions are questions involving numerical summaries about the population (parameters, which are fixed, unknown numbers describing the population). One way to answer a research question is to provide an estimate of the parameter of interest. As discussed, a statistic from a representative sample of the population might provide a good guess or estimate of the parameter. Unfortunately, a sample (even a very good representative sample) is very unlikely to provide a statistic that is exactly the parameter. In fact, it is so unlikely that the statistic is assumed never to be exactly the same as the parameter. The reason is that the statistic and the parameter are the same *size*, that is, they are both just numbers or points. The numerical summary of the sample (the statistic) has essentially no chance of perfectly hitting the numerical summary of the population (the parameter). However, if the statistic (point estimate) is made into something larger than the parameter, the larger quantity has a pretty good chance that it could actually hit the parameter. If a statistic is an estimate of a point, then the larger quantity used to estimate the parameter is a collection of points, or an interval estimate.

The method for creating the interval estimate so that the interval has a good chance of hitting the parameter of interest involves statistical inference. The statistic (point estimate) from a single sample can be made bigger by adding and subtracting an amount

Point to Ponder

If a statistic provides an estimate for a parameter, why does it matter that the statistic might not exactly hit the parameter? It's only an estimate, after all. The problem with a point estimate is that the parameter is unknown; so knowing whether the statistic is just shy of the parameter or not even in the same ballpark is not possible. Interval estimates are constructed so that, in addition to providing a set of possible values for the parameter, they also provide a level of comfort that the interval will contain a value that is the parameter—a hit.

(the **margin of error**) on either side of the point estimate. The sampling distribution can be used to determine how much needs to be added or subtracted on either side of the estimate to hit the true parameter.

The sampling distribution consists of all possible statistics and how often these statistics occur. As an example, if many random samples of 610 children attending public schools are selected and the mean weight of the children in each sample is calculated, these sample means would pile up so that the sampling distribution (Figure 1-12) would be normally distributed and centered at the parameter (the true population mean of children's weights).

Because the sampling distribution is a normal distribution, the empirical rule can be used to determine the number of observations (statistics) that are one, two, and three standard errors from the mean. (Remember that the standard deviation of a sampling distribution of means is the standard error.) If the center of the sampling distribution is the parameter (the true population mean), then

- 68% of all sample means are within one standard error of the parameter.
- 95.4% of all sample means are within two standard errors of the parameter.
- 99.7% of all sample means are within three standard errors of the center the parameter.

By the empirical rule, 95.4% of all statistics are within two standard errors of the true population mean (the parameter). In other words, if two standard errors are added and subtracted to every possible sample mean, 95.4% of the statistics (point estimates) would result in interval estimates that would hit or include the true population mean. Hence, the interval estimate provides a range of plausible values for the parameter as well as a level of comfort (95.4%) that the interval estimate will hit the parameter. Accordingly, these interval estimates are often known as **confidence intervals**, where the level of comfort is called the *confidence level*.

Common confidence levels are 90%, 95%, and 99%. For a normally distributed sampling distribution:

- 90% of all statistics are within 1.645 standard errors of the true parameter.
- 95% of all statistics are within 1.96 standard errors of the true parameter.
- 99% of all statistics are within 2.58 standard errors of the true parameter.

These confidence intervals can be calculated as:

90% confidence interval: point estimate $\pm$ (1.645 $\times$ standard error)

95% confidence interval: point estimate $\pm$ (1.96 $\times$ standard error)

99% confidence interval: point estimate $\pm$ (2.58 $\times$ standard error)

Even when the sampling distribution is not normally distributed, the principle that interval estimates cover the true parameter holds.

Figure 1-12 An application of the Empirical Rule.
© *Cengage Learning, 2012.*

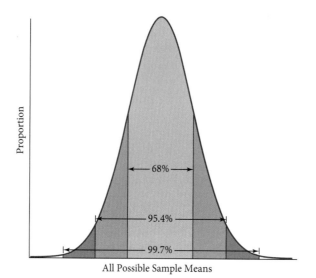

All Possible Sample Means

Hypothesis Testing (*p*-Values)

Although providing an estimate of the parameter helps in answering a research question for estimation, investigators may have a hypothesis to test. Statistical hypotheses involve a claim about the value of a parameter. Therefore, testing the hypothesis means testing whether a parameter is a particular value, a null parameter. The *null parameter*, is a possible parameter. It is not necessarily the true parameter, but it is referred to as a parameter because it is a numerical summary that *may* describe the population. To distinguish between null and true parameters, the notations are different. A null parameter is typically notated in the same way as the true parameter, but a zero (0) subscript is added. For example, if the true parameter is μ, then the null parameter is presented as μ_0.

A study may be conducted because an investigator wants to test whether the true parameter is a hypothesized value, the null parameter. The data collected in a study are used to provide empirical evidence for testing the hypothesis, or claim, about the parameter. If the summary of the sample data (statistic) is very different from the proposed (null) parameter, then there is evidence that the hypothesis is not true.

In hypothesis testing, a statement claiming that the null parameter is the true parameter is called the *null hypothesis*. The goal of a hypothesis test is to determine if the data provide evidence against the null hypothesis. Recall that a statistic is an estimate of the parameter and should be similar to the parameter. Therefore, when a statistic is obtained that is very different from the null parameter, the null hypothesis can be rejected. An alternative, or *research hypothesis*, is a hypothesis that states that the true parameter is not (or is less than or is greater than) the null parameter. It is so named because it is the hypothesis that corresponds to the research question. Hence the goal of a hypothesis test is to reject the null hypothesis in favor of the research hypothesis.

The sampling distribution can be used to determine whether there is sufficient evidence against the null hypothesis. As an example, suppose that the parameter of interest for this study is the mean weight of the children. If the null hypothesis were true, the null parameter (the hypothesized population mean weight) would be the true parameter (the true population mean weight). In other words, when the null hypothesis is true, all the statistics of all the samples will pile up around the null parameter, and the center of the sampling distribution will be the null parameter. The sampling distribution of the mean when the null hypothesis is true is provided in Figure 1-13 as an example.

The sampling distribution with the null parameter (the hypothesized population mean) at the center can be used to see whether the statistic obtained from a single sample is expected. If the null parameter is the true parameter, the observed statistic in the sample should be relatively close to the null parameter, a common statistic under the null claim. If the null parameter is not the true parameter, a statistic near the null

Point to Ponder

Confidence intervals use sampling distributions to estimate the true parameter, and hypothesis tests use sampling distributions to determine whether there is evidence against a null parameter.

The sampling distribution used in hypothesis testing is the sampling distribution that *would* exist *if* the null hypothesis were true. On the other hand, the sampling distribution used for confidence intervals is the sampling distribution that does exist, centered at the true parameter.

Figure 1-13 Sampling distribution of the mean under the null hypothesis.
© Cengage Learning, 2012.

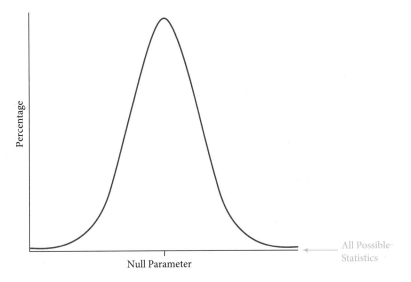

All Possible Statistics

Null Parameter

parameter is not expected. In this case, the statistic will be fairly far from the center of a sampling distribution centered at the null parameter—a rare statistic under the null claim. Rare statistics provide evidence against the null hypothesis.

To reject the null parameter as the true parameter, the observed statistic needs to be far enough away from the center so that the observed statistic clearly came from a sampling distribution that was not centered at the null parameter (Figure 1-14). On the other hand, when the observed statistic is very close to the null parameter, claiming that this statistic would not be expected from a sampling distribution centered at the null parameter would be difficult (Figure 1-15). In these examples, it is fairly obvious that the observed statistics either do not (Figure 1-14) or do (Figure 1-15) belong to the sampling distribution centered at the null parameter. What happens when the evidence is not as strong? Is the statistic in Figure 1-16 far enough away from the null parameter to reject the null hypothesis?

Instead of measuring distances away from the null parameter, distance is quantified as the proportion of statistics that are even farther away from the observed statistic.

- If the proportion of statistics even farther away from the null parameter than the observed statistic is small (Figure 1-14), then the statistic is not expected (rare) to be from the sampling distribution centered at the null parameter.
- If the proportion of statistics even farther from the center than the observed statistic is large (Figure 1-15), then the statistic is considered common to the sampling distribution centered at the null parameter.

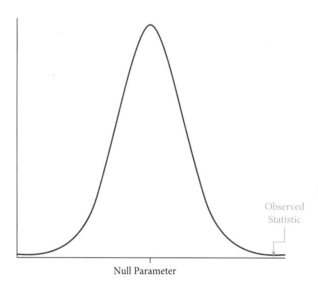

Observed
Statistic

Null Parameter

Figure 1-14 Statistic close to the tails.
© *Cengage Learning, 2012.*

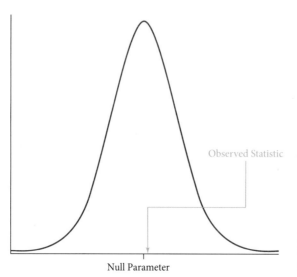

Observed Statistic

Null Parameter

Figure 1-15 Statistic close to the null parameter.
© *Cengage Learning, 2012.*

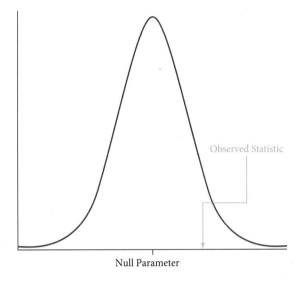

Figure 1-16 Statistic between the null parameter and the tails.
© *Cengage Learning, 2012.*

The proportion of statistics that are even farther from the null parameter than the observed statistic is called the ***p*-value**.

- When the *p*-value is small, the observed statistic is rare and provides evidence against the null hypothesis.
- When the *p*-value is large, the observed statistic is common and does not provide sufficient evidence against the null hypothesis.

The farther the statistic is from the null parameter, the smaller the proportion of statistics that are even farther from the null parameter. Generally, *p*-values that are smaller than 0.05 are considered small enough to reject the null hypothesis. When studies are observational or exploratory, researchers may consider *p*-values smaller than 0.10 as small enough to reject the null hypothesis. In contrast, when the researcher wants to be really sure that the null parameter is not the true parameter, 0.01 or even 0.001 is defined as small enough to reject the null hypothesis.

The sampling distribution example presented here was normally distributed. This may not always be the case depending on the parameter of interest. Although other types of sampling distributions exist, most hypothesis tests involve sampling distributions that resemble common distributions in statistics (normal, *t*-, *F*-, chi-square, binomial, or Poisson). In fact, the calculations for a hypothesis test involve transforming numerical summaries obtained from a sample into a value (test statistic) that belongs to one of these commonly used distributions. When the sampling distribution is one of these commonly used distributions, statistical tables or online probability calculators can be used to determine the proportion of statistics that are farther away than the one observed (*p*-value).

Type 1 Error

Even when a small *p*-value is obtained, the null hypothesis may still really be true. In the sampling distribution, not all statistics will be next to the parameter; some will be farther away. Therefore, a statistic may be far away from the null parameter but still come from the null sampling distribution. When a statistic provides evidence against the null parameter, but the null parameter is really the true parameter a **type 1 error** is made. A type 1 error occurs when the null hypothesis is rejected even though it is really true.

One way to reduce the chance of making a type 1 error is to make rejecting the null hypothesis difficult. By making rejecting the null hypothesis very hard, a lot of evidence is required against the null parameter. If the evidence has to be very convincing to reject, the *p*-value must be very small.

If the cutoff for defining a small enough *p*-value to reject the null is set at 0.05, or 5%, then 5% of the possible statistics in the sampling distribution are far enough away to reject the null parameter even though it is really the true parameter.

Therefore, there is a 5% chance that a type 1 error will be made because these are rare statistics from a sampling distribution centered around the null parameter. Similarly, if the cutoff for defining a small p-value is 1%, rare statistics are defined as the farthest 1% of all possible statistics in the sampling distribution. This means that there is a 1% chance of observing a rare statistic that is actually from the null sampling distribution.

The cutoff for defining how small a p-value needs to be to reject the null is based on the chance of making a type 1 error. The chance of a type 1 error is defined as the **significance level**, which is the proportion of statistics that are far away from the null parameter but still come from the null sampling distribution. Therefore, it represents the probability of making a type 1 error. The significance level is often set at 5% (0.05) and is represented as α.

The significance level is sometimes confused with the p-value, but the two are not the same. The p-value is the proportion of statistics that are farther from the null parameter than the observed statistic. The significance level is often used as the cutoff for how small the p-value has to be before the null parameter can be rejected. The rule for when to reject the null parameter as the true parameter is often written as when p-value $< \alpha$; for example, p-value < 0.05.

Type 2 Error

To prevent type 1 errors, the significance level could be set to an extremely small value, such as $\alpha = 0.000001$. If only the very farthest statistics are evidence that the null parameter is not the true parameter, rejecting the null hypothesis will be very hard. If so, then a different kind of mistake could be made: not rejecting the null hypothesis when it is false. Some other value (an alternative parameter), not the null parameter, may be the true parameter. If the statistic is so far away from the null parameter that it cannot be the true parameter, the alternative parameter (suggested by the research hypothesis) may be the true parameter.

If the research hypothesis is true and the null hypothesis is not rejected, a mistake is made. This mistake is called a **type 2 error**. When the significance level (α) is set to a very small value, then it is more likely that a type 2 error will be made. Thus, as the chance of a type 1 error decreases, the chance of a type 2 error increases. A type 2 error occurs when the null parameter is not the true parameter, but the null hypothesis is not rejected. The probability of a type 2 error is presented less often than the significance level (probability of a type 1 error). When it is provided, it is represented as β and generally ranges from 10% to 20%.

Power

The goal of any hypothesis test is to have a sample with good power, that is, a sample with a good chance of supplying enough evidence so that an incorrect null parameter can be rejected as the true parameter. The probability that the null hypothesis will be rejected when it is indeed false is called **power**. Power is the opposite of the probability of a type 2 error and can be written as $1 - \beta$. A study with good power has power of 80–90%. If a study has 90% power, this means that there is a 90% chance that a false null parameter will be rejected as the true parameter.

Power, type 1 error, and type 2 error all work together. The probabilities of type 1 and type 2 errors are inversely related (when one increases the other decreases). Because the probability of a type 2 error and power are opposites, they are also inversely related. Hence, when the probability of a type 1 error increases, then the power also increases. Figure 1-17 demonstrates the relationships of power and the probabilities of type 1 and type 2 errors for two normally distributed sampling distributions.

Notice that the proximity of the null and alternative distributions is linked to how difficult it is to determine whether a statistic came from the null or alternative distribution. If the two distributions are skinnier and more separated, determining which sampling distribution the statistic belongs to is much easier. When the sample size of a

Figure 1-17 Relationship of power, α, and β.
© Cengage Learning, 2012.

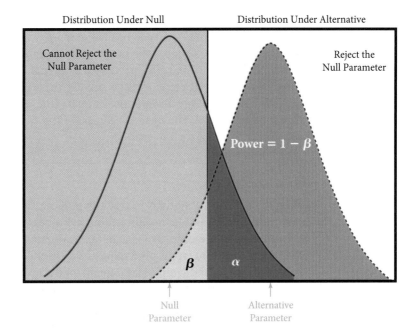

study is larger, the variability between samples is reduced, making the sampling distribution appear skinnier because even more of the statistics pile up at the true parameter. Hence, if the sample size is increased, then the null and alternative distributions get skinnier and become more separated, making it easier to discern between the null and alternative sampling distributions. As the sample size increases, a false null hypothesis becomes more likely to be rejected. In other words, as the sample size increases, the power increases.

PLANNING STUDIES

Planning a study not only involves determining whom to study but how many subjects to study. Conducting a study with too many or too few subjects wastes resources. A study with more subjects than needed is wasteful because the study could be conducted with fewer participants. A study with too few subjects is wasteful because useful inferences and generalizations will be limited. Designing a study with the appropriate number of subjects depends on the research question (or the outcome) and on the purpose of the study.

If the purpose of the study is *estimation*, then the goal is to provide a precise estimate of the outcome, and confidence intervals can be used to determine sample size. This is often the case in exploratory or observational studies. If, however, the purpose of the study is *testing*, then the goal is to test some hypothesis; significance levels and power are necessary for estimating the sample size. This is often the case in clinical trials, experiments, and confirmatory studies.

Estimation Study

When the goal of the study is estimation, the study is likely to involve only one group of interest. In these studies, the objective is generally to estimate a mean, proportion, or rate. Providing an estimate of the parameter means providing a confidence interval. The precision of the confidence interval is the same as its width.

- A parameter is estimated with high precision when the confidence interval is narrow.
- A parameter is estimated with low precision when the confidence interval is wide.

Determining an appropriate sample size when estimation is the goal means utilizing the confidence interval, specifically the margin of error. The *margin of error* of the confidence interval is simply the number of standard errors to add and subtract from the point estimate to make it an interval estimate. The larger the sample size is, the smaller the margin of error and the smaller the width will be. Hence, a sample size calculation using the precision of the estimate (the width of the confidence interval) is fairly straightforward. You need (1) a guess of the variability and (2) an estimate of the precision or width of the interval.

Testing Study

When the goal of the study is to test a hypothesis, the study is likely to involve more than one group. In public health, testing hypotheses often entails comparing groups. In these studies, the objective is generally to perform a test to determine whether a parameter is different from some value: the difference in means is not 0 or a ratio is not 1. Calculations for the sample size depend on the research question and the parameter of interest. However, regardless of the parameter of interest, all sample size estimation when the objective is testing involves the relationship of power (type 2 error), type 1 error, and effect size.

In hypothesis testing, two errors can be made:

- When the decision is to reject the null hypothesis, an error means that it should not have been rejected (type 1).
- When the decision is to fail to reject the null hypothesis, an error means that it should have been rejected (type 2).

The goal of any hypothesis test is to reject the null hypothesis when it should be rejected (power). Because type 1 and type 2 errors are inversely related, making it very hard to reject the null hypothesis is not possible without increasing the chance that the null hypothesis will not be rejected when it should be. The goal is to design a study so that the probability of a type 1 error is reduced and the power (the opposite of the type 2 error) is as large as possible.

Determining an appropriate sample size when testing is the goal requires decisions to be made about power and type 1 error. In general, potential power values are 80–90%. Although greater than 90% power is desirable, a study with less than 80% power should not be considered. Furthermore, the possible values of the probability of a type 1 error range from 1% to 0.1%. Observational, exploratory studies, where a type 1 error is not as critical, can handle larger probabilities of type 1 error ($\alpha = 0.1$). However, most studies use a two-sided probability of a type 1 error of 0.05. If the study is very concerned with making a type 1 error, a lower value is used ($\alpha = 0.01$).

Once decisions are made for power and the probability of a type 1 error, the only other piece that is needed is the effect size. Typically, testing involves being able to detect a difference between groups. The size of this difference is the *effect size*. Studies trying to detect very small effects require a large sample size. On the other hand, studies trying to detect large effects do not require as large a sample size.

SUMMARY

Many research questions remain to be answered in public health. Statistical methods can be utilized in the development of the question, deciding whom or what to study, determining what to measure, summarizing the measurements, and testing hypotheses. After the research question has been posed, the sample selected, and the measurements made, statistical methods provide a strategy for moving from datapoints to answers.

This chapter provided an overview of the primary statistical concepts encountered in public health research: describing the data, estimating the parameter, and testing the hypothesis. There are many statistical procedures for implementing these elements; trying to determine which one to use can sometimes be daunting. However, organizing the methods according to the research question (or the type of variable measured) simplifies choosing the appropriate statistical method. In the chapters that follow, statistical methods appropriate for specific types of research questions are discussed in greater detail.

- Chapter 2 provides details on statistical methods when the research question involves a comparison of groups and the outcome is continuous.
- Chapter 3 continues investigating continuous outcomes by discussing methods for investigating relationships between multiple variables and a continuous outcome.
- Chapters 4 and 5 describe statistical methods for discrete outcomes. Comparing categorical outcomes is the focus of Chapter 4. Chapter 5 provides further details for studies involving a dichotomous outcome.
- Chapters 6 and 7 involve research questions for event rates. The emphasis of Chapter 6 is on count data, while Chapter 7 deals with research questions for the time until an event.

KEY TERMS

population	continuous variables	sampling variability
census	count variables	sampling distribution
sample	parameter	confidence intervals
biased sample	statistic	test statistic
random sample	distribution	margin of error
sampling frame	symmetric	p-value
categorical variables	point of curvature	type 1 error
ordinal variables	skewed	significance level
nominal variables	percentiles	type 2 error
dichotomous variables	reliability	power

1. Consider the population of children ages 6–10 who attend public schools. How could a representative sample of this population be obtained? Identify the problems with using the following methods to obtain a sample of this population:
   a. Send a survey (with a stamped return envelope) to every public elementary school. The students who return the survey are the sample.
   b. The investigator has worked with educational leaders in states in the Southeast and knows that the schools in this region will be motivated to participate. The investigator collects data only on children from these schools.
   c. Children attending elementary schools with high test scores may be more likely to participate, so the investigator chooses only children from schools in the top 10%.
   d. The investigator conducts a random sample using home telephone number of parents with children ages 6–10 in public schools.

2. Describe a scenario when it would be preferable to present the distribution with a count on the vertical axis? With a proportion?

3. Suppose you were conducting a study to investigate the effects of an exercise program on a participant's weight. The participants will be coming in weekly to be weighed. Describe how reliability might be a factor in this study.

4. You collect information on a random sample of women and obtain estimates on vitamin D exposure. However, the results that you find are different than those conducted at another study site. Should you be concerned? Explain your answer using the concept of sampling variability.

5. You are reviewing a publication, and the authors provide a statistic in the results section. It has a large p-value. The discussion section states that, even though the p-value indicates that the null parameter cannot be rejected, the research hypothesis may still be true because the study had low power. Why does low power cause the authors to contradict the conclusion provided by the p-value?

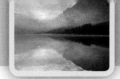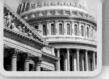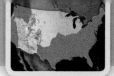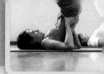
continuous data
making comparisons

Data are considered to be *continuous* when every value is possible; that is, gaps between values do not occur naturally. Continuous data are likely to occur when measuring clinical outcomes: hemoglobin, blood pressure, weight, temperature, gene expressions, or levels of a biomarker. A variable like hemoglobin, for example, is considered continuous because every possible value between 10.1 and 10.2 is possible. The hemoglobin measure of one subject could be 10.1111, and that of another subject could be 10.1999. Typically, hemoglobin is not measured at this level of detail, and the hemoglobin measures for these two subjects would be reported as 10.1 and 10.2.

For a continuous variable, the level of detail is limited only by how precisely the instrument measures. Most methods for collecting data have limited precision, and continuous variables result with some amount of gaps. Depending on the variable, some gaps are bigger than others, but these outcomes are still treated as continuous variables due to the many possible values. For example, age (measured in whole years), the number of calories consumed (measured in whole calories), or income (measured in $1000 increments) are variables that have gaps between possible values but that are still frequently analyzed using the methods for continuous variables. Regardless of how much detail the instrument measures, the analyses of continuous variables in public health include summaries and comparisons.

Summaries that combine the many different values of a continuous variable were introduced in Chapter 1, but this chapter will focus on some of the common statistical methods unique to research questions requiring comparisons when the outcome is continuous.

Continuous data often arise in public health applications, especially when clinical outcomes are measured. The methods for analyzing continuous outcomes constitute the foundation for many of the methods discussed later in this text. In general, the statistical analysis of continuous outcomes involves straightforward calculations and requires limited mathematical manipulations. For this reason, this text starts the investigation of statistical applications in public health at the analysis of continuous data.

LEARNING OBJECTIVES

How do I describe continuous data?

Identify, create, and present appropriate descriptive statistics and figures specific for continuous data.

How do I make comparisons?

Identify appropriate statistical tests for comparison in one, two, or more samples.

Interpret the results of the statistical tests.

How do I make comparisons without assuming the distribution is normal?

Identify appropriate nonparametric tests for comparison in one, two, or more samples.

Interpret the results of the statistical tests.

How do I plan for a study when the outcome is continuous and I need to make a comparison?

Understand the roles that power, effect size, and sample size play in designing a study.

What method do I use?

Identify the most appropriate method for describing the data, numerically and graphically.

Identify the most appropriate method for making comparisons.

Public Health Application

The U.S. EPA estimates that 76–85 million pounds of atrazine (6-chloro-N_2-ethyl-N_4-isopropyl-1,3,4-triazine-2,4-diamine), a triazine herbicide, is produced annually with approximately 76.5 million pounds applied within the United States, making it one of the most widely used pesticides in the country (Cooper, et al., 2007; Gammon, Aldous, Carr, Sanborn, & Pfeifer, 2005; U.S. Environmental Protection Agency, 2008a). Atrazine's main use is to control broadleaf and grassy weeds with the most common sites of application being corn, sugarcane, and sorghum. (Cooper, et al., 2007). Other uses include maintenance of a myriad of crops, golf courses, rangeland, residential lawns, landscapes, forests, recreational areas, and industry (U.S. Environmental Protection Agency, 2008a). Once introduced into the environment, atrazine is not easily broken down and has been shown to persist for long periods (U.S. Environmental Protection Agency, 2008b). In areas such as subsurface soil or aquifers, no biodegradation of atrazine has been shown. This persistence provides ample opportunity for water system contamination (Agency for Toxic Substances and Disease Registry, 2003).

Current research shows that atrazine exposure may pose a significant threat to human health with drinking water providing the most widespread route of exposure (Villanueva, Durand, Coutte, Chevrier, & Cordier, 2005). Triazines in general are considered to be endocrine disrupters (Gammon, et al., 2005). A large number of animal studies have been conducted that demonstrate mixed results concerning the link between atrazine and several adverse health effects including reproductive outcomes and cancer ("EXTOXNET," 1996; Gammon, et al., 2005; Hayes, 2005). (Rinsky et al., 2011)

Data Description

To investigate the impacts of herbicides on maternal health, a longitudinal study was conducted to determine whether drinking water exposed to herbicides would have adverse outcomes on the mother during pregnancy. A **longitudinal study** is a study where subjects are followed for a period of time and the outcome is measured multiple times throughout the study.

A sample of 995 pregnant women from a large farming community was recruited for this study during their initial prenatal visits (approximately week 9). Often an initial measurement is referred to as a *baseline* measurement because it serves as a reference point before the treatment, intervention, condition, or disease occurs. In this study, week 9 measurements serve as baseline measurements because the pregnancy has just begun.

The groundwater in the region is known to be exposed to herbicides. At this initial visit, the women were surveyed about their planned drinking habits for the duration of the pregnancy. In particular, women were asked whether they plan to drink water "only from the tap," "only from bottled water," or "from both the tap and bottle." For the purposes of this study, filtered water was grouped with bottled water. Of the 995 pregnant women, 275 planned to drink only from the tap, 320 were going to drink only bottled water, and 400 intended to drink from both sources. In addition to water source, information on the number of previous births (parity), prepregnancy smoking status, income, and education was also obtained at the initial visit. After that visit, hemoglobin measurements were taken from these women throughout their pregnancy: week 12 (hgb12), 24 (hgb24), and 36 (hgb36). In addition to hemoglobin measures, measures of weight gain (lb) were also obtained. Only women who had resided in the region for the last 10 years, had singleton births after week 36 (full-term), and were compliant with their water consumption plans were included in the analysis, resulting in a final sample of 270 who drank only from the tap, 315 who drank only bottled water, and 394 who drank from both sources. The primary goal of this study is to understand how hemoglobin changes differ for the women who were exposed to herbicides in the water versus those who were not. The outcome of interest is the change in hemoglobin from week 9 to week 36 or hgb9–hgb36.

DESCRIBING THE DATA

RESEARCH QUESTION:

Does exposure to herbicides in drinking water impact changes in hemoglobin?

Because measuring continuous variables can result in many possible values, describing the data typically includes providing a summary of the center and the spread of the observed values. The most common numerical summaries of center are mean and median, and the most common numerical summaries of spread are standard deviation and range, respectively. Graphically, histograms are very useful for describing continuous data, box and whisker plots are effective when comparing distributions of continuous data, and plots of the means with standard error bars are helpful when comparing means.

In this study, several variables can be classified as continuous variables: age, weight gain, week 9 hemoglobin, week 36 hemoglobin, and the change in hemoglobin from week 9 to week 36.

Numerical Summaries: Measures of Center and Spread

Numerical summaries are very helpful for describing continuous data, and the most common numerical summary is the mean. The *mean* represents the center of the continuous variable by summing all the values and dividing by the number of subjects that contributed values. The *population mean* is typically represented by μ. Using a sample, the population mean μ is estimated by the sample mean $\bar{x}$. The *sample mean* is a statistic; it is simply the sum of the values observed in the sample divided by the number of subjects that contributed data.

Application of Formula: SAMPLE MEAN

$$\bar{x} = \frac{\sum_{i=1}^{n} x_i}{n}$$

x_i = The value of the continuous variable for subject i

n = The total number of subjects with values

What you need to calculate the mean:

1. *The sample size:* In this example, the hemoglobin change in 979 women was measured. Therefore, $n = 979$.
2. *The sum of the values of the continuous variable:* In this example, the sum of all the hemoglobin change values is 2890.7.

To calculate the mean: Divide the sum of the values (2) by the sample size (1). In this example, the sample mean is $\frac{2890.7}{98179} = 2.95$, $\bar{x} = 2.95$ g/dL.

With continuous data, simply describing the center of the distribution is not sufficient; a measure of spread is also needed. When the mean is chosen to describe the center, the variance or standard deviation is the appropriate measure to describe the spread of values. The **variance** is the average squared distance that each observation is from the mean. The **standard deviation** is simply the square root of the variance.

The standard deviation is always positive. Suppose one of the hemoglobin change values for a subject is 2.25 g/dL. This value is 0.70 g/dL below the mean (-0.70 g/dL). Another hemoglobin change value may be 3.65 g/dL. This value is 0.70 g/dL above the mean ($+0.70$ g/dL). If these two distances from the mean were averaged, the value would be 0.0 g/dL, indicating that there was no variation in the change scores (i.e., the observed hemoglobin change scores were all the same). This is obviously not the case. To prevent the cancellation that occurs when considering observations that are bigger or smaller than the mean, the distances from the mean are squared. Squaring the distances from the mean makes all the values positive. The squares of these distances are 0.49 each and sum to 0.98.

The sum of the squared differences from the mean is called the *total sum of squares.* The total sum of squares is then divided by $n - 1$ to obtain the sample variance. The sample variance is a statistic represented by s^2. It is used to estimate the population variance (σ^2). The sample standard deviation is the square root of the sample variance.

The standard deviation is also a statistic, represented by s, and is used to estimate the population standard deviation (σ). The standard deviation is often reported in lieu of the variance because the units of the standard deviation are the same as the units of the mean. In this study, the units associated with the variance for the change in hemoglobin are $(g/dL)^2$, whereas the units of the mean and standard deviation are g/dL.

Application of Formula: SAMPLE VARIANCE

$$s^2 = \frac{\text{Total sum of the squares}}{n - 1}$$

x_i = The value of the continuous variable for subject i

$\bar{x}$ = The sample mean for the continuous variable

n = The total number of subjects with values

What you need to calculate the sample variance:

1. *An easier equation:* $s^2 = \frac{\sum_{i=1}^{n} x_i^2 - n\bar{x}^2}{n - 1}$
2. *The sample size:* $n = 979$.
3. *The sample mean:* $\bar{x} = 2.95$ g/dL.
4. *Square the sample mean and multiply by the sample size:* $n\bar{x}^2 = 979 \times (2.95^2) = 979 \times 8.70 = 8{,}519.7$.
5. *Uncorrected Sum of Squares: Square each value for each subject and sum,* $\sum_{i=1}^{n} x_i^2 = 9{,}108.1$.
6. *Corrected Sum of Squares: Subtract (4) from (5),* $\sum_{i=1}^{n} x_i^2 - n\bar{x}^2 = 9{,}108.1 - 8{,}519.7 = 588.4$.

To calculate the variance: Divide (6) by [(2) − 1], $588.4/979 = 0.60$.
To calculate the standard deviation: Take the square root of the variance, $s = \sqrt{0.60} = 0.77$ g/dL.

Hemoglobin measures are not expected to be highly skewed. Therefore, the mean is an appropriate measure of the center. However, the mean is not always the most appropriate measure of the center. With some continuous data, the values are either right- or left-skewed so that there is a longer tail to either the right or the left, respectively. The mean is not a robust numerical summary because it is pulled toward the extreme data (tail). A numerical summary is considered *robust* if it is not easily pulled toward the tail; extreme values are less likely to affect them. The median provides a robust numerical summary of the center. The median is a more robust measure of the center because it is at the middle of the values. Even if the tails contain extreme values, the middle value is less likely to be pulled toward the extreme values than a sum of all the values (which is a critical part of the calculation of the mean). When the data are not heavily skewed, the mean and median will be fairly close.

The median represents the center of the continuous variable by sorting all the possible values and dividing those values in half. The median is the value of the continuous variable at the halfway point; 50% of the values are smaller than the median and 50% of the values are larger. The population median is represented by M. Using a sample, the population median M is estimated by the sample median, $\bar{m}$. The *sample median,* a statistic, is simply the middle value of the sorted observed values.

Application of Formula: SAMPLE MEDIAN

$\overline{m}$ = The 50th percentile of the data

What you need to calculate the median:

1. *Sorted data:* Sorted from smallest to largest.
2. *The sample size:* $n = 979$
3. *Divide the data in half:* This provides the position of the median. With 979 subjects, the position of the median is 490.

To calculate the median: This is the value of the continuous variable in the position found in entry 3. The estimated median change in hemoglobin for this sample is $\overline{m} = 3.12$ g/dL.

Just as the mean is not sufficient for describing continuous data, merely describing the center of the distribution with a median is not adequate either; a measure of spread is also needed. When the median is chosen to describe the center, however, the variance and the standard deviation are not appropriate because they involve describing distances from the mean. The interquartile range or range, on the other hand, is an appropriate measure to describe the spread of values. The *range* is the difference between the minimum and maximum values; it truly represents the range of values in the distribution. The *interquartile range* is a condensed version of the range; it is the difference between the first and third quartiles or the difference between the values at the 25th and 75th percentiles. The interquartile range represents the range of values that belong to the middle 50% of the subjects.

Application of Formula: SAMPLE RANGE

Estimated range $= x_{(n)} - x_{(1)}$

$x_{(n)}$ = The smallest value of the continuous variable (maximum)

$x_{(1)}$ = The largest value of the continuous variable (minimum)

What you need to calculate the estimated range:

1. *Sorted data:* Sorted from smallest to largest.
2. *The smallest value:* $x_{(1)} = \min = 0.65$ g/dL.
3. *The largest value:* $x_{(n)} = \max = 4.77$ g/dL.

To calculate the estimated range: This is the difference between the largest (3) and the smallest (2) values: $x_{(n)} - x_{(1)} = 4.12$ g/dL. In this example, the hemoglobin change of the women ranges from 0.65 to 4.77 g/dL, a range of 4.12.

Application of Formula: SAMPLE INTERQUARTILE RANGE (IQR)

Estimated interquartile range $= \hat{q}_3 - \hat{q}_1$

$\hat{q}_3$ = The value in the 75th percentile, the midpoint of the upper half of the data

$\hat{q}_1$ = The value in the 25th percentile, the midpoint of the lower half of the data

continues

continued

What you need to calculate the sample interquartile range:

1. *Sorted data:* Sorted from smallest to largest.
2. *The median:* $\overline{m} = 3.12$.
3. *Divide the data into an upper and lower half using the median as the dividing point:*
   a. The lower half of the data are any points less than the median
   b. The upper half of the data are any points greater than the median
4. *Find the median of each half of the data:*
   a. The median of the lower half of the data is $\hat{q}_1 = 2.36$ g/dL.
   b. The median of the upper half of the data is $\hat{q}_3 = 3.56$ g/dL.

To calculate the interquartile range: Subtract (4a) from (4b): $3.56 - 2.36 = 1.2$ g/dL. In this example, the middle 50% of the women have a hemoglobin change ranging from 2.36 to 3.56 g/dL, a sample IQR of 1.2 g/dL.

Graphical Summaries for a Continuous Outcome

Graphical summaries of continuous outcomes are also an important part of describing the data. Continuous outcomes provide a lot of information; and for a continuous variable, every subject could have a different value. Summarizing all this information graphically is very helpful. The three most common graphical summaries for a continuous outcome are histograms, box-and-whisker plots, and plots of means with error bars.

Histograms

Graphical representations of the distribution of continuous variables are often done with histograms. As described in Chapter 1, *histograms* are created by grouping similar values and describing the number of subjects within the groups as bars, resulting in a bar graph with bars that touch. Because histograms group the many possible values of a continuous variable, they are perfect for presenting a quick picture of the shape, center, and spread of the distribution of a continuous variable. Furthermore, histograms are particularly suited for continuous outcomes because, like a continuous outcome, the horizontal axis and the arrangement of the bars have a defined order.

In this example, as expected with hemoglobin values, the shape is relatively symmetric, and the center appears to be around 11.3 g/dL (Figure 2-1). Recall from Chapter 1 that a distribution is considered *symmetric* when an imaginary line can be drawn down the center and the bars on either side of the line are roughly the same. In a symmetric histogram, the center represents the average (summarized by either the

Figure 2-1 Distribution of baseline hemoglobin (g/dL). © *Cengage Learning, 2012.*

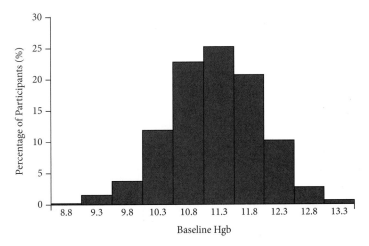

mean or the median). In Figure 2-1, the women at week 9 are, on average, nonanemic (the average hemoglobin is greater than 10 g/dL), but some women have hemoglobin as low as 8.8 g/dL. The distribution of the hemoglobin values is fairly symmetric and *unimodal (one peak)*. In Chapter 1, these types of distributions were identified as *normal distributions*.

It may be of interest to investigate the separated distributions of women who drink only from the tap and of those who drink only bottled water. To do that, the researcher would create a histogram for each drinking category (Figure 2-2), providing a visual comparison of the two distributions. In the figure, women who drink only from the tap tend to have lower initial hemoglobin measures than those who drink only bottled water.

Figure 2-2 Distribution of baseline hemoglobin (g/dL) by water group.
© *Cengage Learning, 2012.*

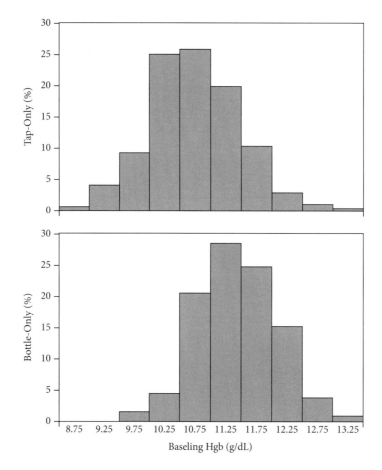

Figure 2-3 Distribution of hemoglobin change (g/dL).
© *Cengage Learning, 2012.*

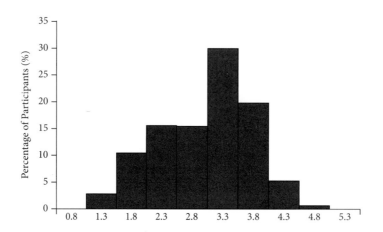

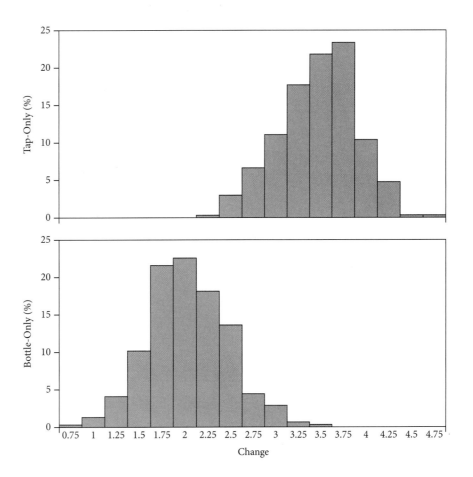

Figure 2-4 Distribution of hemoglobin change by water group.
© Cengage Learning, 2012.

Similarly, the histogram for the change in hemoglobin from week 9 to week 36 also has a symmetric distribution (Figure 2-3). The distribution of hemoglobin change is centered at approximately 3 g/dL. The separated histograms for women who drink only from the tap and for women who drink only bottled water indicate that women who drink only from the tap have larger changes than women who drink only bottled water (Figure 2-4).

Box-and-Whisker Plots

When the goal is compare, the box-and-whisker plot may be a more appropriate graphical summary than creating a separate histogram for each group. A box-and-whisker plot incorporates the **five number summary:** the median, first and third quartile, and minimum and maximum. Although there are variations to the box-and-whisker plot, a basic plot (Figure 2-5) consists of:

- Box containing the median and first and third quartiles.
- And whiskers that extend to the minimum and maximum.

Unlike histograms, box-and-whisker plots are not useful when describing one group or sample. The purpose of box-and-whisker plots is to provide a visual comparison of the distribution of a continuous variable. When comparing the distribution of two or more groups using box-and-whisker plots, two questions are of interest:

1. *Are the centers of the groups similar?* Similar medians suggest that the centers of the distributions are the same.
2. *How do the spreads compare?* The spread can be described by the length of the box and by the length of the whiskers. The length of the box describes the interquartile range, the middle 50% of the data. A group with a shorter box suggests not as much variability as a group with a longer box. The length of the whiskers, from one end to the other, represent the full range of the data. Like the length of the box, the length of the whiskers can describe how spread out the data are.

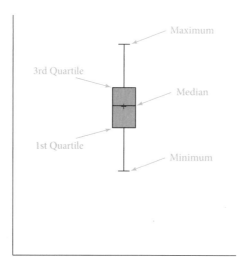

Figure 2-5 Box-and-whisker plot.
© *Cengage Learning, 2012.*

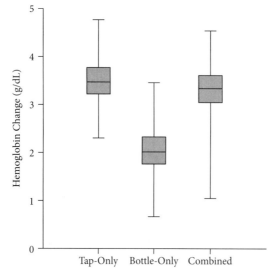

Figure 2-6 Box-and-whisker plot for comparing three groups.
© *Cengage Learning, 2012.*

For example, consider the box-and-whisker plots created from the hemoglobin change data for the three water consumption groups (Figure 2-6). The centers of the tap-only and combined-water use are similar, and both groups are different, on average, from the bottle-only group. In fact, the maximum change in hemoglobin for bottle-only pregnant women is near the median hemoglobin change for the tap-only and combined-water groups. Furthermore, although the spreads of the bottle-only and tap-only groups are similar, the spread of the combined-water group is much larger. However, the larger spread in the combination group may be expected because it potentially represents a more diverse group of pregnant women.

By portraying the center and spread of distributions, box-and-whisker plots not only provide a description of the distributions but also suggest whether differences between groups exist.

Plotting Means

Sometimes describing the distribution of the continuous variable may not be sufficient to portray comparisons of continuous outcomes for different groups. Because research questions often involve comparing means, a visual depiction of means is useful. To show how the means of different groups compare, bar graphs are used. In these plots, however, the vertical axis represents the mean of the continuous variable, each group has a separate bar, and the height of the bar represents the value of the mean for

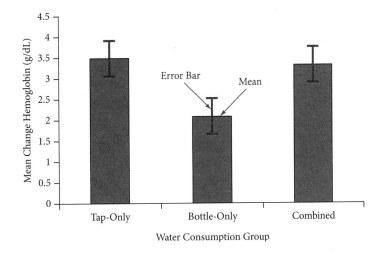

Figure 2-7 Plot of means and standard deviations for water groups.
© *Cengage Learning, 2012.*

that group. In contrast to a histogram, the bars do not touch, and the horizontal axis (groups) may not have a pre-defined order. Moreover, the vertical axis is also different because it represents the mean of the continuous variable.

However, merely providing a description of the center (mean) without also providing a description of the spread is not sufficient. Therefore, plots of the means are often presented with lines to represent the variability, called *error bars*. Generally, the error bars represent the mean plus or minus the standard deviation or the standard error. Choosing between the standard error or the standard deviation for the plot depends on the purpose of the graphical summary. Standard deviations are used when describing the variability in the sample, and standard errors are generally used for statistical inference.

These plots provide a quick comparison of the means for each group and show how variable the responses are within a group. In this example, the hemoglobin mean changes for the three water consumption groups are different, but the standard deviations (error bars) are similar (Figure 2-7).

ONE-GROUP STUDIES WITH A CONTINUOUS OUTCOME

Sometimes only one group of subjects is of interest: for example, suppose only women who drink water from the tap, the exposed group, are analyzed. When only one group of subjects is of interest, the study is often referred to as a *one-sample study*.

Table 2-1 displays examples of numerical summaries or descriptive statistics in a one-sample study. The pregnant women in the exposed sample tend to be young (average age 25, SD = 1.9), report a median household income of $33K with a range of $8.7K, and have a low educational level (only 41% have a high school degree). On average, the week 9 hemoglobin of these pregnant women is low (10.7 g/dL, SD = 0.74 g/dL). Based on the median, half of the women have week 9 hemoglobin values of less than 10.8, indicating that half of the women are already at anemic levels (<11 g/dL) at week 9. The primary outcome for this research question, is the change in hemoglobin (Table 2-2). The pregnant women in this sample who drink water only from the tap have an average decrease in hemoglobin of 3.5 g/dL (SD 0.43 g/dL) from week 9 to week 36.

One-sample studies are conducted for two reasons:

- Obtaining an additional group or sample for comparisons is not practical.
- The change (such as the difference between before and after a condition or pre- and post-test) is of primary interest.

A one-sample study does not have an independent comparator or control group. On the other hand, if the one-sample study is employed because a change is of interest, the subjects in the study serve as their own control. One-sample studies with a change

TABLE 2-1 **CHARACTERISTICS OF THE SAMPLE**

	Tap Only (*N* = 270)
Age (years)	*n* = 270
Mean (SD)	25.03 (1.907)
Median (min, max)	25.1 (18.9, 30.7)
Household Income ($10K)	*n* = 270
Mean (SD)	3.75 (1.434)
Median (min, max)	3.3 (2.2, 10.9)
Weight Gain (lb)	*n* = 270
Mean (SD)	41.60 (4.106)
Median (min, max)	41.5 (29.5, 56.4)
Adequate Prenatal Care	
No	175 (64.8%)
Yes	95 (35.2%)
Smoked Prior to Pregnancy	
No	183 (67.8%)
Yes	87 (32.2%)
Education	
Less HS	149 (55.2%)
HS/GED	111 (41.1%)
College +	10 (3.7%)
Number of Previous Births (parity)	
None	45 (16.7%)
One	137 (50.7%)
Two	78 (28.9%)
Three or More	10 (3.7%)

© Cengage Learning, 2012.

TABLE 2-2 **SUMMARY OF HEMOGLOBIN OUTCOMES**

	Tap Only (*N* = 270)
Week 9 Hemoglobin (g/dL)	*n* = 270
Mean (SD)	10.73 (0.739)
Median (min, max)	10.8 (8.6, 13.2)
Final Hemoglobin (g/dL)	*n* = 270
Mean (SD)	7.26 (0.856)
Median (min, max)	7.3 (5.3,10.1)
Change in Hemoglobin (g/dL)	*n* = 270
Mean (SD)	3.47 (0.423)
Median (min, max)	3.5 (2.3, 4.8)

Note: The change in hemoglobin represents initial (week 9) less final (week 36) hemoglobin.
© Cengage Learning, 2012.

outcome are generally conducted when the investigator expects considerable individual differences. If a one-sample study is being conducted because an independent comparator group is not practical, then historical information or historical controls are used for comparison. **Historical controls** are estimates of the true parameter that were found using data from a different study, such as studies from a different time period, a different region, different population, or a different kind of exposure. Historical controls come into play when the control data are not collected concurrently within the same study.

One-Sample Hypothesis Test: Historical Controls

In this example, women who drank water only from the tap might have been exposed to herbicides found in the region's groundwater. Suppose it is of interest to compare the changes in hemoglobin in women exposed to herbicides to changes in women who have been exposed to other environmental factors. For example, mercury has been found in groundwater in areas close to manufacturing centers. Suppose investigators want to compare the mean hemoglobin change in pregnant women exposed to herbicides in water to the mean change in pregnant women exposed to mercury in water. To make this comparison, the mean hemoglobin change in mercury-exposed pregnant women has to be obtained. Suppose the average change in hemoglobin in pregnant women in areas exposed to mercury has been reported as 2.0 g/dL. Because this information is obtained from a different study, the mean hemoglobin change for mercury-exposed pregnant women represents a historical control.

Although the observed mean in this study ($\bar{x} = 3.50$ g/dL) is different from the 2.0 g/dL historical control, the sample mean ($\bar{x} = 3.50$ g/dL) could be specific to this particular sample. Because of sampling variability, it is possible that statistics can vary from sample to sample.

- Did it just happen that this sample of women drinking tap water resulted in a value different from 2.0 g/dL?
- Would another sample of women exposed to herbicides have a similar mean change in hemoglobin?
- Is the discrepancy between the statistic (3.5 g/dL) and the historical control (2.0 g/dL) large enough to conclude that the hemoglobin changes in pregnant women exposed to herbicides are different from the hemoglobin changes in pregnant women exposed to mercury?

Hypothesis testing can help answer these questions; providing a conclusion for the research question.

RESEARCH QUESTION: Is the hemoglobin change in pregnant women exposed to herbicides different from that in pregnant women exposed to mercury?

RESEARCH HYPOTHESIS: The true mean (μ) hemoglobin change for pregnant women exposed to herbicides is not 2.0 g/dL.

NULL HYPOTHESIS: The true mean (μ) hemoglobin change for pregnant women exposed to herbicides is 2.0 g/dL.

To test this hypothesis, it must be assumed that the true parameter (the true mean hemoglobin change for pregnant women exposed to herbicides in drinking water) is 2.0 g/dL. In other words, the historical control (the value obtained from a previous study) serves as the null parameter, $\mu_0 = 2.0$ g/dL. The data in the sample ($n = 270$) provide a statistic (an estimate of the mean: $\bar{x} = 3.50$ g/dL), and it must be determined whether this statistic would be expected if the null parameter ($\mu_0 = 2.0$ g/dL) were the true parameter. Therefore, the goal is to use the sample data to provide evidence against the null hypothesis.

Hypothesis tests assume that the null parameter is the true parameter. When a hypothesis is tested, an investigator assumes the null is true. For hypotheses involving means, this implies that the null parameter is the center of the sampling distribution. Statistics close to the center of the sampling distribution are supposed to be common or to occur often. Therefore, when a statistic far away from the null parameter is found, this supplies evidence against the null hypothesis. Hence, hypothesis testing means determining whether the observed statistic is far away from or close to the null parameter. An observed statistic that is far away from the null parameter is considered *rare* and would not be expected if the null parameter really was at the center of the sampling distribution. Therefore, rare statistics result in rejecting the null hypothesis.

In Chapter 1, a sampling distribution was defined as the distribution of all possible statistics obtained from all possible samples of the same size. In this example, the sampling distribution would consist of all possible sample means obtained from samples with 270 pregnant women. Sampling distributions are often standardized to simplify determining whether a statistic is common or rare. When dealing with means, the sample mean is standardized into a test statistic by subtracting the null parameter and then dividing by the standard error (the standard deviation divided by the square root of the sample size). If the null parameter is the true parameter, then the sampling distribution of the test statistics is centered at 0 and has a standard deviation of 1 (Figure 2-8).

When the statistic is a sample mean, the standardized sampling distribution is known as the *t*-distribution (Figure 2-8). The *t*-distribution resembles a normal distribution in shape. The mean and the median are in the center at the peak. However, the tails of the *t*-distribution are a little thicker than those of the normal distribution. Thicker tails imply a greater possibility of observing values in the tails. As the sample size increases, the *t*-distribution more closely resembles a normal distribution.

The *t*-distribution is also characterized by **degrees of freedom**. Degrees of freedom are found in several sampling distributions and can be thought of as the independent pieces of information needed to estimate parameters and variability. In this example, the degrees of freedom are the sample size minus 1 or $(n - 1)$. In a random sample with n subjects, n pieces of independent information are available. If the mean is estimated, then there are $n - 1$ pieces of independent information (or degrees of freedom) left over to estimate the variance. Therefore, for a one-sample study, the degrees of freedom associated with the sampling distribution are $n - 1$.

The hypothesis test involving the mean in a study with only one group is called a *one-sample t-test*.

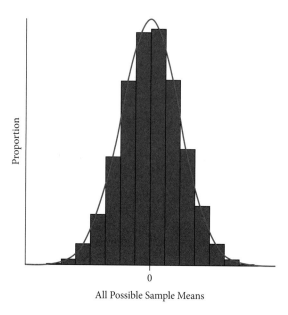

Proportion

0

All Possible Sample Means

Figure 2-8 Standardized sampling distribution for sample means. © *Cengage Learning, 2012.*

Test statistic $(t) = \dfrac{\bar{x} - \mu_0}{\frac{s}{\sqrt{n}}}$

$\bar{x}$ = The sample mean

μ_0 = The null parameter (the guess of the population mean)

s = The standard deviation of the sample

n = The sample size

What you need for a one-sample *t*-test:

1. *The difference between the sample mean and the null parameter:* In this study, the sample mean is 3.5 g/dL, and the null parameter is 2 g/dL. The difference is 1.5 g/dL.
2. *The standard error:* The estimate of the standard error of the mean is the sample standard deviation divided by the square root of the sample size. In this study, the standard error is $0.423/\sqrt{270} = 0.026$.

To calculate the test statistic (t) for the one-sample t-test: Divide (1) by (2): $1.5 \div 0.026 = 57.7$. Now, is this value far enough away from the center of the standardized sampling distribution? The standardized sampling distribution is a *t*-distribution with 269 degrees of freedom centered at 0 (because the null parameter of 2 has been subtracted). The larger the magnitude of the test statistic is, the farther away the test statistic is from 0, or the center of the sampling distribution. As a general rule, test statistics that are bigger than 3 or smaller than -3 are considered to be far enough away from the center of the sampling distribution; so a test statistic of 57.7 is very large or is very far away from 0 and would be considered very rare.

In Chapter 1, *p-values* were described as a different, but equivalent, way to measure the distance from the center of the sampling distribution. Instead of counting by standardized distances, *p*-values measure how far a test statistic is away from the center by providing the proportion of test statistics that are even farther away. In this example, the test statistic that results from a one-sample *t*-test is 57.7 and is considered to be very large. The exact proportion of test statistics that are even farther away than 57.7 is <0.0001. This proportion represents the *p*-value and can be found by using statistical software (Table 2-3) or statistical tables. Because the *p*-value is so small, this test statistic is considered rare and would not be expected if the true parameter was the null parameter.

TABLE 2-3 **RESULTS FROM THE ONE-SAMPLE *t*-TEST**

Variable: Hemoglobin Change		Results of *t*-Test		
N	270	*t*-value	DF	Pr > |t|
Mean	3.4689			
Std Dev	0.4234	56.94	269	<0.0001
Std Error	0.0258			

Note: Values may be slightly different from Application of Formula calculations due to rounding.

© Cengage Learning, 2012.

CONCLUSION: There is sufficient evidence to reject the null hypothesis that the true parameter is 2 g/dL. Hence, there is a difference in the hemoglobin change for pregnant women exposed to herbicides compared to pregnant women exposed to mercury in the water.

One-sample studies may be conducted when the research question involves a change or a difference within subjects. In these studies, the subjects in the sample serve as their own control because having an independent control group does not provide a good comparison. These studies are appropriate when more variability is expected between subjects than within a subject; in other words, subjects are too different to make useful comparisons. Weight loss studies, educational interventions, or implementation of lifestyle changes are all such situations. Using the subject's "before" measurement as the control is more logical than comparing the "after" measurements of two independent subjects. For example, comparing the before and after hemoglobin values of a participant in a pregnancy study makes more sense than comparing the final hemoglobin of one participant to another control participant. The before and after measurements are compared by calculating the change for each subject and determining whether the mean change is different from 0. The difference or change between measurements made on the same subject is often referred to as a paired difference.

A **paired difference** is the difference between a pair of measurements. Data are considered paired when two measurements are related. Therefore, pre- and post-measurements are paired data because they are obtained from the same subject; the two measurements are related. Although pre- and post values are a common source of paired differences, research questions involving paired differences are not limited to studies that measure before and after results. For example:

- A study investigating the effects of pesticides on plants may divide the plant leaf into two parts and compare two parts on the same leaf instead of having a control plant and treated plant.
- A study on hands may use one hand as the control and the other hand for the intervention and compare differences between the hands rather than having one person supply a treatment hand and another person supply a control hand.

Paired data is used whenever the variability between subjects is so great that meaningful comparisons require using the subject as its own control.

Usually, the goal of a paired difference analysis is to determine whether the paired difference is equal to 0; a difference of 0 means that the two measurements are the same. Hence, the statistical methods for paired differences are really the same methods as those using a historical control. The observations are just differences (the difference between before and after measurements, for example) and 0 is used as the null parameter.

Suppose investigators wanted to determine whether the hemoglobin in pregnant women exposed to herbicides changed during pregnancy. In a study to determine hemoglobin changes in pregnancy, taking initial and final measurements on the same pregnant woman and having her serve as her own control is the appropriate approach. Therefore, the week 9 and week 36 hemoglobins represent a pair of observations on a single subject. Because the week 36 hemoglobin is dependent on the week 9 hemoglobin, the change in hemoglobin (the difference between week 9 and week 36 hemoglobin) represents a paired difference.

Although the observed mean change (paired difference) in this study ($\bar{x} = 3.5$ g/dL) is different from 0, this sample mean may be specific to this sample. Is the difference between 3.5 and 0 related to this sample, or is 3.5 g/dL different enough from 0 g/dL to state that herbicide-exposed pregnant have changes in hemoglobin? Hypothesis testing can help.

> **RESEARCH QUESTION:** Is there a change in hemoglobin for pregnant women exposed to herbicides?

RESEARCH HYPOTHESIS: The true mean (μ) hemoglobin change for pregnant women exposed to herbicides is not 0 g/dL.

NULL HYPOTHESIS: The true mean (μ) hemoglobin change for pregnant women exposed to herbicides is 0 g/dL.

In the hypothesis test, it is assumed that the true parameter (the true mean hemoglobin change for pregnant women exposed to herbicides in drinking water) is 0 g/dL. In other words, a no-difference value serves as the null parameter, $\mu_0 = 0$ g/dL. The data in the sample ($n = 270$) provide a statistic (an estimate of the mean: $\bar{x} = 3.5$ g/dL), and it must be determined whether this statistic would be expected if the null parameter ($\mu_0 = 0$ g/dL) was the true parameter. Therefore, the goal is to use the sample data to provide evidence against the null hypothesis.

When the mean is obtained from the paired differences of one sample, the test to determine whether there is sufficient evidence against the null hypothesis is called a *one-sample paired t-test*.

Application of Formula: PAIRED *t*-TEST

$$\text{Test statistic } (t) = \frac{\bar{x}_d - 0}{\frac{s_d}{\sqrt{n}}} = \frac{\bar{x}_d}{\frac{s_d}{\sqrt{n}}}$$

$\bar{x}_d$ = The sample mean of the paired differences

s_d = The sample standard deviation of the paired differences

n = The sample size

What you need for a one-sample *t*-test:

1. *The sample mean of the paired differences:* $\bar{x}_d = 3.5$ g/dL.
2. *The standard error:* The estimate of the standard error of the mean differences is the sample standard deviation of the differences divided by the square root of the sample size. In this study, the standard error is $0.423/\sqrt{270} = 0.026$.

To calculate the test statistic (t) for the paired t-test: Divide (1) by (2): $3.5 \div 0.026 = 134.6$.

Is this value far enough away from the center of the standardized sampling distribution? The standardized sampling distribution is a *t*-distribution with 269 degrees of freedom centered at 0. The larger the magnitude of the test statistic is, the farther away the test statistic is from 0, or the center of the sampling distribution. As a general rule, test statistics that are bigger than 3 or smaller than -3 are considered to be far enough away from the center of the sampling distribution; so a test statistic of 134.6 is very large and would be considered very rare.

In this example, the test statistic that results from the paired *t*-test is 134.6 and is considered to be quite large. In fact, the proportion of test statistics that are even farther away than 134.6 is <0.0001 (*p*-value) and can be found by using statistical software (Table 2-4) or by using statistical tables.

Because such a small percentage of statistics are even farther away, this test statistic is considered rare. It would not be expected at all if the true parameter was the null parameter.

TABLE 2-4 **RESULTS FROM THE PAIRED *t*-TEST**

Variable: Hemoglobin Change		Results of t-Test		
N	270	*t*-value	DF	Pr > |*t*|
Mean	3.4689			
Std Dev	0.4234	134.47	269	<0.0001
Std Error	0.0258			

Note: Values may be slightly different from Application of Formula calculations due to rounding.

© Cengage Learning, 2012.

CONCLUSION: There is sufficient evidence to reject the null hypothesis that the true parameter is 0 g/dL. Hence, for pregnant women exposed to herbicides, hemoglobin does change throughout pregnancy.

One-Sample Confidence Intervals for the Mean

Although hypothesis tests are helpful for determining whether the null hypothesis can be rejected, they do not provide an estimate for the true parameter. Based on the one-sample tests (one-sample *t*-test and paired *t*-test), the true mean change in hemoglobin for pregnant women exposed to herbicides is neither 2.0 g/dL nor 0.0 g/dL. However, to estimate the true mean change in hemoglobin, confidence intervals must be used.

Like hypothesis tests, confidence intervals also use sampling distributions and the fact that not all samples will result in the same statistics. The estimate of $\bar{x} = 3.5$ g/dL is a point estimate and describes only this sample. Interval estimates are needed to make statistical inferences and to better estimate the true mean change.

Both confidence intervals and hypothesis tests use the sampling distribution; if many more samples of the same size are randomly selected and the mean is found in each sample, the statistics (estimates of the mean) should all pile up fairly close to the true parameter (μ). In contrast to hypothesis testing, where the null parameter is assumed to be at the center of the sampling distribution, confidence intervals are calculated assuming the true parameter is at the center.

In this example, the sampling distribution is a *t*-distribution with $270 - 1 = 269$ degrees of freedom. All sample mean changes in hemoglobin are assumed to pile up at the true mean change in hemoglobin. Therefore, most statistics are going to be close to the true mean (the parameter μ), and a few statistics will be farther away. In fact, using the number of standard deviations as a measure of the distance from the center of the sampling distribution, it is possible to determine just how many statistics will be close to the true parameter, the true mean change in hemoglobin. For this particular *t*-distribution, 90% of all statistics are within 1.65 standard deviations of the true parameter, 95% of all statistics are within 1.97 standard deviations of the true parameter, and 99% of all statistics are within 2.59 standard deviations of the true parameter. This means that most of the statistics in the sampling distribution are close enough to the true parameter that increasing a single statistic from a point estimate to an interval estimate by adding and subtracting a little to each side results in an interval estimate that covers the true parameter.

Application of Formula: ONE-SAMPLE CONFIDENCE INTERVAL FOR THE MEAN

C% confidence interval for the mean: $\bar{x} \pm t^*(SE)$

$\bar{x} =$ The sample mean

$C =$ The confidence level for a C% confidence interval

$t^* =$ The number of standard deviations from the center of the sampling distribution

$SE =$ The standard error of the mean

continues

continued

What you need to calculate the confidence interval:

1. *The sample mean or the point estimate of the mean:* $\bar{x} = 3.5$ g/dL.
2. *The standard error:* The sample standard deviation divided by the square root of the sample size, $SE = 0.423/\sqrt{270} = 0.026$.
3. *The confidence level:* C% is typically 95%, but 90% and 99% are also common.
4. *The number of standard deviations from the center of the sampling distribution:* This depends on C% (3) and the sampling distribution. In this case, where the sampling distribution is a *t*-distribution with 269 degrees of freedom, the t^* for a 90% confidence interval is 1.65, the t^* for a 95% confidence interval is 1.97, and the t^* for a 99% confidence interval is 2.59. Therefore, confidence intervals can be calculated as

90% confidence interval: $\bar{x} \pm (1.65 * SE)$

95% confidence interval: $\bar{x} \pm (1.97 * SE)$

99% confidence interval: $\bar{x} \pm (2.59 * SE)$

To calculate the 95% confidence interval: The number of standard errors from the mean is $1.97*(0.423/\sqrt{270}) = 1.97*0.026 = 0.051$ and is also known as the *margin of error*. Adding and subtracting the margin of error from the point estimate results in the 95% confidence interval: $[3.5 - 0.051, 3.5 + 0.051]$ or $[3.45, 3.55]$.

The 95% confidence interval for the true mean change in hemoglobin for pregnant women who drink only from the tap in the region exposed to herbicides is $[3.5 - 0.051, 3.5 + 0.051]$ or $[3.45, 3.55]$. Interpreting a confidence interval, which represents a set of plausible values for the true parameter, is straightforward. In addition to providing an interval estimate for the true mean change in hemoglobin, it can also be used to make inferences about the true mean change in hemoglobin. The fact that this interval does not cover 0 or 2.0 g/dL gives reason to believe that there is change in the hemoglobin and that the change in hemoglobin is not the same as pregnant women exposed to mercury. In other words, neither 0 nor 2.0 g/dL is a plausible value for the true mean change in hemoglobin for pregnant women exposed to herbicides in drinking water. Since the confidence interval provides an interval estimate for the true parameter, the true mean change in hemoglobin, the true parameter can be estimated *and* guesses of the true parameter can be rejected.

Point to Ponder

How do you know that the one statistic obtained from a sample is going to have a confidence interval that covers the true parameter? You will not know for certain. However, in a 95% confidence interval, 95% of all statistics are close enough to the true parameter that their interval estimates cover the true parameter. This means that 95% of all interval estimates cover the true parameter. For that reason, it is reasonable to assume the one interval estimate calculated from this one sample covers the true parameter. This is why a confidence interval represents a set of plausible values for the true parameter.

Planning a One-Sample Study

Planning a study with the appropriate number of subjects depends on the research question (or the outcome) and the purpose of the study. When the outcome is continuous, research questions typically involve a population mean. The goal of the study may be to compare the mean to some value (either a historical control or a value of 0 change) or simply to estimate the population mean. In either case, even though the emphasis is on the mean, sample size estimation requires finding a reasonable estimate of the variability or the standard deviation. Unfortunately, in continuous, normally distributed data, the mean and standard deviation are not related. Therefore, having a good estimate of the mean provides no information on an estimate of variability E.

Too often published works and preliminary studies do not provide adequate estimates of variability. This is especially true for research involving a change, where the mean and standard deviation at baseline and final are typically reported but the standard deviation of the change is not. When the planned study is novel and no historical information for the standard deviation is available, researchers may obtain an estimate of variability from preliminary data. One difficulty, however, with using preliminary data is that the sample size is often small. A small sample size may lead to a larger estimate of variability than is needed. In summary, finding an estimate of the variability can be troublesome. Often investigators have no idea what to use to estimate the variability and too often have to just guess.

Planning for Estimating a Mean

When the goal of the study is estimation, a precise estimate of the true mean is needed. The precision translates to the width of the confidence interval. A parameter is estimated with high precision when the confidence interval is narrow and with low precision when the confidence interval is wide. Determining an appropriate sample size when estimation is the goal is as simple as calculating a confidence interval, specifically the margin of error. The margin of error of the confidence interval is the number of standard errors to add and subtract from the point estimate to make it an interval estimate. Therefore, determining the sample size when the goal of the study is to estimate the mean is fairly straightforward. Two items are needed:

- A guess of the variability
- An estimate of the precision or width of the interval

A guess of the variability or of the standard deviation is necessary because it indicates how similar the responses in the sample will be. Highly variable responses require a larger sample size to precisely estimate the mean; responses that are fairly consistent (i.e., having small standard deviation) do not require such a large sample. For example, suppose a study is planned for estimating the mean change in hemoglobin. A confidence interval for the true mean change in hemoglobin will be very different if the expected standard deviation of the change in hemoglobin is 0.05 g/dL compared to 5.0 g/dL.

A guess of the width of the interval is a little easier to manage because it is somewhat investigator dependent. If an investigator wants to estimate the mean change in hemoglobin within 0.5 g/dL, then the width of the interval is ±0.5 g/dL. Sometimes the width of the interval is determined by what the investigator can afford. A larger width (less precision) requires fewer subjects. However, care must be taken when making a width too large. Suppose the width of the interval is 5.0 g/dL. This is a large change in hemoglobin. In fact, it is so large that it will not be helpful in providing an estimate of the true mean change in hemoglobin.

Table 2-5 provides a summary of how the sample size estimate changes with increased standard deviation estimates and increased precision (smaller width). Decreasing the precision of the estimate has the effect of decreasing the sample size; increasing the variability (standard deviation) requires an increased sample size (Figure 2-9).

Planning for Making Comparison with a Mean

When the goal of the study is to make a comparison using a hypothesis test, sample size estimation depends on the relationships among power, type 1 error, type 2 error, and effect size. Power, type 1 error, and type 2 error were discussed in Chapter 1. The goal

TABLE 2-5 **SAMPLE SIZE ESTIMATES (95% CONFIDENCE INTERVAL OF A MEAN)**

Proposed Sample Size	Estimate of Standard Deviation	Width of the Interval
246	2	
554	3	
984	4	0.25
1537	5	
62	2	
139	3	
246	4	0.50
385	5	

Sample size estimates are based on a two-sided 95% confidence interval.

© Cengage Learning, 2012.

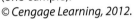
Figure 2-9 Sample size estimates based on widths and variability (one-sample).
© *Cengage Learning, 2012.*

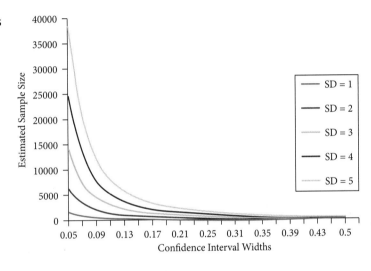

is to plan the study with a sufficient number of subjects so that the null hypothesis can be rejected when it should be rejected (high power) and to minimize the chance of rejecting it when it should not be (type 1 error).

Hence, when testing a hypothesis, determining an appropriate sample size requires decisions to be made about power and type 1 error. In general, potential power values are 80–90%. Although greater than 90% power is desirable, a study with less than 80% power should not be considered. Furthermore, possible values of the probability of a type 1 error often range from 0.01–0.1. Observational, exploratory studies, where a type 1 error is not as critical, can handle larger probabilities of type 1 error ($\alpha = 0.1$). However, most studies use a two-sided probability of a type 1 error of 0.05. If the study is very concerned with making a type 1 error, a lower value is used ($\alpha = 0.01$).

The effect size must next be determined. In a one-sample study, the effect size is the difference between the null mean and an alternative mean, standardized by the standard deviation:

$$\text{Effect size} = \frac{\text{Null mean} - \text{Alternative mean}}{\text{Standard deviation}}$$

Determining the effect size involves finding an estimate of the difference between the means *and* a measure of the standard deviation. A small effect size suggests that the true mean is not very far from the null mean; a large effect size implies that the true mean is very far from the null mean. However, a large effect size is not simply a large difference in means. If the difference in means is large but the standard deviation is also large, the effect size can end up being moderate or even small. However, if the standard deviation is very low, then the effect size could be large even if there was not a large difference in means. Studies trying to detect very small effects require a large sample size. On the other hand, studies trying to detect large effects do not require as large a sample size.

Although investigators typically have an expectation of how different the alternative mean will be from the null mean, rarely do they have a good estimate of the standard deviation. Because the mean and standard deviation are not related, an estimate of the mean difference provides no information on an estimate of variability. Luckily, having an explicit estimate of the mean difference or the variability to propose sample sizes is not necessary. All that is needed is potential effect sizes.

Table 2-6 provides a summary of how the sample size estimates change with increased effect size estimates, increased power, and smaller significance level (probability of a type 1 error). As the significance level is made small and power increases, the estimated sample size increases as well. Furthermore, smaller effect sizes result in larger sample size estimates (Figure 2-10).

TABLE 2-6 **SAMPLE SIZE ESTIMATES (TESTING WITH A MEAN)**

Proposed Sample Size	Effect Size	Significance Level	Power
128	0.25		
34	0.50	0.05	0.80
16	0.75		
171	0.25		
44	0.50	0.05	0.90
21	0.75		
191	0.25		
51	0.50	0.01	0.80
25	0.75		
242	0.25		
63	0.50	0.01	0.90
30	0.75		

Sample size estimates are based on conducting a one-sample *t*-test.

© Cengage Learning, 2012.

Figure 2-10 Sample size estimates based on power and significance level (one-sample). © *Cengage Learning, 2012.*

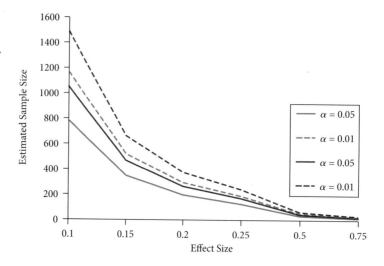

Although it is not necessary to have an estimate of the difference in means and/or standard deviation to perform the sample size calculation, the effect size has to be justified. Merely stating that only 30 subjects per group are needed when the effect size is 0.75 is not appropriate. A justification has to be given as to why an effect size of 0.75 is reasonable. Generally, this justification comes from having an estimate of the difference in means and/or standard deviation. Therefore, even though mean and standard deviation estimates are not necessary for the calculation of the sample size, they are necessary for justifying it.

One-Sample Median: Nonparametric Hypothesis Test

So far, the continuous outcome in this one-sample study was assumed to conform to a symmetric, bell-shaped distribution, suggesting that the data were normally distributed. This assumption was based on the histogram of hemoglobin outcomes and on knowledge about the distribution of hemoglobin values. Means and standard deviations were used to describe the sample numerically, and sampling distributions following t-distributions were used to create confidence intervals and to perform hypothesis tests. However, continuous outcomes do not always conform to normal distributions. Good examples of public health outcomes that may not arise from a normal distribution are count data (the number of fractures experienced, the number of visits to the hospital, etc.) and financial data (dollars spent on prescription medication, the cost of in-home care, income, etc.). Additionally, ordinal data (health perception, quality of life, pain scales) is not generally referred to as continuous because of the gaps between values. However, because these variables have rank or order, investigators may still want to investigate center and spread as they would any other continuous variable. Unfortunately, methods that assume a normal distribution may no longer be appropriate in these cases.

When the data come from a symmetric distribution but no other assumptions are made about the distribution, a *nonparametric* or *distribution-free test* might be of interest. Suppose that investigators are interested in changes in hemoglobin but that they do not want to make assumptions about the distribution of change values. Specifically, they do not want to assume that the hemoglobin changes are normally distributed. Without assuming normality, a one-sample t-test or a paired t-test is no longer appropriate. The nonparametric equivalent to these tests can help to answer the same research questions.

RESEARCH QUESTION: Is the change in hemoglobin in pregnant women exposed to herbicides different from that in pregnant women exposed to mercury?

Suppose investigators still want to explore the change in hemoglobin for women exposed to herbicides. They are still interested in whether mercury exposure is the same as herbicide exposure, but now the distribution of hemoglobin changes does not come from a normal distribution.

Assume that pregnant women exposed to mercury in water have a median hemoglobin change of 2.0 g/dL. The research question is exactly the same as when the data were assumed to be normally distributed, but now the average change is expressed as a median. The observed median change (the median of the paired difference) in this study ($\overline{m} = 3.5$ g/dL) is different from 2.0 g/dL, but is this sample median specific to this sample? The question of whether 3.5 g/dL is different enough from 2.0 g/dL must be answered to state that herbicide-exposed pregnant have different changes in hemoglobin from those in mercury-exposed pregnant women. Just as when the data were assumed to be normally distributed, hypothesis testing can help, except now, instead of a test that involves means, (a one-sample t-test) a test of the median is used.

RESEARCH HYPOTHESIS: The true median (M) hemoglobin change for pregnant women exposed to herbicides is not 2 g/dL.

NULL HYPOTHESIS: The true median (M) hemoglobin change for pregnant women exposed to herbicides is 2 g/dL.

RESEARCH HYPOTHESIS: The hemoglobin values for week 9 and week 26 have different distributions.

NULL HYPOTHESIS: The hemoglobin values for week 9 and week 26 have the same distribution.

The *signed rank test* is the nonparametric test used when there is only one sample, either because a pair of observations are of interest (within-subject controls) or because there is only one group of interest (historical controls). Hence, the signed rank test essentially translates into a one-sample test about a median (Table 2-7). The *p*-value that results from the signed rank test for this study is <0.0001.

TABLE 2-7 **TEST FOR LOCATION: MEDIAN = 2.0**

Test	Statistic	*p*-value
Signed Rank	18292.5	<0.0001

© Cengage Learning, 2012.

CONCLUSION: This is sufficient evidence ($p < 0.0001$) to reject the null hypothesis. Hence the median hemoglobin changes from week 9 to week 36 for pregnant women exposed to herbicides in drinking water is different from 2 g/dL (the median change for pregnant women exposed to mercury).

RESEARCH QUESTION: Is there a change in hemoglobin for pregnant women exposed to herbicides in drinking water?

This is an example of a one-sample nonparametric test where the research question involved comparing the median value to a historical control. Like the parametric tests, these nonparametric tests can also be used to determine whether there is a difference between a pair of observations. When using subjects as their own control and testing for paired differences, the same nonparametric test is used but the hypothesis involves testing whether the median is 0.

RESEARCH HYPOTHESIS: The true median (*M*) hemoglobin change for pregnant women exposed to herbicides is not 0 g/dL.

NULL HYPOTHESIS: The true median (*M*) hemoglobin change for pregnant women exposed to herbicides is 0 g/dL.

When dealing with nonparametric tests, investigators are often interested in determining whether distributions are similar. Therefore, instead of considering the median change, an equivalent way to present these hypotheses is to compare the distributions at week 9 and week 36.

RESEARCH HYPOTHESIS: The hemoglobin values for week 9 and week 36 have different distributions.

NULL HYPOTHESIS: The hemoglobin values for week 9 and week 36 have the same distribution.

The signed rank test is again appropriate because only one sample is of interest. Hence, the signed rank test again translates into a one-sample test about a median, except now the question is whether the true median is 0 (Table 2-8). The *p*-value that results from the signed rank test for this study is <0.0001.

TABLE 2-8 **TEST FOR LOCATION: MEDIAN = 0**

Test	Statistic	*p*-value
Signed Rank	18292.5	<0.0001

© Cengage Learning, 2012.

CONCLUSION: This is sufficient evidence ($p < 0.0001$) to reject the null hypothesis. Hence, the median hemoglobin changes from week 9 to week 36 for pregnant women exposed to herbicides is not 0 g/dL. Furthermore, this significant *p*-value suggests that the distribution of hemoglobin values for week 9 is different from the distribution of hemoglobin values for week 36.

TWO-SAMPLE STUDIES WITH A CONTINUOUS OUTCOME

RESEARCH QUESTION: Is there a difference in the change in hemoglobin for women who are exposed to herbicides (tap water only) versus those who are not (bottle water only)?

Many times the research question involves comparing the outcome of one group to another group, resulting in two groups or cohorts. One group generally serves as the exposed or treatment group, and the other group serves as the unexposed or control group. This design is often preferred over using historical controls (one-sample study) because data on the comparison group is collected concurrently, in the same study, and under similar conditions. For example, to determine the maternal effects of exposure to herbicides in the water, data are collected on an additional group of pregnant women who have not been exposed to herbicides in drinking water (the bottle-only group). Comparing the outcomes of the two groups of women (unexposed and exposed) would help to determine whether exposure to herbicides is associated with adverse maternal outcomes.

These two groups consist of completely different pregnant women, and the measurements obtained from one group have nothing to do with those obtained from the other group. Therefore, these two groups are considered **independent groups**. Because two groups or two independent samples are of interest, the study is often referred to as a *two-sample study*.

Because this is a two-sample study, there is now an independent comparator or control group: the pregnant women who drink only bottled water. Descriptive statistics can be provided to describe the sample of pregnant women who drink only from the tap as well as the those who drink only bottled water (Tables 2-9 and 2-10). In this example, tap-only drinkers, compared to bottle-only drinkers tend to be older (average age 25, SD 1.9 vs. average age 27, SD 1.5). When compared to bottle drinkers, tap drinkers report lower incomes (the median income for tap only pregnant women is $20K less than bottle-only pregnant women) and lower rate of high school graduation (41% vs. 76%).

On average, the baseline hemoglobin of tap-only pregnant women is low (10.7 g/dL, $SD = 0.74$ g/dL). Based on the median, half of the women have baseline hemoglobin values less than 10.8, indicating that half of the women are already at anemic levels (<11 g/dL) at baseline. This is in contrast to bottle-only pregnant women who, on average, report baseline hemoglobin measures above the anemia cutoff (average hemoglobin 11.4 g/dL $SD = 0.65$ g/dL). Of particular interest for this study is the comparison of changes in hemoglobin. The tap-only pregnant women have an average decrease in hemoglobin of 3.5 g/dL (SD 0.42 g/dL), whereas the bottle-only group has an average change of 2.0 ($SD = 0.43$ g/dL) from baseline to week 36. The difference between these two groups is 1.4 g/dL ($SD = 0.43$ g/dL), suggesting that on average the tap-only group has a 1.4 g/dL greater decline in hemoglobin over the course of the pregnancy.

TABLE 2-9 **CHARACTERISTICS OF THE SAMPLE**

	Tap Only (N = 270)	Bottle Only (N = 315)
Age (years)		
Mean (SD)	25.03 (1.907)	27.11 (1.467)
Median (min, max)	25.1 (18.9, 30.7)	27.1 (22.9, 31.0)
Income ($10K)	n = 270	n = 312
Mean (SD)	3.75 (1.434)	4.06 (1.775)
Median (min, max)	3.3 (2.2, 10.9)	3.5 (2.2, 12.2)
Weight Gain (lb)		
Mean (SD)	41.60 (4.106)	42.01 (4.152)
Median (min, max)	41.5 (29.5, 56.4)	42.1 (30.0, 51.7)
Adequate Prenatal Care		
No	175 (64.8%)	52 (16.5%)
Yes	95 (35.2%)	263 (83.5%)
Smoked Prior to Pregnancy		
No	183 (67.8%)	261 (82.9%)
Yes	87 (32.2%)	54 (17.1%)
Education		
Less HS	149 (55.2%)	46 (14.6%)
HS/GED	111 (41.1%)	238 (75.6%)
College +	10 (3.7%)	31 (9.8%)
Number of Previous Births (parity)		
None	45 (16.7%)	48 (15.2%)
One	137 (50.7%)	167 (53.0%)
Two	78 (28.9%)	92 (29.2%)
Three or More	10 (3.7%)	8 (2.5%)

© Cengage Learning, 2012.

TABLE 2-10 **SUMMARY OF HEMOGLOBIN OUTCOMES**

	Tap Only (N = 270)	Bottle Only (N = 315)	Difference (Tap − Bottle)
Baseline Hemoglobin (g/dL)	n = 270	n = 315	
Mean (SD)	10.73 (0.739)	11.42 (0.647)	−0.69 (0.691)
Median (min, max)	10.8 (8.6, 13.2)	11.4 (9.7, 13.3)	
Final Hemoglobin (g/dL)	n = 270	n = 315	
Mean (SD)	7.26 (0.856)	9.39 (0.753)	−2.13 (0.802)
Median (min, max)	7.3 (5.3, 10.1)	9.3 (7.1, 11.7)	
Change in Hemoglobin (g/dL)*	n = 270	n = 315	
Mean (SD)	3.47 (0.423)	2.03 (0.433)	1.4 (0.429)
Median (min, max)	3.5 (2.3, 4.8)	2.0 (0.7, 3.5)	

*The change in hemoglobin represents baseline-final hemoglobin.

© Cengage Learning, 2012.

If the groups had the same change in hemoglobin, the expected difference would be 0. Although an observed difference in means of 1.4 (SD=0.43) exists between the groups, is this enough evidence to show that herbicide exposure through tap-water leads to a greater change in hemoglobin?

- Is a 1.4 g/dL mean different enough from 0 g/dL to state that pregnant women exposed to herbicides in the water have a change different from that of unexposed pregnant women?
- Would another sample have a similar difference between the two groups?
- Is the discrepancy between the statistic (1.4 g/dL) and the expected difference of 0 g/dL so great that it could not have just happened by chance?

Hypothesis tests and confidence intervals help to answer these questions.

Two Sample Means: Equal Variances

RESEARCH QUESTION:
Is there a difference in the hemoglobin change in women who are exposed to herbicides (tap water only) versus those who are not (bottle water only)?

One of the goals of this study is to better understand the association between herbicide exposure and hemoglobin changes in pregnant women. A comparison of the mean changes in hemoglobin for pregnant women who do and do not drink tap water helps in answering this question. Specifically, the aim is to determine whether the mean change in hemoglobin for pregnant women exposed to herbicides via tap water (μ_{tap}) is different from the mean change in hemoglobin for women who have not been exposed (μ_{bottle}). Because this is a two-sample study, the difference between the means of the two groups can be calculated. A difference other than 0 suggests that the two groups experience different hemoglobin changes. In this example, the sample mean difference in hemoglobin change is $\bar{x}_{tap} - \bar{x}_{bottle} = 1.4$ g/dL and can be used to make inferences about the population mean difference ($\mu_{tap} - \mu_{bottle}$).

Just comparing the means of the two samples is not sufficient. The change in hemoglobin is a continuous variable and cannot be described by a measure of center alone; a measure of the spread is also necessary. Unfortunately, although subtracting the sample means is easy, finding a combined standard deviation (a measure of spread) is not as simple as subtracting the two sample standard deviations.

Standard deviations are calculated differently from means. Although means are just the sum of the observations divided by the sample size, standard deviations are more complicated. Calculating a standard deviation means finding the difference between the mean and each observation, squaring this difference, adding up all the squared differences, dividing by the sample size, and then taking the square root. Therefore, the standard deviation of the differences cannot be obtained just by subtracting the standard deviation of group 1 from the standard deviation of group 2. A standard deviation that represents the combination of the two samples must be found.

The distributions of the hemoglobin changes for each of the two groups (Figure 2-4) are quite similar. Except for the fact that the tap-only group seems to be shifted to the right, which is consistent with a sample mean difference of 1.4 g/dL, the two samples appear to have similar shapes and spreads. This is confirmed with the standard deviation estimates (SD = 0.423 and SD = 0.433). To have a measure of spread for the difference in means, the variances (and standard deviations) from the two samples must be combined. Because the two samples have fairly similar spreads; a single numerical summary of the variance can be obtained by averaging or pooling the variances of the two distributions.

Application of Formula: POOLED SAMPLE VARIANCE

$$\text{Estimate of pooled variance} = \frac{\sum_{i=1}^{n_1}(x_{1i} - \bar{x}_1)^2 + \sum_{j=1}^{n_2}(x_{2j} - \bar{x}_2)^2}{(n_1 - 1) + (n_2 - 1)}$$

$\bar{x}_1$ = The sample mean for group 1

$\bar{x}_2$ = The sample mean for group 2

x_{1i} = The value of the continuous variable for subject i in group 1

continues

x_{2j} = The value of the continuous variable for subject j in group 2

n_1 = The sample size for group 1

n_2 = The sample size for group 2

What you need to calculate the pooled variance:

1. *The total sums of squares for each group:*

    a. The total (corrected) sums of squares for the tap water group: $\sum_{i=1}^{n_1}(x_{1i} - \bar{x}_1)^2 = 48.3$.

    b. The total (corrected) sums of squares for the bottle water group: $\sum_{j=1}^{n_2}(x_{2j} - \bar{x}_2)^2 = 58.8$.

2. *The numerator:* This the sum of the two total sums of squares: (1a) + (1b) = 107.1.
3. *The degrees of freedom:* The sum of the two sample sizes -2: $n_1 + n_2 - 2 = 585 - 2 = 583$.

To calculate the estimate of the pooled variance: The numerator (2) divided by the degrees of freedom (3): $107.1 \div 583 = 0.184$.

To calculate the pooled standard deviation: Take the square root of the pooled variance: $\sqrt{0.184} = 0.43$.

To calculate the pooled standard error: Multiply the pooled standard deviation by the square root of sum of the inverses of the two sample sizes: $\sqrt{\left(\frac{1}{n_1} + \frac{1}{n_2}\right)} = \sqrt{\left(\frac{1}{270} + \frac{1}{315}\right)} = \sqrt{(0.004 + 0.003)} = \sqrt{0.007}$. So, the pooled standard error is $0.43 * \sqrt{0.007} = 0.43 * 0.084 = 0.036$.

With an estimate of the pooled variance and the mean difference, inferences can be made using hypothesis tests and confidence intervals.

Hypothesis Test

In this example, the sample mean difference in hemoglobin change is $\bar{x}_{tap} - \bar{x}_{bottle} = 1.4$ g/dL. If the two groups do not have different outcomes, then the difference in the mean change should be 0. A hypothesis test can be used to determine whether there is enough evidence from the data to claim that the two groups (tap-only versus bottle-only) have different mean changes in hemoglobin.

RESEARCH HYPOTHESIS: The average difference in the hemoglobin changes in pregnant women who are exposed to herbicides (via tap water) versus those who are not (bottled water) is not 0 g/dL, or $\mu_{tap} - \mu_{bottle} \neq 0$ g/dL.

NULL HYPOTHESIS: The average difference in the hemoglobin changes in pregnant women who are exposed to herbicides (via tap water) versus those who are not (bottled water) is 0 g/dL, or $\mu_{tap} - \mu_{bottle} = 0$ g/dL.

To test this hypothesis, the null hypothesis is assumed true: the true parameter (the average difference in the hemoglobin change for the two groups, $\mu_{tap} - \mu_{bottle}$) is assumed to be 0 g/dL. Therefore, the goal is to use the sample data to provide evidence against the null hypothesis. Assuming the null parameter (0 g/dL) is the true parameter, would this statistic ($\bar{x}_{tap} - \bar{x}_{bottle} = 1.4$ g/dL) be expected? When data are normally distributed from two independent samples and the variances are equal, the hypothesis test used to determine whether the mean difference is different from 0 is called a *two-sample t-test with equal variances.*

Test statistic for difference in means $(t) = \dfrac{(\bar{x}_1 - \bar{x}_2) - 0}{\text{Standard error}} = \dfrac{\bar{x}_1 - \bar{x}_2}{\text{Standard error}}$

$\bar{x}_1$ = The sample mean for group 1

$\bar{x}_2$ = The sample mean for group 2

Standard error = The pooled standard error

What you need for a two-sample *t*-test with equal variances:

1. *The difference between the two sample means:* In this study, the sample mean for tap water only is 3.47 g/dL; for bottled water only, it is 2.03 g/dL. The difference is 1.44 g/dL.
2. *The standard error:* In this study, the pooled standard error is 0.036.

To calculate the test statistic (t) for the two sample t-test with equal variances: This the difference (1) divided by the standard error (2): $1.44 \div 0.036 = 40.0$.

Is this value far enough away from the center of the standardized sampling distribution? This test statistic comes from a *t*-distribution with $(n_1 - 1) + (n_2 - 1)$ degrees of freedom. Therefore, for this study, the sampling distribution is a *t*-distribution with 583 degrees of freedom. The test statistic of 40.0 is pretty far from the center of the standardized sampling distribution, suggesting that a statistic was obtained that was very far away from the null parameter.

The exact proportion of test statistics that are even farther away than 40.0 (*p*-value) can be found by using statistical software (Table 2-11) or statistical tables.

The *p*-value from this test is <0.0001. Because the *p*-value is so small, the test statistic is considered rare. This test statistic would not be expected at all if the true parameter was the null parameter.

TABLE 2-11 RESULTS FROM THE TWO-SAMPLE *t*-TEST (EQUAL VARIANCES)

Variable: Hemoglobin Change			
	Group 1	Group 2	Difference (Group 1 − Group 2)
N	270	315	
Mean	3.4689	2.0325	1.4364
Std Dev	0.4234	0.4334	0.4288
Std Error	0.0258	0.0244	0.0356
Results of *t*-Test				
Method	Variances	*t*-value	DF	Pr > |*t*|
Pooled	Equal	40.39	583	<0.0001

Note: Results may differ from Application of Formula calculations due to rounding

© Cengage Learning, 2012.

CONCLUSION: There is sufficient evidence to reject the null hypothesis. Hence, there is a difference in the mean hemoglobin change for pregnant women who drink only tap water (exposed) versus women who drink only bottled water.

Confidence Intervals

While the hypothesis test indicates that there is a difference in the mean hemoglobin changes between pregnant women exposed to herbicides and those not exposed, it does not provide an estimate for the true mean difference. The point estimate of

1.4 g/dL indicates that this sample of tap-only subjects has a greater change than that of the bottle-only sample. However, to use this point estimate to estimate the true population mean difference, confidence intervals are needed.

Confidence intervals provide a range of plausible values for the true parameter. In this case, the true parameter is the true mean difference in hemoglobin changes in pregnant women drinking only bottled water versus tap water. Calculating a confidence interval for the difference in the mean change in hemoglobin will provide an interval estimate for the parameter that can be used to determine whether the true parameter is 0.

Confidence intervals are based on the idea that if different samples of the same size are selected, not all samples will result in exactly the same statistics. For example, another sample of 585 pregnant women is not likely to have exactly the same difference in sample means ($\bar{x}_{1tap} - \bar{x}_{1bottle} = 1.4$ g/dL). However, different statistics obtained from different samples should all be fairly similar. In fact, if many random samples of the same size are taken over and over again, the statistics (estimates of the mean difference) from the samples may be expected to all pile up fairly close to the true parameter (the true mean difference).

This pile of statistics, the sampling distribution, is the same as the sampling distribution used for the two-sample t-test with equal variances: a t-distribution with $(n_1 + n_2) - 2 = 585 - 2 = 583$ degrees of freedom. Unlike hypothesis tests, confidence intervals assume that the sampling distribution is centered at the true parameter, not at the null parameter. Therefore, most of the statistics will be close to the true parameter (the true difference in means), and a few statistics will be farther away. Specifically, by counting with standard deviations of the sampling distribution, it can be determined just how many statistics will be close to the true parameter. A sampling distribution that follows a t-distribution with 583 degrees of freedom will have:

- 90% of all statistics within 1.65 standard deviations of the true parameter.
- 95% of all statistics within 1.96 standard deviations of the true parameter.
- 99% of all statistics within 2.58 standard deviations of the true parameter.

Therefore, most of the statistics are close enough to the true parameter that increasing a statistic from a point estimate to an interval estimate by adding and subtracting a little to each side will often result in an interval estimate that covers the true parameter.

Application of Formula: CONFIDENCE INTERVAL FOR THE MEAN DIFFERENCE

$C\%$ confidence interval for the mean difference: $\bar{x}_1 - \bar{x}_2 \pm t^* (\text{SE}_{pooled})$

$\bar{x}_1 - \bar{x}_2 = $ The difference between the sample means

$C = $ The confidence level for a $C\%$ confidence interval

$t^* = $ The number of standard deviations from the center of the sampling distribution

$\text{SE}_{pooled} = $ The pooled standard error

What you need to calculate the confidence interval:

1. *The difference of the sample means or the point estimate of the mean difference:* $\bar{x}_{tap} - \bar{x}_{bottle} = 1.4$ g/dL.
2. *The pooled standard error:* $\text{SE}_{pooled} = 0.036$.
3. *The confidence level:* $C\%$ is typically 95%, but 90% and 99% are also common.
4. *The number of standard deviations from the center of the sampling distribution:* This depends on $C\%$ (3) and the sampling distribution. In this case, where the sampling distribution is a t-distribution with 583 degrees of freedom, the t^* for a 90% confidence interval is 1.65, the t^* for a 95% confidence interval is 1.96, and the t^* for a 99% confidence interval is 2.58.

continues

Public Health Professional

continued

Therefore, confidence intervals can be calculated as:

90% confidence interval: $\bar{x}_1 - \bar{x}_2 \pm (1.65 * SE_{pooled})$

95% confidence interval: $\bar{x}_1 - \bar{x}_2 \pm (1.96 * SE_{pooled})$

99% confidence interval: $\bar{x}_1 - \bar{x}_2 \pm (2.58 * SE_{pooled})$

To calculate a 95% confidence interval: The number of standard errors from the mean (margin of error) is $1.96 * (0.036) = 1.96 * 0.036 = 0.071$. Adding and subtracting the margin of error from the point estimate results in the confidence interval: $[1.4 - 0.071, 1.4 + 0.071]$, or $[1.33, 1.47]$.

The 95% confidence interval for the true mean difference in hemoglobin changes in pregnant tap-only women versus those who drink only bottled water is $[1.4 - 0.071, 1.4 + 0.071]$, or $[1.33, 1.47]$. This interval estimate represents a set of plausible values for the true parameter, the true mean difference in hemoglobin changes ($\mu_{tap} - \mu_{bottle}$). Because this interval does not cover $0\,g/dL$, $0\,g/dL$ is not a plausible value for the true mean difference between the tap-only group and the bottle–only group. Furthermore, because the difference was calculated as the mean for the bottle group subtracted from the mean for the tap group, the fact that the interval includes only positive values for the difference suggests that the true mean hemoglobin change in bottle-only pregnant women is smaller than that in tap-only pregnant women. Given that the confidence interval provides an interval estimate for the true parameter, the true mean difference in the change in hemoglobin, the true parameter is estimated *and* guesses of the true parameter are rejected.

Two Sample Means: Unequal Variances

The two-sample confidence interval and *t*-test assuming equal variances pools the variances of the two groups for a single estimate of the variance. However, these methods assumed that the variances of the groups were equal. If the variation or the spreads of the two samples are different, then combining the variances into a single, pooled estimate would not make sense.

Suppose that the distribution of the change in hemoglobin for the tap-only group was more spread out than the change in hemoglobin for the bottle-only group (Figure 2-11). Although both distributions are still somewhat normally distributed, the distribution for bottle-only pregnant women has much less variability than (the hemoglobin change values are not as spread out as) the distribution for tap-only group. In fact, the standard deviation for the change in hemoglobin for the tap-only sample is $0.57\,g/dL$ whereas the standard deviation for the change in hemoglobin for the bottle-only sample is $0.43\,g/dL$. A smaller standard deviation suggests less variability. Because the standard deviations differ, the variances of the two distributions will also differ.

When two things are different, trying to average or pool them is not correct. When the variances for the two samples are unequal, both variances and not a combined estimate must be used in the calculation of the standard error. In determining whether the two groups in fact have different variances, graphical representations (histograms) and statistics (sample variances) can be very helpful. However, a hypothesis test can also be used to decide whether the two populations have similar spreads around the mean or not.

RESEARCH HYPOTHESIS: The two groups have different variances; the ratio of variances $\left(\dfrac{\sigma^2_{tap}}{\sigma^2_{bottle}}\right)$ is different from 1.

NULL HYPOTHESIS: The two groups have equal variances; the ratio of variances $\left(\dfrac{\sigma^2_{tap}}{\sigma^2_{bottle}}\right)$ is equal to 1.

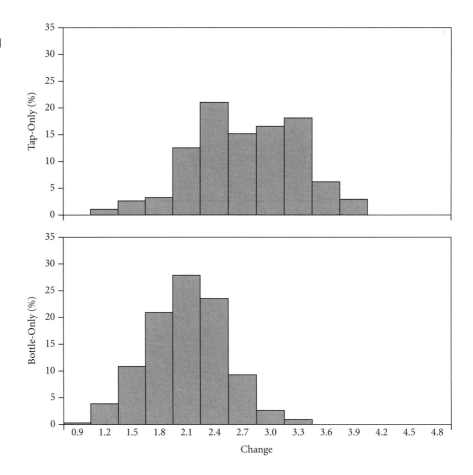

Figure 2-11 Distribution of hemoglobin change (unequal variances).
© *Cengage Learning, 2012.*

In the previous discussions of sampling distributions, means were the parameter of interest. Now variances are of interest and the appropriate test statistic for comparing two variances is simply the ratio of variances. Just as the test statistics for comparing means have a special sampling distribution, the ratio of variances has a specific sampling distribution as well. However, the shape of the sampling distribution when investigating means is different from the sampling distribution for the ratio of variances. Variances (and the ratio of variances) can never be negative, and so the sampling distribution must reflect this. If many random samples of two groups are selected over and over again, two pairs of variances would result. The ratio of sample variances can be calculated for each sample by dividing one sample variance by the other (e.g. the variance of the tap water sample divided by the variance of the bottled water sample $= s^2_{tap}/s^2_{bottle}$). The distribution of all possible ratios of sample variances is right-skewed and is a special distribution called the **F-distribution** (Figure 2-12).

Just as the *t*-distribution is dependent on degrees of freedom for its shape, so is the F-distribution. The *t*-distribution had only one set of degrees of freedom, but the *F*-distribution has two sets. The degrees of freedom for the variance in the numerator ($n_1 - 1$) and the degrees of freedom for the variance in the denominator ($n_2 - 1$) dictate the shape of the distribution. The *F*-distribution starts at 0 and is skewed to the right. How skewed it is depends on how large the degrees of freedom are in the numerator and the denominator.

The sampling distribution of the ratio of the two variances can be used to test whether the true population variances are equal or not. A small *p*-value obtained from this test is evidence that the ratio of the population variances is not 1 and that the two variances are assumed to be unequal. Otherwise, if the sample ratio is close to 1 (a large *p*-value), then the two variances are assumed to be equal.

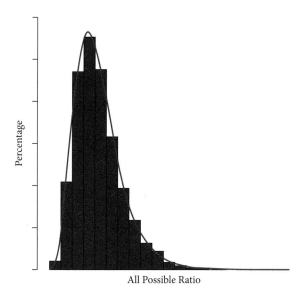

Figure 2-12 Example of the sampling distribution (*F*-distribution). © *Cengage Learning, 2012.*

All Possible Ratio

Application of Formula: EQUALITY OF VARIANCES TEST

Test statistic $(F) = \dfrac{s_1^2}{s_2^2}$

$s_1^2 =$ The sample variance in group 1

$s_2^2 =$ The sample variance in group 2

What you need to calculate the test statistic:

1. *The sample variance for group 1:* $s_{\text{tap}}^2 = 0.57^2 = 0.33$.
2. *The sample variance for group 2:* $s_{\text{bottle}}^2 = 0.43^2 = 0.19$.
3. *The numerator degrees of freedom:* $n_{\text{tap}} - 1 = 315 - 1 = 314$
4. *The denominator degrees of freedom:* $n_{\text{bottle}} - 1 = 270 - 1 = 269$

To calculate the test statistic (F): The (1) is divided by (2). The ratio of these two sample variances is $0.188 \div 0.179 = 1.74$. Using an *F*-distribution with 314 and 269 as the numerator and denominator degrees of freedom, the *p*-value is <0.001.

The resulting *p*-value is smaller than 0.001 (Table 2-12) and indicates that a ratio of 1.74 would not be expected or is considered rare if the variances were equal (or if the ratio of the variances is 1).

TABLE 2-12 **RESULTS OF A TEST FOR EQUALITY OF VARIANCES**

Method	Num DF	Den DF	*F* Value	Pr >*F*
Folded F	314	269	1.74	<0.0001

© Cengage Learning, 2012.

CONCLUSION: There is sufficient evidence to reject the null hypothesis that the variances are equal. The standard error used to determine whether there is a difference in the means cannot be obtained from a pooled estimate of the variances.

When the variances are unequal, the standard error of the test statistic to compare the means is simply the square root of the sum of the sample variances divided by each of the sample sizes.

$$\text{Standard error} = \sqrt{\frac{s_1^2}{n_1} + \frac{s_2^2}{n_2}}$$

$s_1^2 =$ The sample variance in group 1

$s_2^2 =$ The sample variance in group 2

$n_1 =$ The sample size for group 1

$n_2 =$ The sample size for group 2

What you need to calculate the standard error:

1. *The sample variances:*
   a. The sample variance of group 1: $s_{tap}^2 = 0.33$.
   b. The sample variance of group 2: $s_{bottle}^2 = 0.19$.
2. *The sample variances divided by the respective sample sizes:*

   a. $\dfrac{s_{tap}^2}{n_{tap}} = \dfrac{0.33}{270} = 0.001$.

   b. $\dfrac{s_{bottle}^2}{n_{bottle}} = \dfrac{0.19}{315} = 0.0006$.

3. *Sum of 2a and 2b:* $\dfrac{s_{tap}^2}{n_{tap}} + \dfrac{s_{bottle}^2}{n_{bottle}} = 0.001 + 0.0006 = 0.0016$.

To calculate the standard error: Take the square root of the sum of the sample variances (3): $\sqrt{0.0016} = 0.04$.

This standard error can now be used in the hypothesis test and the confidence interval for the mean difference. The sampling distribution for this test is very similar to the one used for the two-sample *t*-test and confidence interval when the variances are equal. However, when the variances are unequal, the calculation of the degrees of freedom is not as simple. A formula (Satterthwaite's method) is used to calculate the degrees of freedom. The sampling distribution is still a *t*-distribution, but now it uses Satterthwaite's method for the degrees of freedom.

Hypothesis Test

The fact that the variances are not equal does not change the research question or the hypotheses, which is still whether the groups have similar mean changes in hemoglobin.

RESEARCH QUESTION: Is there a difference in the hemoglobin change in women who are exposed to herbicides (tap water only) versus those who are not (bottle water only)?

RESEARCH HYPOTHESIS: The average difference in the hemoglobin change for pregnant women who are exposed to herbicides (via tap water) versus those who are not (bottled water) is not 0 g/dL, or $\mu_{tap} - \mu_{bottle} \neq 0$ g/dL.

NULL HYPOTHESIS: The average difference in the hemoglobin change for pregnant women who are exposed to herbicides (via tap water) versus those who are not (bottled water) is 0 g/dL, or $\mu_{tap} - \mu_{bottle} = 0$ g/dL.

The purpose of the hypothesis test is still to determine whether the sample data provides sufficient evidence against the null hypothesis, that is, that the true mean difference is 0 g/dL. When data come from two independent samples and the variances are not equal, the hypothesis test used to determine whether the mean difference is different from 0 is called a two-sample *t*-test with unequal variances.

Test statistic for difference in means $(t) = \dfrac{(\bar{x}_1 - \bar{x}_2) - 0}{\text{Standard error}} = \dfrac{\bar{x}_1 - \bar{x}_2}{\text{Standard error}}$

$\bar{x}_1$ = The sample mean for group 1

$\bar{x}_2$ = The sample mean for group 2

What you need for a two-sample *t*-test with unequal variances:

1. *The difference between the two sample means:* In this study, the sample mean for tap-only group is 3.5 g/dL, and the sample mean for bottle-only group is 2.03 g/dL. The difference is 1.44 g/dL.

2. *The standard error:* In this study, the sample variances are not equal, and so the standard error is the square root of the sum of the two variances divided by their respective sample sizes. In this study, the standard error is $\sqrt{\left(\frac{0.57^2}{270}\right) + \left(\frac{0.43^2}{315}\right)} = 0.04$.

3. *The degrees of freedom:* Because the variances are unequal, Satterthwaite's method must be used to calculate the degrees of freedom. The Satterthwaites's degrees of freedom are 492.87.

To calculate the test statistic (t) for the two-sample t-test with unequal variances: This the difference between the two sample means (1) divided by the standard error (2): $0.64/0.04 = 16.0$.

Is the test statistic is far enough away from the center of the standardized sampling distribution? The standardized sampling distribution is a *t*-distribution with 493 degrees of freedom. The test statistic of 16.0 is pretty large, suggesting that the null parameter of 0 is not the true parameter. However, the exact percentage of test statistics that are even farther away than 16.0 can be found by using statistical software or statistical tables. The proportion of test statistics that are even farther away from the null parameter than 16.0 is <0.0001.

The *p*-value that results from the two sample *t*-test for this study is <0.0001 (Table 2-13). Therefore, this test statistic would not be expected at all if the true parameter was the null parameter.

TABLE 2-13 **RESULTS OF TWO-SAMPLE *t*-TEST**

Variable: Hemoglobin Change			
	Group 1	Group 2	Difference (Group 1 − Group 2)
N	270	315	
Mean	2.7326	2.0897	0.6429
Std Dev	0.5695	0.4272	0.4980
Std Error	0.0347	0.0241	0.0413
Results of *t*-Test			
Method	Variances	*t*-value	DF	Pr > |*t*|
Satterthwaite	Unequal	15.24	492.87	<0.0001

© Cengage Learning, 2012.

CONCLUSION: There is sufficient evidence to reject the null hypothesis that the null parameter is 0 g/dL. Hence, there is a difference in the hemoglobin changes in pregnant women who drink only tap water (exposed) versus those who drink only bottled water.

Confidence Interval

The hypothesis test determined whether there is enough evidence to claim that the means of two groups are different , but hypothesis tests do not provide an estimate for the parameter, the true mean difference. Confidence intervals offer a set of possible values for the true parameter. Previously, confidence intervals were used to estimate the true mean difference in hemoglobin changes in pregnant women who drank tap water versus bottled water. However, these confidence intervals used a standard error based on a pooled estimate of the variance. If the two groups have different variances, then pooling the variances is no longer appropriate.

When the goal is to estimate the true mean difference between two groups, but it is no longer reasonable to assume that the variances of the two groups are the same, the sampling distribution must reflect the fact that the variances are different. The sampling distribution used to find the confidence interval, is the same as the sampling distribution used for the two-sample t-test with unequal variances, that is, a t-distribution with degrees of freedom obtained using Satterthwaites's method. However, confidence intervals depend on the sampling distribution being centered at the true parameter, not at the null parameter. Therefore, calculating the confidence interval for the true difference in means depends on the fact that most of the statistics in the sampling distribution are going to be close to the true parameter (the center of the distribution) and that very few will be far away.

In this example, where the variances are assumed to be unequal, a sampling distribution with 493 degrees of freedom will have:

- 90% of all statistics within 1.65 standard deviations of the true parameter.
- 95% of all statistics within 1.96 standard deviations of the true parameter.
- 99% of all statistics within 2.58 standard deviations of the true parameter.

So clearly most of the possible statistics are close enough to the true mean difference that increasing a statistic from a point estimate to an interval estimate by adding a little to each side results in an interval estimate that is likely to cover the true parameter.

Application of Formula

C% confidence interval for the mean difference: $\bar{x}_1 - \bar{x}_2 \pm t^*SE$.

$\bar{x}_1 - \bar{x}_2 =$ The difference between the sample means

$C =$ The confidence level for a C% confidence interval

$t =$ The number of standard deviations from the center of the sampling distribution

$SE =$ The standard error

What you need to calculate the confidence interval:

1. *The difference of the sample means or the point estimate of the mean difference:* $\bar{x}_{tap} - \bar{x}_{bottle} = 0.64$ g/dL.
2. *The standard error:* $SE = 0.04$. The standard error when the variances are unequal is $\sqrt{\frac{0.33}{270} + \frac{0.19}{315}} = 0.04$.
3. *The confidence level:* C% is typically 95%, but 90% and 99% are also common.
4. *The number of standard deviations from the center of the sampling distribution:* This depends on C% (3) and the sampling distribution. In this case, where the sampling distribution is a t-distribution with 493 degrees of freedom, the t^* for a 90% confidence interval is 1.65, the t^* for a 95% confidence interval is 1.96, and the t^* for a 99% confidence interval is 2.58. Therefore, confidence intervals can be calculated as

90% confidence Interval: $\bar{x}_1 - \bar{x}_2 \pm (1.65^*SE)$

95% confidence Interval: $\bar{x}_1 - \bar{x}_2 \pm (1.96^*SE)$

99% confidence Interval: $\bar{x}_1 - \bar{x}_2 \pm (2.58^*SE)$

To calculate the 95% confidence interval: The number of standard errors from the mean (the margin of error) is $1.96^*(0.04) = 1.96^*0.04 = 0.078$. Adding and subtracting the margin of error from the point estimate results in the 95% confidence interval: $[0.64 - 0.078, 0.64 + 0.078]$, or $[0.56, 0.72]$.

Assuming unequal variances, the 95% confidence interval for the true mean difference in hemoglobin changes for tap-only pregnant women versus the bottle-only group is [0.64 − 0.078, 0.64 + 0.078], or [0.56, 0.72]. This interval estimate represents a set of plausible values for the true parameter, that is, the true mean difference in hemoglobin changes ($\mu_{tap} - \mu_{bottle}$). Since this interval does not cover 0 g/dL, 0 g/dL is not a plausible value for the true mean difference.

In addition to eliminating candidate values for the true parameter, confidence intervals also offer additional insights into the size of the mean difference. For example, because the difference was calculated as the mean for the bottle-only group subtracted from the mean for the tap-only group, the fact that the interval includes only positive values for the difference suggests that the true mean change in hemoglobin for bottle water pregnant women is smaller than the true mean change in hemoglobin for the tap water pregnant women. Hence, with confidence intervals, the true parameter can be estimated *and* guesses of the true parameter can be rejected.

Planning a Two-Sample Study

When planning a two-sample study, the goal is usually to try to estimate the difference in means or to determine whether the means of the two groups are different. A key piece to planning any study is identifying an appropriate sample size, and in the case of a two-sample study, a sample size for each group is needed. Before planning a two-sample study, two issues need to be discussed: the size of the groups and the spread in the groups.

Given that a two-sample study involves two independent groups of subjects, the sample sizes of the two groups may be the same or different. Generally, a two-group study uses a **balanced design**, that is, a design in which both groups have an equal number of subjects. In a balanced design, the sample size of one of the groups is simply half the size of the entire study. Although investigators may intend to have two equally sized groups, the actual sizes of the two groups could, in practice, differ. A large difference in sample size impacts the researcher's ability to estimate the difference in means or to compare the means of the two groups. If the groups are likely going to be of different sizes, then the planning of the study should take this possibility into account.

After it has been determined whether the two groups will be the same size, the variability of the two groups have to be addressed. Regardless if the goal is to estimate or to compare, when the mean is of interest, estimates of the variability have to be incorporated. In a two-sample study, this means that it has to be decided whether equal variances are reasonable to assume. Unfortunately, getting a good estimate of the variance is not easy, and determining whether two variances will be equal may not be a simple task.

When the outcome is continuous and normally distributed, the mean and standard deviation are not related. So, having a good estimate of the mean for each group provides no information on an estimate of variability for each group and does not suggest whether the groups have similar spreads. Previously published works might give investigators an idea of the variability in the groups to expect. If estimates for the standard deviation are provided for the two groups, these might be reasonable to use in planning a study. Estimates of variability may also be obtained from preliminary data. One difficulty, however, with using preliminary data is that the sample size is often small. A small sample size may lead to a larger estimate of variability than is needed. In summary, finding estimates of the variability can be troublesome. Often investigators have no idea of what to use to estimate the variability, and too often they have to just guess.

Planning for Estimating a Mean

A study whose goal is estimation requires a precise estimate of the true mean difference. Estimating suggests providing an interval estimate, and the precision of the estimate translates to the width of the confidence interval. The true mean difference is estimated with high precision when the confidence interval is narrow. By focusing on the margin of error (how wide the confidence interval is), sample sizes can be justified. Recall that the margin of error is simply the number of standard errors to add and subtract from the point estimate to make it an interval estimate. The larger the sample size is, the smaller the margin of error will be and the smaller the width of the interval. As discussed in this section, however, the determination of the standard error depends on whether assuming that the variances are equal is appropriate. Calculating the sample size requires:

- A guess of the standard error (choose between pooled and unequal).
- A level of precision (width of the interval).

A guess of the standard error provides a description of how similar the responses in the samples will be. Highly variable responses require a larger sample size to estimate the mean difference precisely. Again, estimating the variability in the samples is not always a simple task. An estimate of the width of the interval, on the other hand, is a little easier to manage because the estimate tends to be investigator dependent. If an investigator wants to estimate the difference in the mean change in hemoglobin within 0.05 g/dL, then the width of the interval is $+/-0.05$ g/dL. Generally, it is up to the investigator to determine the appropriate width or precision needed. However, care must be taken when making a width too large. Suppose the width of the interval is 5.0 g/dL. This is a large difference in the mean hemoglobin changes. In fact, it is so large that it will not be helpful in providing an estimate of the true mean difference of hemoglobin change.

To demonstrate the sample size requirements for estimating a mean difference, suppose a two-sample study with groups of the same size is proposed, a balanced design. Furthermore, assume that the variances are equal and that a common, single standard deviation can be used to estimate the variability for both samples. For estimating a mean difference in a two-sample study with equal variances, all that is needed is an estimate of the common standard deviation and the width of the interval (precision). Table 2-14 provides a summary of how the sample size estimate changes with increased common standard deviation estimates and increased precision (smaller width). Decreasing the precision of the estimate decreases the sample size, and increasing the variability (standard deviation) requires an increased sample size.

Planning for Making a Comparison with a Mean

When the goal of the study is to make a comparison with a hypothesis test, sample size estimation depends on the relationship of power, type 1 error, type 2 error, and effect size. Power, type 1 error, and type 2 error were discussed in Chapter 1. Essentially, the

TABLE 2-14 **SAMPLE SIZE ESTIMATES (95% CONFIDENCE INTERVAL OF A MEAN)**

Proposed Sample Size (Per Group)	Estimate of Common Standard Deviation	Width of the Interval
492	2	
1107	3	
1967	4	0.25
3074	5	
123	2	
277	3	
492	4	0.50
769	5	

Sample size estimates are based on a two-sided 95% confidence interval.

© Cengage Learning, 2012.

goal is to reject the null hypothesis while avoiding mistakes or errors: rejecting the null hypothesis when it is true (type 1 error) and keeping the null hypothesis when it is false (type 2 error). The goal is to design a study so that the probability of a type 1 error is reduced and so that the power (the opposite of a type 2 error) is as large as possible.

Hence, determining an appropriate sample size when testing a hypothesis requires decisions about power and type 1 error. In general, potential power values are 80–90%. Typical values of the significance level (probability of a type 1 error) range from 0.1 to 0.01. Observational, exploratory studies, where a type 1 error is not as critical, can handle larger significance levels ($\alpha = 0.1$). However, most studies use a two-sided significance level of 0.05. If the study is very concerned with making a type 1 error, a lower value is used ($\alpha = 0.01$).

Determining sample size estimates for continuous data where the goal is to compare two means is actually quite easy. The only thing needed is a level of power, significance level, and the effect size. If an investigator already wants 80% power with a two-sided significance level of 0.05, all that is needed is an effect size. Assuming that the variances of the two groups are equal, the effect size is a standardized difference of means.

$$\text{Effect size of mean} = \frac{\text{Difference between means}}{\text{Common standard deviation}}$$

Determining the effect size involves finding an estimate of the difference between the means *and* a measure of the standard deviation. When the effect size is larger, the sample size required to detect this effect is smaller. However, a large effect size is not simply a large difference in means. Given a large difference in means but a large standard deviation, the effect size can end up being small. Similarly, the difference in means could be moderate to small. But, if the standard deviation is low, then the effect size could end up being large. Many consider an effect size of 0.8 to be large, 0.5 to be moderate, and 0.2 to be small (Cohen, 2003).

Typically, the planned study has not been conducted before, and no historical information for what difference in means and/or standard deviation estimates to expect are available. However, even if published works are available, rarely do authors publish the pooled standard deviation. When the pooled standard deviation is not provided, one option for the common standard deviation is to use an estimate of the standard deviation from one of the groups or simply average the two standard deviations. Larger estimates for the common standard deviation will result in larger sample sizes. However, having explicit estimates of the mean difference or the variability to propose sample sizes is not necessary. All that is needed is potential effect sizes.

In this example, with an estimate of effect size, power, and probability of type 1 error, sample size estimates can be obtained. Table 2-15 provides a summary of how the sample size estimate changes with increased effect size estimates, increased power, and decreased significance level (probability of a type 1 error), assuming a comparison of means with equal variances.

Although having an estimate of the difference in means and/or standard deviation to perform the sample size calculation is not necessary, the effect size has to be justified. Stating that only 20 subjects per group are needed when the effect size is 1.0 is not sufficient. A justification has to be given as to why an effect size of 1.0 is reasonable. Generally, this justification comes from having an estimate of the difference in means and/or standard deviation. Therefore, although estimates of the means and standard deviation are not necessary for the calculation of the sample size, they are necessary for justifying the sample size.

In this example, the groups were assumed to be of equal size. When the groups are not equal, sample sizes can be estimated (not provided in Table 2-15). Furthermore, when the two groups cannot be assumed to have equal variances, sample sizes can also be calculated. In this case, however, sample size calculators typically require an estimate for the difference in means *and* an estimate of each of the standard deviations for the groups.

TABLE 2-15 **SAMPLE SIZE ESTIMATES (TESTING FOR A DIFFERENCE IN MEAN)**

© Cengage Learning, 2012.

Point to Ponder

The sample size estimates for the two-sample study are larger than estimates for the one-sample study, which would be expected because there are now two populations of interest. However, the sample size estimates for the two-sample study are more than double that of the one-sample study. When planning a two-sample study, why is it not appropriate to simply perform sample size calculations for two one-sample studies?

Proposed Sample Size (per Group)	Effect Size	Significance Level	Power
66	0.5		
30	0.75	0.05	0.80
18	1.0		
89	0.5		
40	0.75	0.05	0.90
23	1.0		
98	0.5		
45	0.75	0.01	0.80
26	1.0		
125	0.5		
57	0.75	0.01	0.90
33	1.0		

Sample size estimates are based on conducting a two-sample t-test (equal variances).

Two Samples: Nonparametric Hypothesis Test

The methods used for estimating and testing the mean difference in hemoglobin changes between the two samples assumed that the outcome came from a normal distribution. This assumption was based on the histogram of hemoglobin outcomes and on knowledge about the distribution of hemoglobin values. Means and standard deviations were used to numerically describe the samples; sampling distributions following t-distributions were used to create confidence intervals and to perform hypothesis tests. However, continuous outcomes do not always conform to symmetric, unimodal distributions for the groups.

Suppose that investigators are interested in changes in hemoglobin, but they do not want to make assumptions about the distribution of change values. Specifically, the only assumption the investigators are willing to make about the outcome is that there is an order to the data, e.g. a change of 1.2 is smaller than a change of 3.2. Without assuming normality, a two-sample t-test (equal or unequal variances) is no longer appropriate. The nonparametric equivalent to these tests can help to answer the same research questions.

The two-sample t-tests address the research question by comparing the means of the two groups. When dealing with nonparametric tests, however, differences between groups are often determined based on whether the distributions are similar.

RESEARCH QUESTION:
Is there a difference in the hemoglobin change in women who are exposed to herbicides (tap-only) versus those who are not (bottle-only)?

RESEARCH HYPOTHESIS: The hemoglobin change values for pregnant women exposed to herbicides (tap-only) has a different distribution than the hemoglobin change values for pregnant women who are not exposed (bottle-only).

NULL HYPOTHESIS: The hemoglobin change values for pregnant women exposed to herbicides (tap-only) has the same distribution as the hemoglobin change values for pregnant women who are not exposed (bottle-only).

When assuming that the dependent variable comes from a normal distribution is unreasonable but it is still of interest to make comparisons between two groups, the *Wilcoxon or Mann-Whitney U test* can be used. This example involves two independent groups: those with exposure to herbicides in the water and those without. Investigating this research question with nonparametric tests, makes no assumption about the distribution of the outcome. The only requirement is that the outcome has an order, which is true of change in hemoglobin values. In this test, a significant p-value ($p < 0.0001$) results (Table 2-16).

TABLE 2-16 **RESULTS FROM THE WILCOXON OR MANN-WHITNEY U TEST**

Wilcoxon Two-Sample Test	
Statistic	120611.0000
Normal Approximation	
Z	20.36
One-sided Pr $> Z$	<0.0001
Two-sided Pr $>|Z|$	<0.0001
t-approximation	
One-sided Pr $> Z$	<0.0001
Two-sided Pr $>|Z|$	<0.0001

© Cengage Learning, 2012.

CONCLUSION: There is sufficient evidence to reject the null hypothesis. Hence, there is a difference in the underlying distributions of the two groups.

Unlike the one-sample nonparametric test, the Wilcoxon Mann-Whitney U test is not simply a test to compare to group medians. Therefore, the conclusion from a small p-value is that there is sufficient evidence to reject the null hypothesis: The underlying distribution of the change in hemoglobin values is different for tap-only pregnant women versus those who drink only bottled water.

MULTIPLE GROUP STUDIES WITH A CONTINUOUS OUTCOME

So far, the methods for comparing one group to a value (one-sample) and comparing the difference in outcomes between two groups (two-sample) have been discussed. However, many times investigators are interested in comparing multiple groups. Suppose investigators decide to include the additional group of pregnant women ($n = 394$) who drank a combination of tap and bottled water during pregnancy. They may be interested in comparing the outcomes not only for pregnant women who drink only from the tap ($n = 270$) and pregnant women who drink only bottled water ($n = 315$), but also for women who drink from both sources ($n = 394$). Investigating these three groups might help explain what severe (tap-only) and moderate (tap-and-bottle) exposures have on maternal outcomes. In this example, tap drinkers and tap-and-bottle drinkers have similar ages and tend to be younger than bottled water drinkers (Table 2-17). On the other hand, tap-and-bottle drinkers and bottle-only drinkers are similar when it comes to income, having median incomes $20K higher than tap-only drinkers. Those who drink bottled water have the highest high school graduation rates (76%), followed by tap-and-bottle drinkers (55%) and by tap-only drinkers (41%). A similar pattern is observed for previous smoking status, with bottle-only drinkers reporting the lowest prepregnancy smoking rates (17%), followed by tap-and-bottle drinkers (25%) and tap water only drinkers (32%). Furthermore, most (84%) of the bottle-only women have had adequate prenatal care, unlike tap-and-bottle drinkers (58%) and tap-only drinkers (35%), who have lower percentages with adequate prenatal care. Bottled-only pregnant women have higher incomes and educational attainment in this sample. In addition, they smoked less prior to pregnancy and were more likely to receive adequate prenatal care during pregnancy.

On average, the baseline hemoglobin of tap-only pregnant women is low (Table 2-18). Based on the median, half of the women have baseline hemoglobin values of less than 10.8, indicating that half of them are already at anemic levels (<11 g/dL) at baseline. This is in contrast to bottle-only and tap-and-bottle pregnant women who, on average, report baseline hemoglobin measures above the anemia cutoff (average hemoglobin 11.4 g/dL SD = 0.65 g/dL and 11.3 SD = 0.69).

Of particular interest for this study is the comparison of changes in hemoglobin. The pregnant women who drink water only from the tap in this sample have an average decrease in hemoglobin of 3.5 g/dL (SD 0.42 g/dL). Pregnant women who drink water

TABLE 2-17 **CHARACTERISTICS OF THE SAMPLE**

	Tap Only (*N* = 270)	Bottle Only (*N* = 315)	Both (*N* = 394)
Age (years)	*n* = 270	*n* = 315	*n* = 394
Mean (SD)	25.03 (1.907)	27.11 (1.467)	25.00 (1.335)
Median (min, max)	25.1 (18.9, 30.7)	27.1 (22.9, 31.0)	25.0 (21.3, 28.9)
Income($10K)	*n* = 270	*n* = 312	*n* = 393
Mean (SD)	3.75 (1.434)	4.06 (1.775)	3.92 (1.702)
Median (min, max)	3.3 (2.2, 10.9)	3.5 (2.2, 12.2)	3.5 (2.2, 11.8)
Weight Gain (lb)	*n* = 270	*n* = 315	*n* = 394
Mean (SD)	41.60 (4.106)	42.01 (4.152)	41.91 (3.909)
Median (min, max)	41.5 (29.5, 56.4)	42.1 (30.0, 51.7)	42.0 (30.5, 52.9)
Adequate Prenatal Care			
No	175 (64.8%)	52 (16.5%)	167 (42.4%)
Yes	95 (35.2%)	263 (83.5%)	227 (57.6%)
Smoked Prior to Pregnancy			
No	183 (67.8%)	261 (82.9%)	297 (75.4%)
Yes	87 (32.2%)	54 (17.1%)	97 (24.6%)
Education			
Less HS	149 (55.2%)	46 (14.6%)	141 (35.8%)
HS/GED	111 (41.1%)	238 (75.6%)	218 (55.3%)
College +	10 (3.7%)	31 (9.8%)	35 (8.9%)
Number of Previous Births (Parity)			
None	45 (16.7%)	48 (15.2%)	57 (14.5%)
One	137 (50.7%)	167 (53.0%)	211 (53.6%)
Two	78 (28.9%)	92 (29.2%)	115 (29.2%)
Three or More	10 (3.7%)	8 (2.5%)	11 (2.8%)

© Cengage Learning, 2012.

TABLE 2-18 CHARACTERISTICS OF HEMOGLOBIN MEASURES

	Tap Only (N = 270)	Bottle Only (N = 315)	Both (N = 394)
Baseline Hemoglobin (g/dL)	n = 270	n = 315	n = 394
Mean (SD)	10.73 (0.739)	11.42 (0.647)	11.29 (0.693)
Median (min, max)	10.8 (8.6, 13.2)	11.4 (9.7, 13.3)	11.3 (9.0, 13.3)
Final Hemoglobin (g/dL)	n = 270	n = 315	n = 394
Mean (SD)	7.26 (0.855)	9.39 (0.753)	7.96 (0.798)
Median (min, max)	7.3 (5.3, 10.1)	9.3 (7.1, 11.7)	8.0 (5.1, 9.9)
Change in Hemoglobin (g/dL)	n = 270	n = 315	n = 394
Mean (SD)	3.47 (0.423)	2.03 (0.427)	3.33 (0.420)
Median (min, max)	3.5 (2.3, 4.8)	2.0 (0.7, 3.5)	3.3 (1.1, 4.5)

Note: The change in hemoglobin represents baseline–final hemoglobin.

© Cengage Learning, 2012.

RESEARCH QUESTION:
Do differences exist in the hemoglobin change in women who are exposed (tap-only), marginally exposed (tap-and-bottle), and not exposed (bottle-only) to herbicides in water?

from both sources have an average decrease of 3.3 g/dL (SD 0.42 g/dL). In contrast, the bottle-only group has an average change of 2.0 (SD = 0.43 g/dL) from baseline to week 36. These differences suggest that the more tap water that is consumed, the greater the decrease is in hemoglobin over the course of the pregnancy.

Both groups of pregnant women who consume water from the tap may be exposed to herbicides, but those who also drank bottled water would have less exposure. The bottle-only pregnant women would not be exposed to herbicides and would still serve as a control group. The descriptive statistics (Table 2-18) suggest that differences in hemoglobin changes may exist between the groups. If the outcomes differ among the three groups, perhaps the differences can be attributed to the differences in water sources.

Because this is a multisample study, there is now a control group (bottle-only drinkers), a marginally exposed group (tap-and-bottle drinkers), and an exposed group (tap-only drinkers). Specifically of interest is determining whether there are any differences in the mean hemoglobin changes in pregnant women exposed to herbicides (via tap water), exposed to herbicides to a lesser degree (both tap and bottled water), or unexposed to herbicides (bottled water only).

With three groups, if differences exist, then one or more of the following could be true:

1. The mean hemoglobin change is different for tap- and bottle-only drinkers,
2. The mean change in hemoglobin for bottle-only and tap-and-bottle drinkers is different.
3. The mean change in hemoglobin for tap-only and tap-and-bottle drinkers is different.

In this multiple group sample, the following mean differences were observed:

1. The mean difference in hemoglobin change between the bottle-only and tap-only groups is 1.5 g/dL, indicating that on average tap-drinkers have a 1.5 g/dL larger drop in hemoglobin over the course of the pregnancy.
2. The mean difference in hemoglobin change between the bottle-only and tap-and-bottle groups is 1.3 g/dL, indicating that on average combination drinkers have a 1.3 g/dL larger drop in hemoglobin over the course of the pregnancy.
3. The mean difference in hemoglobin change between the tap-only and tap-and-bottle groups is 0.2 g/dL, indicating that on average tap-only drinkers have a 0.2 g/dL larger drop in hemoglobin over the course of the pregnancy.

Do these differences in sample means support the claim that differences exist between the groups?

Once the groups have been described, the groups can be compared to determine whether the means for the groups are truly different. When there are more than two groups, the comparison of means to determine whether any of the groups are different is known as an ANalysis Of Variance (ANOVA).

The ANOVA is used when the research question involves the comparisons of means from more than two independent groups. It is assumed that:

- The groups are independent.
- The variance for each of the groups is the same.
- The outcome comes from a normal distribution.

These are the same assumptions as in the two-sample *t*-test with equal (pooled) variance. In fact, when there are only two groups, a two-sample *t*-test (with pooled variance) and an ANOVA are equivalent.

It may seem confusing that the method to investigate means between multiple groups is called analysis of *variance*. The ultimate goal is to ascertain whether any of the group means are different; so why not call this method the analysis of means? Outcomes have two sources of variability: variability because the subjects are in different groups and variability that occurs within each group because each subject is unique. If the variability between the groups is greater than the variability within the groups, then the group means would be different. In other words, when a significant amount of variability in the outcome is attributable to group membership, the group means are different (Figure 2-13). However, when the variability within a group is large, then stating that the groups are different is difficult (Figure 2-14).

In an ANOVA analysis, the goal is to take the variability of the outcome and divide it into the variability between the groups and the variability within the groups. Typically, the partitioning of the variability is presented in a table called an *ANOVA table* (Table 2-19).

Recall from the numerical summaries section of this chapter that the sample variance is found by taking the sum of the squared differences from the mean (the total sum of squares) and dividing this by the degrees of freedom ($n - 1$). The total sum of squares (the numerator of the sample variance) can be split into the sums of squares for between the groups and for within the groups. Table 2-19 is structured to demonstrate that the total sum of squares of the outcome is equal to the between sum of squares (SSB) plus the within sum of squares (SSE). Likewise, since the between sum of squares and the within sum of squares must add up to the total sum of squares, the degrees of freedom for the between and within sums of squares must also add up to the total degrees of freedom.

The total variability in the outcome is estimated by dividing the total sum of squares by the degrees of freedom ($n - 1$). Likewise, the between variability in the outcome is estimated by dividing the between sum of squares by its degrees of freedom (number of groups $- 1$). The between sum of squares (SSB) divided by the number of groups $- 1$, or degrees of freedom, is called the *mean squared between (MSB)*. Because dividing by the number of groups $- 1$ creates a calculation that is like the average variability between the groups, the MSB represents the variability between the groups.

TABLE 2-19 **ANOVA TABLE**

Source	Degrees of Freedom	Sum of Squares	Mean Square	F
Between	Number of groups $- 1$	SSB	$MSB = \dfrac{SSB}{\text{Between DF}}$	$\dfrac{MSB}{MSE}$
Within (error)	(Number of observations $-$ Number of groups)	SSE	$MSE = \dfrac{SSE}{\text{Within DF}}$	
Total	Number of observations $- 1$	SST		

© Cengage Learning, 2012.

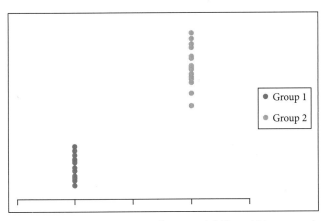

Figure 2-13 Group outcomes (large variability within groups). © *Cengage Learning, 2012.*

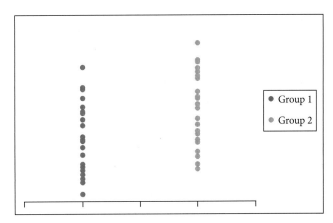

Figure 2-14 Group outcomes (large variability between groups). © *Cengage Learning, 2012.*

Furthermore, the within variability is estimated by dividing the within sum of squares by its degrees of freedom (n − the number of groups). The within (or residual) sum of squares (SSE) divided by its degrees of freedom is called the mean squared within, or *mean squared error (MSE)*. The within sum of squares is often referred to as the error sum of squares because it is the variability that is left over or unexplained by group membership. Because the MSE represents the average variability within the groups and the variability in the groups was assumed to be equal, it is really a measure of the variability within each group. Therefore, the MSE is the value used to estimate the common variance.

Multiple Sample Means: Overall Hypothesis Test

The purpose of using a method like ANOVA is to answer the question, "Are the group means different?" In this example, the goal is to test whether the true mean hemoglobin changes are different for the three groups: tap-only (μ_{tap}), bottle-only (μ_{bottle}), and tap-and-bottle (μ_{both}).

RESEARCH HYPOTHESIS: The true mean hemoglobin changes are different for at least two of the groups; $\mu_{tap} \neq \mu_{bottle}$ or $\mu_{tap} \neq \mu_{both}$ or $\mu_{both} \neq \mu_{bottle}$.

NULL HYPOTHESIS: The true mean hemoglobin changes are the same for all the groups; $\mu_{tap} = \mu_{bottle} = \mu_{both}$.

The ANOVA helps to answer this question by splitting up the sources of variability. If the between variability is larger than the within variability, then the group means are different (Figure 2-13). If the between variability is not large enough, then there is not enough evidence to claim the groups are different (Figure 2-14). To determine whether the between variability is large enough to state that the groups are different, a ratio of the variability between and within the groups is used as the test statistic for the hypothesis test.

Specifically, the ratio of the mean squared between and the mean squared error is calculated and used to conclude whether the between variability is large enough. If the mean squared error is small, then the ratio will be large. If the mean squared error is large, then the ratio is small. Hence, the size of this ratio can help in determining whether there is a difference between the groups. Because this ratio is a test statistic, determining whether the ratio is large enough implies determining whether the test statistic is large enough to reject the null hypothesis.

Whenever a ratio of variances is used, the sampling distribution of the ratios follows an *F*-distribution with degrees of freedom from the numerator and the denominator of the ratio. Therefore, the ANOVA provides for a statistical test, using the *F*-statistic, for determining whether there is enough evidence to reject the null hypothesis that all the means are equal.

$$\text{Test statistic } (F) = \frac{\text{Mean square between}}{\text{Mean square error}}$$

What you need to calculate the test statistic:

1. *The mean square between:* MSB = 198.07.
2. *The mean square error:* MSE = 0.181.
3. *The degrees of freedom:*
   a. MSB, df = 2.
   b. MSE, df = 976.

To calculate the test statistic: The ratio, MSB (1) divided by MSE (2), is the test statistic. MSB/MSE = 198.07 ÷ 0.181 = 1095.50.

Using an *F*-distribution with numerator degrees of freedom of 2 and denominator degrees of freedom of 976, the percentage of ratios that are even farther from the ratio that was observed with this sample is less than 0.01% (*p*-value <0.0001).

Performing an ANOVA analysis in any statistical software program will result in an ANOVA table. In this example, the resulting ANOVA table (Table 2-20) provides the information needed for testing the hypothesis for group differences.

TABLE 2-20 **EXAMPLE OF ANOVA TABLE**

Source	Degrees of Freedom	Sum of Squares	Mean Square	F	p-Value
Between	2	396.15	198.07	1095.50	<0.0001
Within (error)	976	176.46	0.181		
Total	978	572.61			

© Cengage Learning, 2012.

CONCLUSION: Since this *p*-value is small, there is evidence that the ratio is large or that the variability between the groups is large enough to suggest that the group means are different. In other words, there is sufficient evidence to reject the null hypothesis that the three group means are the same. Hence, at least one of the three group means is different from the others.

The ANOVA helped to provide an answer to the question of whether the mean hemoglobin changes were the same between the groups. However, this may not be sufficient to fully answer the research question. The *F*-statistic (the ratio of the variances) is often referred to as the *overall F-test*. The results can be used only to determine whether there is a difference in any of the groups. This test does not indicate specific group differences. The *F*-statistic helps to answer the question of whether the groups are different, but it and the resulting *p*-value do not indicate which groups are different.

In this example the *F*-statistic was large enough that a small *p*-value was found; all three groups (tap-only, bottle-only, and both) could have different true mean changes in hemoglobin or only one group could have a mean different than the others. To determine which groups are actually different, more specific comparisons have to be performed. However, these more specific comparisons can only be performed *after* determining that differences between the groups exist overall. If the ANOVA results in an *F*-statistic that is not significant (the *p*-value is large), then the overall null hypothesis cannot be rejected: There is no evidence that the groups are different. If there is no evidence that the groups are different, then there is no reason to continue searching for differences by looking at specific comparisons.

RESEARCH QUESTION: Is there a difference in the hemoglobin change in pregnant women who are exposed to herbicides (via tap water) versus those who are not (bottled water)?

RESEARCH QUESTION: Is there a difference in the hemoglobin change in pregnant women who are exposed to herbicides (via tap water) versus those who are marginally exposed (via both tap and bottled water)?

RESEARCH QUESTION: Is there a difference in the change in hemoglobin for pregnant women who are marginally exposed to herbicides (via both tap water and bottled water) versus those who are unexposed (via bottled water)?

Once the ANOVA has been performed, two pieces of information are obtained: (1) whether there is evidence that the group means are different and (2) an estimate of the common variance (mean squared error) for the groups. If the overall F-test indicates that differences exist in the group means, the mean squared error can be used as the pooled variance to determine which groups are different. The hypothesis tests to determine which groups are different are two-sample tests with equal variances, where the "pooled" estimate of the variance is the mean squared error.

The goal of this study is to better understand the relationship between herbicides exposure and hemoglobin changes in pregnant women. Although the overall question of whether differences exist is important, investigators are specifically interested in which groups have different mean hemoglobin changes.

After establishing that there is a difference in the mean hemoglobin change among the three exposure groups, two-group comparisons can be made for bottled water versus tap water, for bottled water versus both, and for tap water versus both by investigating the differences in means between two groups at a time. A mean difference between two groups means is not 0 suggests that the two group means are different.

To test these hypotheses, the true parameters (the average differences in the hemoglobin change) are assumed to be 0 g/dL. In other words, a difference of 0 g/dL serves as the null parameter. The data from the sample provides a statistic, and it must be decided whether this statistic would be expected if the null parameter (0 g/dL) was the true parameter. Therefore, to reject the null hypothesis in favor of the research hypothesis, the sample data must provide evidence against the null parameter.

Just as in the two-sample hypothesis test, the comparison of two means involves determining whether the sample supports the null parameter (0 g/dL) as the true parameter. The test statistic is found by dividing the difference between the sample means by the standard error. Because one of the assumptions of the ANOVA is that the groups have a common variance, the same estimate of the variance can be used to calculate the standard error regardless of what groups are being tested. The estimate for the common variance is just the mean square error. The sampling distribution for the difference between the two means divided by the standard error is a t-distribution with the same number of degrees of freedom as the mean squared error: total sample size – the number of groups.

Point to Ponder

In an ANOVA, the mean squared error is used to estimate the variance in the two-group comparisons. Why not just use the variances of each sample as was done in the two-sample t-test?

RESEARCH HYPOTHESIS: The average difference in the hemoglobin change in pregnant women who are exposed to herbicides (via tap water) versus those who are not (bottled water) is *different* from 0 g/dL: $\mu_{tap} - \mu_{bottle} \neq 0$.

NULL HYPOTHESIS: The average difference in the hemoglobin change in pregnant women who are exposed to herbicides (via tap water) versus those who are not (bottled water) is *equal* to 0 g/dL: $\mu_{tap} - \mu_{bottle} = 0$.

RESEARCH HYPOTHESIS: The average difference in the hemoglobin change in pregnant women who are exposed to herbicides (via both tap water and bottled water) versus those who are not (bottled water only) is *different* from 0 g/dL: $\mu_{both} - \mu_{bottle} \neq 0$.

NULL HYPOTHESIS: The average difference in the change in hemoglobin for pregnant women who are exposed to herbicides (via both tap and bottled water) versus those who are not (bottled water only) is *equal* to 0 g/dL: $\mu_{both} - \mu_{bottle} = 0$.

RESEARCH HYPOTHESIS: The average difference in the hemoglobin change in pregnant women who are exposed to herbicides (via tap water) versus those who are not as exposed (bottled water and tap water) is *different* from 0 g/dL: or $\mu_{tap} - \mu_{both} \neq 0$.

NULL HYPOTHESIS: The average difference in the hemoglobin change in pregnant women who are exposed to herbicides (via tap water) versus those who are not as exposed (bottled water and tap water) is *equal* to 0 g/dL: $\mu_{tap} - \mu_{both} = 0$.

In this study, the degrees of freedom associated with the mean square error is $(979 - 3) = 976$. So the t-distribution with 976 degrees of freedom can be used to calculate the p-value for the three hypothesis tests. Hence, the comparison of every two group means is another type of t-test.

Application of Formula: TWO-GROUP COMPARISON

$$\text{Test statistic } (t) = \frac{\bar{x}_i - \bar{x}_j}{\sqrt{\text{MSE}\left(\frac{1}{n_i} + \frac{1}{n_j}\right)}}$$

$\bar{x}_i - \bar{x}_j$ = The difference in the sample means for group i and j

n_i = The sample size for group i n_j = The sample size for group j

MSE = mean squared error (comes from the ANOVA table)

What you need for the specific two-group comparisons in an ANOVA:

1. *The difference between two sample means:* In this study, the sample mean for tap water only is 3.5 g/dL, the sample mean for bottled water only is 2.0 g/dL, and the sample mean for both sources is 3.3 g/dL. The difference between tap and bottled is 1.5 g/dL, the difference between both and bottled is 1.2 g/dL, and the difference between tap and both is 0.2 g/dL.
2. *The square root of the* MSE: The MSE for this example is 0.181, $\sqrt{0.181} = 0.44$
3. *The standard error:* The standard error is the square root of the mean squared error (2) multiplied by the square root of (1 divided by the sample size of one group + 1 divided by the sample size of another group) (3).

    a. For the tap and bottled water comparison, the standard error is $0.44 * \sqrt{\left(\frac{1}{270}\right) + \left(\frac{1}{315}\right)} = 0.0365$.

    b. For the comparison of tap-and-bottle versus bottle-only, the standard error is $0.44 * \sqrt{\left(\frac{1}{396}\right) + \left(\frac{1}{315}\right)} = 0.0332$.

    c. For the tap-only versus tap-and-bottle comparison, the standard error is $0.44 * \sqrt{\left(\frac{1}{270}\right) + \left(\frac{1}{396}\right)} = 0.0347$.

To calculate the test statistic (t): Divide (1) by the standard error (3).

    a. Tap-only versus bottle-only: The test statistic is $1.5 \div 0.04 = 41.1$.
    b. Tap-and-bottle versus bottle-only: The test statistic is $1.2 \div 0.0332 = 36.1$.
    c. Tap-only versus tap-and-bottle; The test statistic is $0.2 \div 0.0347 = 5.8$.

For each test statistic, the decision has to be made as to whether the test statistic is far enough away from the center of the t-distribution with 976 degrees of freedom. All of these test statistics are large. However, the exact proportions of test statistics (p-values) that are even farther away than each test statistic can be found by using statistical software or statistical tables.

The p-values that result from the three two-way comparisons for this study are <0.0001, <0.0001, and <0.0001 (Table 2-21). Because the p-values are so small, these test statistics are considered rare and would not be expected at all if the true parameters were the null parameters (0 g/dL).

TABLE 2-21 RESULTS FROM POST HOC COMPARISONS OF MEANS

Group	P-values for comparing group means		
	Compared to Group		
	1	2	3
Tap-Only		<0.0001	<0.0001
Bottle-Only	<0.0001		<0.0001
Tap-and-Bottle	<0.0001	<0.0001	

© Cengage Learning, 2012.

CONCLUSION: There is sufficient evidence to reject the null hypothesis is all three comparisons, suggesting that all three group means are different. Hence, the mean change in hemoglobin depends on whether a pregnant woman drinks tap water only, bottle water only, or both.

Point to Ponder

For comparisons of multiple means, why perform the overall F-test? Why not just start with comparing two groups at a time? Is there ever a time when it would be reasonable to skip the overall F-test?

All the means do not have to be significantly different when the overall F-test is statistically significant. Getting a significant p-value from the overall F-test with only one statistically significant two-group comparison is quite possible.

Multiple Sample Means: Multiple Comparisons

In this case the three groups resulted in three comparisons: the comparison between tap-only and bottle-only, the comparison between tap-only and tap-and-bottle, and the comparison between bottle-only and tap-and-bottle. Although three comparisons are not that many, suppose there had been four groups instead of three. In that case, comparisons could be made between group 1 versus group 2, group 1 versus group 3, group 1 versus group 4, group 2 versus group 3, group 2 versus group 4, and group 3 versus group 4. As the number of groups increases, so do the number of comparisons. The more comparisons that are performed, the greater the chance of rejecting the null hypothesis. Whenever there is an increased chance of rejecting the null hypothesis, there is an increased chance of rejecting the null hypothesis when it should not be rejected, or making a type 1 error.

Sometimes making multiple comparisons are unavoidable, so how can multiple groups be compared without increasing the chances of a type 1 error? The first step to prevent inflating the type 1 error rate is to make only the planned or necessary comparisons. If the comparison of bottled water and combination is not important, then do not test for the difference. Generally, clinical trials require that analysis plans be in place prior to the collection of data so that only planned comparisons are made. However, in more exploratory or observational studies, interesting comparisons might not be clear at the outset.

Point to Ponder

Caution: Making it very hard to reject the null hypothesis decreases the chance of a type 1 error but increases the chance of a type 2 error. A type 2 error occurs when the null hypothesis should have been rejected but was not. If the goal of the study is exploratory, which outcome is worse?

- Rejecting the null hypothesis when you should not, which means stating something is significant when it really is not.
- Failing to reject a null hypothesis when you should, which means stating something is not significant when it really is.

Depending on the answer to this question, an investigator may decide not to make adjustments for multiple comparisons.

If multiple comparisons are necessary, one solution is to make the significance level (α) quite small so that it is very difficult to reject the null hypothesis. This is what is done when investigators use a *Bonferroni adjustment*, by which the significance level is reduced by the number of tests to be performed. If investigators want an overall type 1 error rate of 0.05 and want to perform five hypothesis tests, then they would reject null hypotheses only when the p-values are less than 0.01, or 0.05/5. If a p-value has to be very, very small to reject the null hypothesis, then a type 1 error is less likely.

When making corrections to reduce the probability of a type 1 error, statistical software packages have several options. Details on how these methods make adjustments to correct for multiple comparisons can be found in the documentation of the specific software packages. For purposes of illustrating the adjustments, unadjusted p-values as well as Bonferroni, Tukey, and Scheffe adjusted p-values are presented in Table 2-22.

TABLE 2-22 **ADJUSTMENTS FOR MULTIPLE COMPARISONS**

	Group	Change LSMEAN	Standard Error	LSMEAN Number
	Tap-Only	3.46888331	0.02587768	1
	Bottle-Only	2.03253083	0.02395808	2
	Tap-and-Bottle	3.33469379	0.02142196	3

		P-values for comparing group means		
		Compared to Group		
	Group	1	2	3
Unadjusted	1		<0.0001	<0.0001
	2	<0.0001		<0.0001
	3	<0.0001	<0.0001	
Bonferonni	1		<0.0001	0.0002
	2	<0.0001		<0.0001
	3	0.0002	<0.0001	
Tukey	1		<0.0001	0.0002
	2	<0.0001		<0.0001
	3	0.0002	<0.0001	
Scheffe	1		<0.0001	0.0004
	2	<0.0001		<0.0001
	3	0.0004	<0.0001	

© Cengage Learning, 2012.

Planning a Multiple-Sample Study

Planning a study that involves multiple groups is fairly similar to planning a study of two groups. The same issues involving different sized groups, estimating mean differences, and common standard deviation still apply. However, there is an added complication because for every research question that involves multiple groups there are actually two sets of hypotheses: the overall test and the specific tests.

Suppose that investigators need to estimate a sample size for a study comparing four groups. They would like to enroll 25 subjects in each group. They may have performed a preliminary study or searched the literature to find that, for this study, means of 13.2, 14.5, 17.8, and 13.3 are expected. The investigators may also assume a common standard deviation of 4.4. Using a two-sided significance level of 0.05, they want to know the power of the study. Using a sample size calculator, they can determine that an ANOVA will have 95% power to detect the difference in means that they suggest. However, this corresponds to the overall F-test. It does not provide an estimate for the power for comparing between groups or determining which groups are different.

If the investigators are interested in making comparisons between groups, then they would plan the study around making two-group comparisons. Suppose that the control group has a mean of 13.2 and that the primary research question is to compare the control group to the intervention group where a mean of 14.5 is expected. Assuming a two-sided significance level of 0.05 and a common standard deviation of 4.4, a *t*-test contrasting these two groups in an ANOVA will have only 17% power, and a larger sample size is required. Comparing the group with a mean of 17.8 and the group with a mean of 13.2 has 95% power, but this comparison may not be interesting to the investigators. Moreover, these estimates were based on a two-sided significance level of 0.05. If a smaller significance level is planned due to adjustments for multiple comparisons, it needs to be considered in planning the sample size; that is, a two-sided significance level of 0.01 requires a larger sample size. So be careful when planning multiple-group studies. Like all studies, sample size estimation depends on the research question. When multiple groups are of interest, it is possible to have enough power to make some comparisons but not others.

Multiple Samples: Nonparametric Hypothesis Tests

One of the assumptions of the ANOVA presented in this section is that the outcome must be normally distributed. This was not a concern in this example because assuming normality based on the histograms and the nature of hemoglobin changes is quite reasonable. However, this may not always be the case. Analogous to the one-way ANOVA, the *Kruskal-Wallis test* allows for the comparison of more than two groups without assuming the outcome is normally distributed. Also just as the ANOVA is a generalized version of the two-sample *t*-test, the Kruskal-Wallis test is a generalized version of the Wilcoxon Mann-Whitney test.

Suppose that investigators are studying changes in hemoglobin among the three groups, but they do not want to make assumptions about the distribution of change values. Specifically, the only assumption they are willing to make about the outcome is that there is an order to the data; for example, a change of 1.2 is smaller than a change of 3.2. Without assuming normality, an ANOVA is no longer appropriate, but the Kruskal-Wallis test, the nonparametric equivalent to the ANOVA, can help to answer the same research questions.

While the ANOVA addressed this research question by comparing the means of the three groups, the nonparametric test determines differences based on whether the distribution functions of the population are similar.

> **RESEARCH QUESTION:** Do differences exist in the hemoglobin change among women who are exposed to herbicides (tap-only), those with marginal exposure to herbicides (tap-and-bottle), and those with no exposure (bottle-only)?

RESEARCH HYPOTHESIS: At least one of the three groups comes from a different population.

NULL HYPOTHESIS: All of the three groups come from the same population.

When assuming that the dependent variable comes from a normal distribution is unreasonable, but it is still of interest to compare an ordered outcome among multiple groups, the Kruskal-Wallis test can be used. This example consists of three independent groups: those with exposure to herbicides in the water, those without exposure, and those with marginal exposure. Because this is a nonparametric test, there is no assumption on the distribution of the outcome. The only requirement is that the outcome has an order, which is true of change in hemoglobin values. In this test, a significant *p*-value ($p = <0.0001$) results (Table 2-23).

TABLE 2-23 **RESULTS FROM A KRUSKAL-WALLIS TEST**

Chi-square	DF	Pr >chi-square
609.6	2	<0.0001

© Cengage Learning, 2012.

CONCLUSION: There is sufficient evidence to reject the null hypothesis, indicating that there is a statistically significant difference among the three exposure groups.

SUMMARY

This chapter began with an environmental health problem: groundwater impacted by an herbicide, atrazine. Like the public health application, the data presented in this chapter involved investigating maternal health outcomes for women exposed to water that had been affected by herbicides. The research question involved a continuous outcome, hemoglobin. Specifically, it was of interest to investigate how the change in hemoglobin during pregnancy is altered by exposure to herbicides in the water by making comparisons among exposure groups.

Research questions involving clinical outcomes, like hemoglobin, often result in continuous data. For a continuous variable, the level of detail is limited only by how precisely the instrument measures, resulting in potentially infinite numbers of possible values. Hence, graphical and numerical summaries are particularly important with continuous outcomes because they provide a mechanism for understanding and interpreting the data.

Making comparisons between groups when the outcome is continuous is often done by comparing means, although other, nonparametric methods are available that allow comparisons without assuming that the data are normally distributed. The most common analyses associated with making comparisons between groups on continuous outcomes were explained in this chapter. The following Summary of Methods provides a synopsis of the methods discussed in this chapter.

SUMMARY OF METHODS

RESEARCH QUESTION	GRAPHICAL DESCRIPTIONS	NUMERICAL DESCRIPTIONS	STATISTICAL TESTS	
			Normal Data	*Not Normal Data*
Is the mean different from some known value?	Histogram	Mean (SD) Median (range)	One-sample *t*-test	Signed rank test
Is the change different from 0?	Histogram	Mean (SD) Median (range)	Paired *t*-test	Signed rank test
Are the two groups different?	Plot of means with error bars Box-and-whisker plots	Mean (SD) Median (range)	Two-sample *t*-test	Wilcoxon Mann-Whitney test
Is there a difference between the groups? (More than two groups)	Plot of means with error bars Box-and-whisker plots	Mean (SD) Median (range)	ANOVA	Kruskal-Wallis

© Cengage Learning, 2012.

KEY TERMS

longitudinal study   degrees of freedom   balanced design

historical controls   paired differences   *F*-distribution

t-distribution   independent groups

PRACTICE WITH DATA

1. DESCRIBING THE DATA

a. Provide descriptive statistics for the weight gain observed in this sample.

b. Provide descriptive statistics (n, mean, standard deviation, median, first and third quartiles, and minimum and maximum) for the weight gain observed in the sample of women who drank only bottled water versus those who drank only tap water.

c. Use a box-and-whisker plot to compare the distribution of the weight gain of the three water consumption groups (tap-only, bottle-only, and tap-and-bottle). What does the plot show?

2. ONE-SAMPLE STUDY (TAP-ONLY)

a. Estimate (using a 95% confidence interval) the true mean weight gain. Interpret.

b. Abrams et al. (2000) reported that the healthy pregnant women are generally advised to limit weight gain to approximately 26 pounds. Is the weight gain different in the sample of women who drank only tap water? Use statistical inference to justify your answer.

c. Suppose that a normal distribution could not be assumed for the weight change. Use a signed rank test to determine whether the change in this population is different from the historical control (26 pounds). Provide an interpretation of the results.

3. TWO-SAMPLE STUDY (TAP-ONLY AND BOTTLE-ONLY)

a. Provide the null and research hypotheses (defining all symbols) for comparing the mean weight gain in the two water groups.

b. Use a statistical test to determine whether the variances of the two groups (tap-only and bottle-only) are different.

c. Based on the response to part (b), perform the appropriate two-sample t-test (equal or unequal variances). Interpret the results.

d. Based on the response to part (b), provide an interval estimate for the mean difference in weight gain between the two groups. Interpret.

4. THREE-SAMPLE STUDY (TAP-ONLY, BOTTLE-ONLY, TAP-AND-BOTTLE)

a. Provide the null and research hypotheses (defining all symbols) for comparing the mean weight gain among the three groups.

b. Create an ANOVA table using weight gain as the dependent variable.

c. Using the information from the ANOVA table part (a). Conduct an overall F-test. What conclusions can be made?

d. In this example, is it appropriate to perform specific hypothesis tests to determine where group differences exist? If so, perform these tests and provide conclusions. If not, explain why the specific hypothesis tests cannot be performed.

PRACTICE WITH CONCEPTS

1. Consider the following research questions/study scenarios. For each study, discuss the *most* appropriate methods for describing the data (graphically and numerically) and addressing the research questions? Be sure to provide a justification of the statistical method. When a statistical test is needed, provide appropriate null and research hypotheses.

    a. A study was performed to determine differences in pain experienced by children with sickle cell disease (SCD) in inpatient and outpatient settings. Pain intensity (a visual analog scale) was the primary outcome of interest. A visual analog scale (VAS) provides a visual scale/ruler that subjects can use to indicate their level of pain. This particular scale ranges from 0–10.

    b. Elderly subjects are participating in a trial to investigate the benefits of strength training. One of the outcomes is to investigate the expression levels of inflammatory biomarkers. The post-training expression levels are of interest. These expression levels have traditionally followed a normal distribution. Is there a difference in the average expression levels of those who participated in strength training versus those who did not?

    c. Does the type of instruction patients receive improve? A pediatric dentistry clinic wants to evaluate whether the type of instruction on toothbrushing impacts compliance. A study is conducted where parents receive instruction from either the dentist, a paper information packet to take home, or a DVD to watch. Compliance is measured by recording the proportion of days that parents brush the child's teeth in the 30 days following the visit.

    d. Can greater exposure to fresh fruits and vegetables help type 2 diabetics better manage the disease? A nutritional study has been proposed to determine whether providing farmer's market credits to type 2 diabetes patients can help reduce HbA1c, a continuous, normally distributed outcome. HbA1c is measured prior to the distribution of credits.

    e. To evaluate the effectiveness of a smoking cessation program, subjects expressing a desire to quit smoking were enrolled in a modified counseling program. Cotinine levels will be measured prior to enrollment and 6 weeks after the completion of the program. Does the modified counseling program reduce cotinine levels?

    f. Human resource records of a large corporation were investigated to determine the costs of flu-like illnesses on an employed population involved in different working environments. Employees were categorized by working environment: enclosed office, cubicle, open-space, or mobile. It is of interest to determine whether the working environment is related to sick leave. Sick leave is a continuous variable but does not arise from a symmetric distribution.

2. *Disinfection is an essential measure for interrupting human norovirus (HuNoV) transmission, but it is difficult to evaluate the efficacy of disinfectants due to the absence of a practicable cell culture system for these viruses. The purpose of this study was to screen sodium hypochlorite and ethanol for efficacy against Norwalk virus (NV) and to expand the studies to evaluate the efficacy of antibacterial liquid soap and alcohol-based hand sanitizer for the inactivation of NV on human finger pads.* (Liu, Yuen, Hsiao, Jaykus, & Moe, 2010)
The investigators used one-way ANOVA to compare the NV reduction for dry control, water rinse, hand sanitizer, and liquid soap.

    a. Why was the ANOVA an appropriate method?

    b. What are the assumptions of the ANOVA?

    c. Provide the null and alternative hypotheses associated with the ANOVA in this context. Be sure to define all symbols.

3. *The effects of continuous positive airway pressure (CPAP) for obstructive sleep apnoea (OSA) on insulin resistance are not clear. Forty-two men with known type 2 diabetes and newly diagnosed OSA were randomised to receive therapeutic or placebo CPAP for 3 months. Baseline tests were performed and repeated after 3 months. The table below is adapted from their results. (West, Nicoll, Wallace, Matthews, & Stadling, 2007)*

Group	Baseline HbA1c	HbA1c Change	Confidence Interval for Change
Therapeutic CPAP (*n* = 20)	8.5 (1.8)	−0.02 (1.5)	−0.6 to 0.9
Placebo CPAP (*n* = 22)	8.4 (1.9)	0.1 (0.7)	

© Cengage Learning, 2012.

    a. The baseline HbA1c for the two groups is very similar. Explain why this would be important.

    b. Provide an interpretation of the results associated with the change in HbA1c using the confidence interval provided.

    c. *The study was powered not to miss a difference of 0.8 in HbA1c (assuming a within subject SD of 0.8)19 at a significance level of 5% and with a power of 90%, which required 20 subjects in each treatment group.*
The authors failed to reject the null hypothesis ($p = 0.7$). Should the study have been designed with a larger sample to detect a smaller difference?

4. *Individuals with low literacy and symptoms of depression have greater improvement of depression symptoms when their treatment includes education to enhance literacy skills. The reason why literacy enhancement helps depression symptoms is unknown, but we hypothesize that it might be due to improved self-efficacy. We studied whether providing literacy education to individuals with both depression symptoms and limited literacy might improve their self-efficacy. (Francis, Weiss, Senf, Heist, & Hargraves, 2007)*
The authors reported changes in self-efficacy (GSE) and depression (PHD-9) measures. The following table is adapted from Francis et al.

    a. The signed rank test was used. Why?

    b. Provide an interpretation of their findings for PHQ-9.

    c. Identify a problem with the reporting of the following results.

Measure	Baseline (*n* = 39)	12–15 Months (*n* = 31)	P-value*
GSE			0.019
Mean (SD)	27.9 (3.7)	29.9 (1.9)	
Median	28	30	
PHQ-9			<0.01
Mean (SD)	11.9 (5.2)	6.0 (3.9)	
Median	10	4	

*P-values obtained comparing the change from baseline to (12–15 months) using the signed rank test.

© Cengage Learning, 2012.

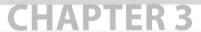
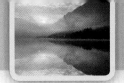
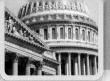
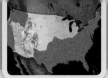
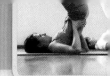

CHAPTER 3

continuous data
correlation and regression

The statistical methods for describing and making group comparisons with continuous outcomes were described in Chapter 2. Briefly, continuous variables consist of variables with many values. Specifically, outcomes are considered continuous when the values are numeric and there are no natural gaps between the values. Numerically, continuous outcomes are summarized with descriptive statistics (sample size, mean, standard deviation, median, first and third quartiles, and minimum and maximum). Graphically, histograms and box-and-whisker plots provide a picture of the distribution. Graphical and numerical summaries of continuous data are particularly helpful because each subject can potentially have different values of the outcome. In Chapter 2, these summaries were discussed, along with research questions involving comparing continuous outcomes, either to a prespecified value or between groups. However, research questions resulting in continuous outcomes are not limited to comparing groups.

Clinical measures like hemoglobin, blood pressure, weight, temperature, gene expressions, or levels of a biomarker are all examples of continuous outcomes found in public health. When multiple continuous variables are measured on a subject, research questions may arise that focus on understanding the relationships between the variables. Examples are how changes in triglycerides impact the HbA1c values in diabetic patients, how weight is related to blood pressure, and how muscle size is related to the expression of inflammatory biomarkers.

This chapter focuses on investigating associations between continuous variables. Simple methods, involving only two variables at a time, will be introduced first. Considerable attention will be given to these methods because they form a basis for understanding many of the more advanced approaches involving multiple variables discussed later in this chapter and text.

LEARNING OBJECTIVES

How do I describe relationships between continuous variables?

Identify, create, and present appropriate descriptive statistics and figures specific for continuous data.

How do I investigate the association of risk factors (continuous and categorical) with the outcome?

Utilize regression techniques to investigate risk factors.

Interpret the results (estimates and statistical tests) of the regression analysis.

How do I compare groups while adjusting for confounders (continuous and categorical)?

Utilize regression techniques to control for confounding.

Interpret the results (estimates and statistical tests) of the regression analysis.

How do I plan for a study when the research question involves two continuous variables?

Understand the roles that power, effect size, and sample size play in designing a study.

What method do I use?

Identify the most appropriate method for describing the data, numerically and graphically.

Identify the most appropriate method for making comparisons.

Public Health Application

The U.S. EPA estimates that 76–85 million pounds of atrazine (6-chloro-N$_2$-ethyl-N$_4$-isopropyl-1,3,4-triazine-2,4-diamine), a triazine herbicide, is produced annually with approximately 76.5 million pounds applied within the United States, making it one of the most widely used pesticides in the country (Cooper et al., 2007; Gammon et al., 2005; U.S. Environmental Protection Agency, 2008a). Atrazine's main use is to control broadleaf and grassy weeds with the most common sites of application being corn, sugarcane, and sorghum (Cooper et al., 2007). Other uses include maintenance of a myriad of crops, golf courses, rangeland, residential lawns, landscapes, forests, recreational areas, and industry (U.S. Environmental Protection Agency, 2008a). Once introduced into the environment, atrazine is not easily broken down and has been shown to persist for long periods (U.S. Environmental Protection Agency, 2008b). In areas such as subsurface soil or aquifers, no biodegradation of atrazine has been shown. This persistence provides ample opportunity for water system contamination (Agency for Toxic Substances and Disease Registry, 2003).

Current research shows that atrazine exposure may pose a significant threat to human health with drinking water providing the most widespread route of exposure (Villanueva et al., 2005). Triazines in general are considered to be endocrine disrupters (Gammon et al., 2005). A large number of animal studies have been conducted that demonstrate mixed results concerning the link between atrazine and several adverse health effects including reproductive outcomes and cancer ("EXTOXNET," 1996; Gammon et al., 2005; Hayes, 2005).

(Rinsky et al., 2011)

Data Description

In Chapter 2 the study to investigate the impacts of herbicide exposure on maternal health was described. For this study, 995 pregnant women from a large farming community were recruited during their initial prenatal visits. The groundwater in the region is known to be exposed to herbicides. At the initial visit (approximately week 9 of the pregnancy), the women were surveyed about their planned drinking habits for the duration of the pregnancy. In particular, women were asked whether they plan to drink water, "Only from the tap," "Only from bottled water," or "From both the tap and bottle." For the purposes of this study, filtered water was grouped with bottled water. Of the 995 pregnant women, 275 planned to drink only from the tap, 320 were planning on drinking only bottled water, and 400 planned to drink from both sources. At the initial visit, the investigators also collected information on the number of previous births (parity), prepregnancy smoking status and weight, income, and education. After the initial visit, hemoglobin measurements were taken from these women throughout their pregnancy: week 12 (hgb12), 24 (hgb24), and 36 (hgb36). In addition to hemoglobin measures, measures of weight gain (lb) were also obtained. Only women who had resided in the region for the last 10 years, had singleton births after week 36 (full-term), and were compliant with their water consumption plans were included in the analysis, resulting in a final sample of 270 who drank only from the tap, 315 who drank only bottled water, and 394 who drank from both sources. The outcome of interest is the hemoglobin change from week 9 to week 36, or hgb9 − hgb36.

Women in the tap-water-only or the both-sources group were also asked to keep records of the amount of tap water consumed throughout the pregnancy. For each woman ($n = 664$), the amount of tap water consumed (L) over the course of the pregnancy was recorded; consumption ranged from 88.6 to 603.6 L.

DESCRIBING THE DATA

In Chapter 2, graphical and numerical summaries that described the center and spread of continuous data were defined, and summaries that displayed comparisons between groups were discussed. When the research question involves more than one continuous variable, descriptions of the relationship of the continuous variables often involve summaries that attempt to explain how changes in one variable impact changes in another. The most common numerical summary for this relationship is correlation, and scatterplots are a very useful for graphical descriptions of it.

Multiple continuous variables in this study are collected: age, weight gain, tap water consumption, week 9 hemoglobin, week 36 hemoglobin, and the hemoglobin change from week 9 to week 36.

Graphical Summaries: Scatterplots

Instead of comparing the hemoglobin change between the groups of pregnant women exposed to herbicides through tap water, it may be of interest to investigate the association of the hemoglobin change values (g/dL) with the actual tap water consumption values (L).

An **association** between two variables is a measure of how much one variable changes when the other variable changes.

- If one variable increases as the other variable increases, the association is *positive*.
- If one variable decreases as the other variable increases, the association is *negative*.

In other words, when the variables move in the same direction, the association is positive, but when they move in different directions, the association is negative.

When investigating the association between two variables, a scatterplot is often used to describe the relationship (Figure 3-1). In a *scatterplot*, each observation is represented by a single point; the point represents a subject's values for each of the variables. If there are two variables, a point represents the measurement of the subject on variable 1 and variable 2. These pairs of measurements are plotted using a horizontal (variable 1) axis and vertical (variable 2) axis to create a single point. The plot of all the pairs (variable 1, variable 2) of measurements for each observation results in a scatterplot.

In Figure 3-1, the tap water consumption variable is on the horizontal axis, and the hemoglobin change variable is on the vertical axis. The picture in this scatterplot reveals that, as the amount of tap water consumed increases, so does the degree of hemoglobin change. Hence, the association between tap water consumption and hemoglobin change is positive. When determining associations, it does not matter which variable

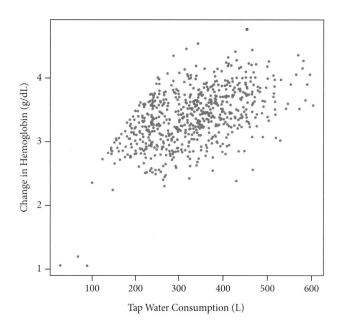

Figure 3-1 Example of a scatterplot.
© *Cengage Learning, 2012.*

Figure 3-2 Example of a scatterplot (axis order reversed).
© Cengage Learning, 2012.

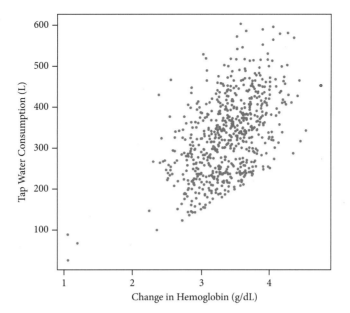

appears on the horizontal or vertical axis. A scatterplot where tap water consumption is on the vertical axis and hemoglobin change is on the horizontal axis still exhibits the same positive association (Figure 3-2).

Numerical Summaries: Correlation

In the scatterplots of Figures 3-1 and 3-2, tap water consumption and hemoglobin change exhibit a positive association. Either scatterplot also shows that the points can be described by a line extending from the smallest hemoglobin change and the smallest tap water consumption to the largest hemoglobin change and the largest tap water consumption. When two variables can be described by a line, their relationship is referred to as being *linear*. To describe the strength of a linear relationship, a numerical summary called *correlation* is used.

The strength of the linear relationship between two variables is measured by the correlation. A correlation ranges from -1 to 1.

- The strongest *positive* relationship results in a correlation of 1.
- The strongest *negative* relationship results in a correlation of -1.
- Two variables that have *no linear association* at all have a correlation of 0.

In a sample, the correlation (statistic) is represented as r. In a population, the correlation (parameter) is represented as ρ.

Application of Formula: CORRELATION COEFFICIENT

$$r = \frac{\text{Estimate of the covariance of } x \text{ and } y}{s_x s_y}$$

x = The explanatory variable

y = The response variable

s_x = The sample standard deviation for the x variable

s_y = The sample standard deviation for the y variable

The *covariance* is a measure of the relationship between the two variables. If the covariance is 0, then the two variables are independent (the value of one has nothing to do with the value of the other). The variance formula can be modified to get the formula for the covariance. If the formula for the variance is $\frac{\sum_{i=1}^{n}(x_i - \bar{x})^2}{n-1} = \frac{\sum_{i=1}^{n}(x_i - \bar{x})(x_i - \bar{x})}{n-1}$, then the formula for the covariance is $\frac{\sum_{i=1}^{n}(x_i - \bar{x})(y_i - \bar{y})}{n-1}$, one of the x's is replaced by the y.

continues

continued

What you need to calculate the correlation:

1. *An estimate of the covariance:*
   a. The difference between the observation and the sample mean for the *x* variable multiplied by the difference between the observation and the sample mean for the *y* variable. This product is obtained for every (*x*, *y*) combination. The products are summed. In this example,

$$\sum_{i=1}^{n}(x_i - \bar{x})(y_i - \bar{y}) = 13200.33.$$

   b. The sample size minus 1: $n - 1 = 664 - 1 = 663$.
   c. The estimate of the covariance is (1a) divided by (1b): $13200.33 \div 663 = 19.91$.
2. *The sample standard deviations for the two variables:*
   a. The sample standard deviation for the *x* variable, tap water consumption, is 94.24 L.
   b. The sample standard deviation for the *y* variable, hemoglobin change, is 0.43 g/dL.

To calculate the estimate of the correlation: Divide (1c) by [(2a) × (2b)]: $19.91 \div (94.24 \times 0.43) = 0.50$.

The correlation estimate in this example is $r = 0.50$. This estimate is positive, indicating that the association between tap water consumption and hemoglobin change is positive. Furthermore, the estimate is relatively large, meaning that the linear relationship between tap water consumption and hemoglobin change is strong. The strength of the linear relationship between tap water consumption and hemoglobin change is visible in the scatterplot because the points so closely resemble a line. The strength and direction of the relationship between two variables corresponds to the value of the correlation and can be seen with scatterplots (Figure 3-3).

Figure 3-3 Examples of correlation.
© *Cengage Learning, 2012.*

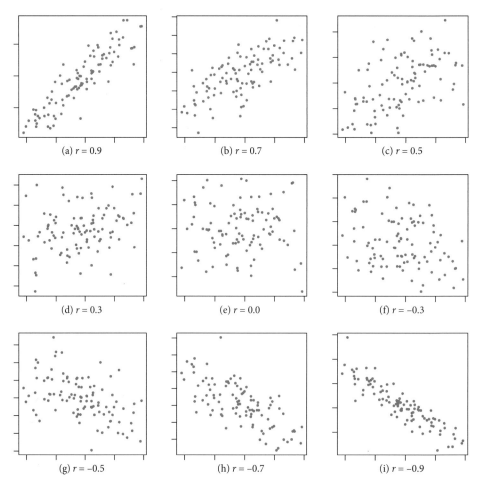

(a) $r = 0.9$ (b) $r = 0.7$ (c) $r = 0.5$
(d) $r = 0.3$ (e) $r = 0.0$ (f) $r = -0.3$
(g) $r = -0.5$ (h) $r = -0.7$ (i) $r = -0.9$

- As the sample correlation r moves toward 1, the strength of the positive linear relationship between the variables increases.
- As the sample correlation r moves toward -1, the strength of the negative linear relationship between the variables increases.
- As the sample correlation r gets closer to 0, the linear relationship (positive or negative) lessens.

This study has multiple continuous variables. In such a case, a table that describes the correlation between the variables is helpful (Table 3-1). All two-variable correlation tables have a similar format. Along the diagonal entries of the table, the correlation estimates are all 1.00 because the correlation of any variable with itself is 1. On either side of the diagonal, the entries are the same; that is, the shaded area in Table 3-1 is a duplicate of the unshaded area. Like the depiction of associations in scatterplots, where the assignment of the vertical and horizontal axes do not matter, it does not matter which variable is considered "first" in the correlation.

The correlation coefficients presented in Table 3-1 are generally referred to as Pearson correlation coefficients. When using this method for estimating the linear relationship between two variables, it is assumed that the two variables are continuous and that each variable is approximately normally distributed. Correlations between variables may be of interest even when the variables are not normally distributed. In fact, a research question could even involve the correlation of two variables when one or both are ordinal. However, when one of the variables is not continuous or does not come from an approximately normal distribution, the Pearson correlation coefficient may not be appropriate. A Spearman rank correlation coefficient, on the other hand, is a nonparametric statistic that does not require assumptions about the two variables of interest (other than that the variables have an order). The Spearman correlation coefficient is easily obtainable in statistical software packages and can be interpreted in the same way as the Pearson correlation coefficient.

Using the data obtained from this study, the Pearson and Spearman correlation estimates are in agreement (Table 3-2).

Point to Ponder

If it is possible to consider the correlation of two ordinal variables, why not talk about the correlation of nominal (categorical variables without order) variables?

TABLE 3-1 **A TABLE OF CORRELATIONS***

	Baseline Hemoglobin (g/dL)	Final Hemoglobin (g/dL)	Hemoglobin Change (g/dL)	Tap Water Consumption (L)
Baseline Hemoglobin (g/dL)	1.00	0.88	−0.04	−0.20
Final Hemoglobin (g/dL)	0.88	1.00	−0.51	−0.40
Hemoglobin Change (g/dL)	−0.04	−0.51	1.00	0.50
Tap Water Consumption (L)	−0.20	−0.40	0.50	1.00

*The correlation estimates presented here are called Pearson correlation coefficients.

© Cengage Learning, 2012.

TABLE 3-2 **TABLE OF SPEARMAN RANK CORRELATIONS**

	Baseline Hemoglobin (g/dL)	Final Hemoglobin (g/dL)	Hemoglobin Change (g/dL)	Tap Water Consumption (L)
Baseline Hemoglobin (g/dL)	1.00	0.86	−0.06	−0.20
Final Hemoglobin (g/dL)	0.86	1.00	−0.52	−0.41
Hemoglobin Change (g/dL)	−0.06	−0.52	1.00	0.49
Tap Water Consumption (L)	−0.20	−0.41	0.49	1.00

© Cengage Learning, 2012.

RESEARCH QUESTION:
Is exposure to herbicides (measured by tap water consumption) in drinking water associated with hemoglobin changes?

Scatterplots and/or correlation coefficients can be very helpful in describing the relationships between two continuous variables. In this example, the scatterplots and correlation estimates suggest that tap water consumption and hemoglobin change have a fairly strong positive linear relationship. However, these summaries describe only the sample. To determine whether there is evidence of an association between tap water consumption and hemoglobin change, hypothesis tests and confidence intervals can be used.

In this study, women who drank water from the tap might have been exposed to herbicides because herbicides have been found in the groundwater of the region. If those who drank tap water were exposed to herbicides, then presumably greater consumption of tap water would result in greater exposure. The expectation is that increasing herbicide exposures results in increasing hemoglobin change—a linear relationship. Hypothesis tests assume no linear relationship between the two variables or that the correlation between the two variables is 0. Therefore, the goal is to determine whether the data support a nonzero correlation between tap water consumption and hemoglobin change.

The observed correlation in this study ($r = 0.50$) is different from 0, but using this value to answer the research question is not appropriate; this sample correlation coefficient may be specific to this particular sample. Because of sampling variability, statistics can vary from sample to sample.

- Did it just happen that this sample of women drinking tap water resulted in a correlation different from 0?
- Would another sample of women exposed to herbicides have a similar correlation between tap water consumption and hemoglobin change?
- Is the discrepancy between the $r = 0.50$ and 0 large enough to conclude that the hemoglobin changes and tap water consumption are linearly related?

Hypothesis testing takes into account the variability that occurs between different samples of the same size and helps in determining whether the statistic merely happened by chance or happened because the true correlation is not 0.

RESEARCH HYPOTHESIS: The true correlation between hemoglobin change and tap water consumption is different from 0: $\rho \neq 0$.

NULL HYPOTHESIS: The true correlation between hemoglobin change and tap water consumption is equal to 0: $\rho = 0$.

In a hypothesis test, the null hypothesis is assumed to be true. In this example, the assumption is that there is no linear relationship between tap water consumption and hemoglobin change or that the parameter is 0 ($\rho_0 = 0$). Using the data in the sample, the hypothesis test helps the investigator to determine whether an assumption of no correlation is reasonable. Samples should result in statistics that are similar to the true parameter, so the most common values in a sampling distribution are the ones closest to the true parameter. If the null parameter ($\rho_0 = 0$) is truly the parameter (ρ), the samples should result in a sample correlation close to 0. If, however, the null parameter ($\rho_0 = 0$) is not the true parameter, the data should produce a statistic that would be not expected or would be rarely observed with a parameter equal to 0. A rare test statistic is evidence that the guess of the true parameter ($\rho_0 = 0$) is wrong.

Test statistic for correlation $(t) = \dfrac{r\sqrt{n-2}}{\sqrt{1-r^2}}$

r = The estimate of the correlation

n = The sample size

What you need to calculate the test statistic:

1. *The square root of (n − 2):* There are 664 pregnant women with tap water consumption and hemoglobin change values, so $\sqrt{n-2} = \sqrt{664-2} = \sqrt{662} = 25.73$.

2. *An estimate of the correlation:* The estimated correlation between tap water consumption and hemoglobin change is $r = 0.50$.

3. *The numerator:* Multiply (2) by (1), so $0.50 \times 25.73 = 12.86$.

4. *The denominator:* This is the square root of 1 − the correlation (2) squared, or $\sqrt{1 - 0.5^2} = \sqrt{0.75} = 0.87$.

To calculate the test statistic: This is the numerator (3) divided by the denominator (4), or $12.86 \div 0.87 = 14.78$. The sampling distribution associated with this test statistic is a *t*-distribution with degrees of freedom $n - 2$. In this example, the test statistic is 14.78, quite large. Using a *t*-distribution with $n - 2 = 662$ degrees of freedom, this test statistic would be considered rare and provides sufficient evidence to reject the null hypothesis. The *p*-value that results from this test is <0.0001.

Because the *p*-value is so small ($p < 0.0001$), this test statistic is considered rare and would not be expected if the null hypothesis were true. This is sufficient evidence to reject the null hypothesis. Therefore, there is a significant linear relationship between tap water consumption and hemoglobin change.

This study has multiple continuous variables. In such a case, a correlation table is helpful for displaying the correlation estimates as well as *p*-values associated with hypotheses of nonzero correlations. Asterisks (*) are typically used to indicate whether the correlations are significantly different from 0 (Table 3-3).

TABLE 3-3 CORRELATIONS WITH STATISTICAL SIGNIFICANCE

	Baseline Hemoglobin (g/dL)	Final Hemoglobin (g/dL)	Hemoglobin Change (g/dL)	Tap Water Consumption (L)
Baseline Hemoglobin (g/dL)	1.00	0.88*	−0.04	−0.20*
Final Hemoglobin (g/dL)	0.88*	1.00	−0.51*	−0.40*
Hemoglobin Change (g/dL)	−0.04	−0.51*	1.00	0.50*
Tap Water Consumption (L)	−0.20*	−0.40*	0.50*	1.00

Note: Correlations are Pearson correlation coefficients.

* indicates p-value <0.05.

© Cengage Learning, 2012.

CONCLUSION: The sample correlations indicate that all hemoglobin outcomes have a linear relationship with tap water consumption. Hemoglobin changes and tap water consumption demonstrate a fairly strong positive relationship ($r = 0.50$, *p*-value < 0.05). This strong, positive correlation indicates that, as tap water consumption increases, so does the hemoglobin change. The small *p*-value ($p < 0.05$) indicates that the null hypothesis can be rejected. However, tap water consumption has a negative relationship with both baseline hemoglobin ($r = -0.20$, $p < 0.05$) and final hemoglobin ($r = -0.40$, $p < 0.05$). These indicate that the higher the tap water consumption, the lower the baseline and final hemoglobin will be.

While hypothesis tests indicate that nonzero correlations exist, they do not suggest possible values for the true correlations. This can be accomplished by providing the interval estimates or confidence intervals for a correlation coefficient. However, the simple t-distribution used for inferences in hypothesis testing is no longer appropriate because the sampling distribution needed for the confidence interval is not necessarily centered at 0 (the sampling distribution used with confidence intervals is centered at the true parameter not the null parameter). Therefore, a transformation must be made to get the confidence interval for the correlation coefficient. Most statistical software packages provide this (Table 3-4). In this example, the 95% interval estimate of the correlation coefficient is (0.44, 0.55), providing a range of plausible values for the true correlation. These values are positive and greater than 0, suggesting a fairly strong, positive, linear relationship between water consumption and hemoglobin change.

TABLE 3-4 **CORRELATION ESTIMATES**

Pearson Correlation Statistics (Fisher's z-Transformation)				
Variable	With Variable	95% Confidence Limits		p-Value for H_0: Rho = 0
hgb9	hgb36	0.859317	0.894339	<0.0001
hgb9	change	−0.117245	0.034667	0.2850
hgb9	water	−0.267171	−0.120755	<0.0001
hgb36	change	−0.568046	−0.455934	<0.0001
hgb36	water	−0.466363	−0.338984	<0.0001
change	water	0.435816	0.550795	<0.0001

© Cengage Learning, 2012.

SIMPLE LINEAR REGRESSION: ONE RESPONSE AND ONE EXPLANATORY VARIABLE

Although determining whether two variables are correlated and estimating the direction of the association is helpful, generally an investigator is trying to explain how one variable impacts another. In public health, research questions often arise when the goal is to try to understand why one person is different from another person. For this study, the goal is to try to understand why one pregnant woman has a different hemoglobin change than another pregnant woman, that is, to understand why outcomes vary. In other words, the tap water consumption is being used to try to explain the variations in hemoglobin changes. Therefore, the tap water consumption variable is referred to as the **explanatory variable** or the independent variable, and hemoglobin change is the **response** (or dependent) **variable**. The goal is to understand the relationship between the response and explanatory variables.

Although these concepts are essentially the same as those discussed with associations and correlations, the distinction now is that one variable is supposed to be making changes in another. Therefore, correlations and scatterplots are still used to describe the relationship, but the scatterplots now have a specific orientation. Usually, the explanatory variable is plotted on the horizontal axis, and the response variable is placed on the vertical axis.

Defining the Linear Relationship

When discussing correlations, the relationship between two variables was described as linear, meaning that a line could be used to represent how the two variables were associated. When two variables appear to demonstrate a linear relationship, a line can be used

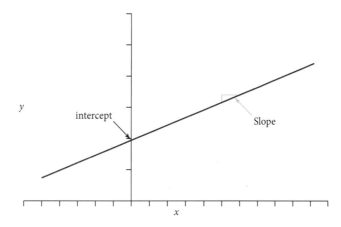

Figure 3-4 Example of a line.
© *Cengage Learning, 2012.*

to model how the response variable relates to the explanatory variable (Figure 3-4). The formula of the line summarizing the relationship between the response and the explanatory variable is:

$$\text{Response variable} = \text{Intercept} + (\text{Slope} \times \text{Explanatory variable})$$

In a scatterplot, the response variable is plotted on the vertical axis, and the explanatory variable is plotted on the horizontal axis. The line intersects the vertical axis at intercept. Therefore, when the explanatory variable is 0 (or has nothing to do with the response), the response is just the value of the intercept.

The slope of the line represents what happens to the response when the explanatory variable increases by 1 unit. When the explanatory variable increases 1 unit, the response changes the amount of the slope.

- If two variables have a positive association, the slope is positive.
- If two variables have a negative association, the slope is negative.
- If two variables are not associated, then the slope is 0 (and the line is horizontal).

Usually, the slope of the line is of the greatest interest because it describes the relationship between the response and explanatory variables. In fact, the *slope* is defined as the change in the response for every 1 unit of change in the explanatory variable. Notice that the interpretation of the slope involves how a 1-unit change in the explanatory variable causes a change in the outcome, not vice versa. The explanatory variable motivates the change in the response variable because changes in the explanatory variable explain differences in the response variable.

Point to Ponder

Notice that the interpretation of the slope, correlation, and association are similar. Would it be possible to have a negative correlation and a positive slope? Are correlation and slope the same thing?

The Model

The line summarizes the relationship of the response and explanatory variables. However, even if the response and explanatory variables have a very strong relationship, the data would not be expected to be arranged perfectly on a line (have a correlation of 1.0). In other words, the line might help to explain part of the relationship between the response and the explanatory variables, but the response variable is unlikely to be simply a function of the explanatory variable. At the very least, there would be some random variation about the line (Figure 3-5). Because of this random variation, the observed response and the response predicted from the formula of the line are different. The distance between the observed and predicted responses is referred to as *error*. Error arises from the fact that the explanatory variable cannot explain all of the variation in the response (unless the correlation between the two variables is 1.0). The leftover variation in the response variable—the part that the explanatory variable cannot explain—is error.

For each observation, the distance between the line and the actual points represents an error. Collectively, these errors are considered to be random; so it is not possible to explain this part of the variation in the response. However, even though the errors

Figure 3-5 Example of the line and random variation.
© Cengage Learning, 2012.

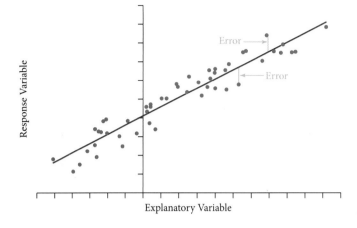

Figure 3-6 Distribution of the errors.
© Cengage Learning, 2012.

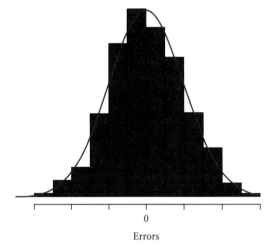

represent unexplained variation, they have certain characteristics. A histogram of all the errors would be symmetric, bell-shaped, and centered at 0 (Figure 3-6). In fact, it is assumed that the errors are independent from each other and that they come from a normal distribution with a mean of 0 and a variance of σ^2.

Hence, the relationship of the explanatory and response variables can be described as the formula of a line plus random error. This forms a statistical model. Statistical models can be used to

- Help us understand relationships in the data and how the data could have been produced.
- Relate a response to an explanatory variable.
- Define how changes in the response variable can be explained by the explanatory variable.
- Provide a mechanism for understanding the random variation that may occur in the relationship between the response and explanatory variables.

To provide a statistical model for the data, the linear relationship of the response and explanatory variable (the line) plus the random variation (the errors) have to be considered. Hence, the line plus the random variation (errors) are used to model how the response variable is produced and how the explanatory and response variables relate to each other.

The statistical model for the linear relationship between the response variable (y) and the explanatory variable (x) can be written as $y = \alpha + \beta x + \varepsilon$, where α represents the intercept, β represents the slop, and ε represent the errors. The model represents what would be true about the relationship of the x (explanatory) and y (response) variables in the population. In this example, the statistical model is *hemoglobin change* $= \alpha + \beta$(tap water consumption) $+ \varepsilon$.

Because the model describes the population, the slope and intercept are parameters and are presented with Greek symbols (α and β). The errors (ε) are also represented with a Greek symbol. Because it is not expected that the data would arise exactly from the line, the errors represent the random variation that might occur in the real data. The random variations are assumed to come from a normal distribution with a mean of 0 and a constant variance (σ^2). Therefore, the assumptions for the statistical model are the assumptions regarding the errors.

Using the data, the true intercept and the true slope in the model ($y = \alpha + \beta x + \varepsilon$) can be estimated. The actual line that summarizes or predicts the data is written as $\hat{y} = a + bx$. This equation for the line has no Greek symbols because it was found using sample data. The intercept (a) and the slope (b) are statistics, not parameters. Also, the y has a hat (^) on it because it is not the response observed in the data, but the response that would result or be predicted by the line. The distances between the observed response (y) and the predicted response ($\hat{y}$) are the observed errors, $e = y - \hat{y}$. Because $\hat{y} = a + bx$, is the equation for the line that best fits the data and not the statistical model, there are no errors (ε) in the equation.

In summary, given a response and an explanatory variable, the linear relationship can be modeled as $y = \alpha + \beta x + \varepsilon$. The assumptions for this model are as follows:

1. The subjects are independent. The hemoglobin change for one pregnant woman has nothing to do with the hemoglobin change for another pregnant woman. If the subjects are independent, then the errors are independent as well. How well one woman's data fit the line has nothing to do with how well another woman's data fit the line.
2. The errors come from a normal distribution that has
    a. A mean of 0
    b. And a constant variance (represented as σ^2)

Using the sample data, estimates for the parameters α and β are obtained by finding the equation of the $\hat{y} = a + bx$ line that best fits the data.

Once it has been established that the relationship between the response (y) and explanatory (x) variables is linear, then any line could be used to "model" the data (Figure 3-7). Clearly, only one line (Line 2) is best for summarizing the relationship of x and y because it does the best job of *fitting* the data.

Line 2 was obtained by minimizing the errors (the difference between the observed points and the predicted line). Actually, the line is obtained by minimizing the sum of the square of the errors. Because some points are above the line, and some are below the line, some errors are positive and some errors are negative, respectively. If these errors are averaged, the positive and negative errors may cancel each other out, and the resulting average would be mistakenly close to 0. To prevent underestimating the errors, these errors (distances between the y and the $\hat{y}$) are squared; the squared differences are all positive. An intercept and a slope are found so that the resulting line has the smallest (least) squared distance between the observed

Figure 3-7 Estimating the regression line.
© *Cengage Learning, 2012.*

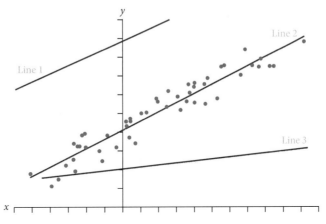

datapoints (y) and the line ($\hat{y}$). Because the line is found using the least squared distance, the method for finding the line that best fits the data is referred to as *ordinary least squares (OLS) regression*.

$$b = \frac{\text{Estimate of the covariance of } x \text{ and } y}{\text{Variance of } x}$$

$$a = \bar{y} - b\bar{x}$$

What you need to calculate the estimates of the line:

1. *An estimate of the covariance of* x *(tap water consumption) and* y *(hgb change):* 19.91.
2. *The sample variance for* x *(tap water consumption):* 8881.74.
3. *The estimate of the slope:* This is (1) divided by (2) = 19.91 ÷ 8881.74 = 0.002.
4. *The sample mean of the response:* $\bar{y}$ = 3.39 g/dL.
5. *The sample mean of the explanatory variable:* $\bar{x}$ = 331.03 L.

To calculate the estimate of the intercept: (4) − [(3) × (5)] = 3.39 − (0.002 × 331.03) = 3.39 − 0.66 = 2.73.
To calculate the estimate of the slope: Divide (1) by (2), or b = 19.91 ÷ 8881.74 = 0.002.
Statistical software packages provide the estimates of the intercept and slope (along with standard errors) as standard output in the linear regression procedure.

Although least squares regression is the method used to obtain the intercept and the slope for a set of data, a and b are just point estimates, or statistics describing this sample. Does a nonzero estimate of the slope indicate that the true slope is not zero (that x and y are linearly related), or is the estimate specific to the sample? Is there evidence to claim that the true parameter, the true slope, is not 0? To determine whether there is a linear relationship between the response (y) and the explanatory variable (x), statistical inference is used to make conclusions about the true parameter (β). Hypothesis tests indicate whether the slope found in this sample is expected when the null is true, and confidence intervals provide a set of plausible values for the true slope.

The ANOVA Table

When comparing multiple groups in Chapter 2, the overall *F*-test was calculated from the ANOVA table, which partitioned the variability in the response into the variability between the groups and the variability within the groups. The within group variability represented the leftover variability in the outcome that could not be explained by group membership. Therefore, the within group variability was referred to as error. The use of the ANOVA table is not limited to just comparisons of groups, however. It can be very helpful in determining how well an explanatory variable accounts for the variability in the response variable. Specifically, the ANOVA can be used to help explain why one pregnant woman has different hemoglobin changes than another pregnant woman. In a linear regression, the ANOVA table describes how the variability observed in the responses (y) is divided into the variability attributable to the explanatory variable (x) and the variability that is unexplained (error).

In an ANOVA analysis, the goal is to divide the variability of the outcome into the variability that can be explained by the explanatory variable and the variability that cannot be explained (error). The partitioning of the variability with linear regression is very similar to the partitioning of the variability when comparing multiple groups (Chapter 2); the term "between" is replaced by "model" (Table 3-5).

The total sums of squares used in the calculation of the sample variance of the response can be split up into the sum of squares for the variability due to the explanatory variable (the model) and the sum of squares for the variability that is left over (the error). Therefore, the total sums of squares (the numerator of the sample variance) of the response

TABLE 3-5 **ANOVA TABLE FOR A LINEAR REGRESSION**

Source	Degrees of Freedom (DF)	Sum of Squares	Mean Square	F
Model	Number of explanatory variables	SSM	$MSM = \dfrac{SSM}{Model\ DF}$	$\dfrac{MSM}{MSE}$
Within (error)	(Total DF − Model DF)	SSE	$MSE = \dfrac{SSE}{Within\ DF}$	
Total	Number of observations − 1	SST		

© Cengage Learning, 2012.

can be split into the model sum of squares and the error sum of squares (Table 3-5). The total sum of squares of the sample is equal to the model sum of squares plus the error sum of squares. The sample variance for the outcome is calculated by dividing the total sum of squares by $n - 1$, or the degrees of freedom. Because the model sum of squares and the error sum of squares must add up to the total sum of squares, the degrees of freedom for the model and error sums of squares must also add up to the total degrees of freedom. The degrees of freedom for the model sum of squares are the number of explanatory variables in the model. For a simple linear regression, there is just one explanatory variable. Consequently, the degrees of freedom for the error sum of squares is what is left over: $(n - 1) -$ (number of explanatory variables), or $n - 2$.

The sample variance for the response is estimated by dividing the total sum of squares by the degrees of freedom $(n - 1)$. Likewise, the model variability is estimated by dividing the model sum of squares by its degrees of freedom (number of explanatory variables), and the within (error) variability is estimated by dividing the within sum of squares by its degrees of freedom: $n -$ the number of explanatory variables $- 1 = n - 2$.

The model sum of squares divided by the number of explanatory variables, or degrees of freedom, is called the *mean squared model*, because dividing by the number of groups creates a calculation that represents the average variability due to the model. Because there is only one explanatory variable, the degree of freedom is just 1. Therefore, in this case, the mean squared model is the same as the model sum of squares. Similarly, the error sum of squares divided by its degrees of freedom is called the *mean squared error*. Because the error represents what is left over, or the residual variability, after accounting for the model, the error is referred to as residuals. Sometimes the error sum of squares and the mean squared error will be noted as residual sum of squares and mean squared residuals. The mean square error (residual) provides an estimate of the overall variability due to error and is used to estimate the common variance of the errors, assumed in the linear regression model.

Variability in the response variable (hemoglobin change) occurs because one pregnant woman has different hemoglobin change than another pregnant woman. If this variability can be explained by the explanatory variable (tap water consumption), then an association between the two variables is established. If a linear relationship exists between two variables, then a line can be used to explain why two subjects are different. Two response values vary or are at different places on the vertical (y) axis because, in part, the two points have different corresponding explanatory values on the horizontal (x) axis (Figure 3-8).

For example, it has been shown that tap water consumption and hemoglobin change exhibit a positive linear relationship. Therefore, if one pregnant woman has a higher consumption of tap water than another, then the woman with the higher tap water consumption may be expected to have a larger hemoglobin change. The tap water consumption (explanatory variable) does not completely explain why two pregnant women have different hemoglobin changes, and some remaining variability in the response variable (hemoglobin change) not explained by tap water consumption exists. A linear model that explains much of the variability in the response implies that the explanatory variable has a strong linear relationship with the response variable. If a lot of the

Point to Ponder

How does splitting up sources of variability (ANOVA) help to answer the question, "Is there a linear relationship between the response and explanatory variable?" If more of the variability in the response can be attributed to the model than to the error, then the explanatory variables are helping to explain why subjects have different response values.

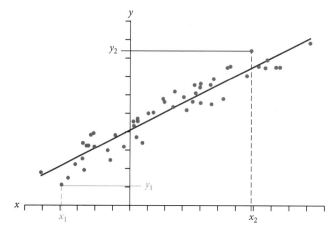

Figure 3-8 Example of explained and unexplained variability.
© *Cengage Learning, 2012.*

variability in the response is unexplained or attributed to error), then the model does not do an adequate job of explaining the different response values, and the explanatory variable has a weaker linear relationship with the response.

The ANOVA table can provide information on how well the model explains changes in the response. Ideally, the model (explanatory variable) explains much of the variation in the response, and very little is left over for the errors. In other words, a good model is able to explain a large proportion of the variability in the response. The proportion of variability explained by the model (the explanatory variable) out of the total variability is defined as R^2.

The R^2 value is obtained by dividing the model sum of squares by the total sum of squares. It represents the proportion of the total variability explained by the model. The maximum R^2 is 1, or 100%. An $R^2 = 0.9$ indicates that the model can explain 90% of the variability in the response variable (total variability). An $R^2 = 0.01$, on the other hand, indicates that the model does a poor job because only 1% of the total variability can be explained by the model. The relationship between total sum of squares, model sum of squares, error sum of squares, and R^2 can be described visually (Figure 3-9). The rectangle represents the total sum of squares, the circle represents the model sum of squares, the remaining part of the rectangle not covered by the circle represents the error sum of squares. Visually, as the circle (amount of variability explained by the model) in Figure 3-9 increases, a greater amount of the rectangle (total sum of squares) is covered. As the area covered by the circle (the model sum of squares) increases, R^2 increases, and the space remaining for the error sum of squares decreases. In simple linear regression, the R^2 is simply the correlation squared. Hence, if the response and explanatory variables are highly correlated, R^2 will be close to 1.

Total Sum of Squares

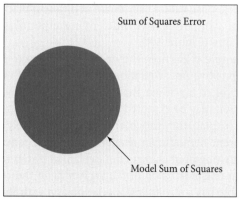

Figure 3-9 Visualization of R^2.
© *Cengage Learning, 2012.*

Overall Hypothesis Test

If the model does a good job of explaining the variability in the response, the variability attributable to the model is larger than the variability of the errors, suggesting the explanatory variable has a linear relationship with the response (Table 3-6). To determine whether the variability explained by the model is large enough to claim that the there is a linear relationship, the ratio of the mean squared model and the mean squared error is calculated. If the mean squared error is small compared to the model, then the ratio will be large. If the mean squared error is large compared to the model, then the ratio is small. The ratio can be used to determine whether the variability explained by the model is large enough to claim that the explanatory variable is linearly related to the response.

RESEARCH HYPOTHESIS: The model explains enough variability in the response.

NULL HYPOTHESIS: The model does not explain enough variability in the response.

Application of Formula: OVERALL *F*-TEST

$$\text{Test statistic } (F) = \frac{\text{Mean square model}}{\text{Mean square error}}$$

What you need to calculate the test statistic:

1. *The mean square model:* MSM = 29.58.
2. *The mean square error:* MSE = 0.14.
3. *The degrees of freedom:*
    a. MSM, DF = the number of explanatory variables = 1
    b. MSE, DF = the number of observations − 1 − (3a) = 664 − 1 − 1 = 662

To calculate the test statistic (F): The ratio is the MSM (1) divided by the MSE (2): $29.58 \div 0.14 = 215.72$. Using an *F*-distribution with numerator degrees of freedom of 1 and denominator degrees of freedom of 662, the percentage of ratios that are even farther from the ratio observed in this sample is less than 0.01% (p-value < 0.0001).

TABLE 3-6 **ANOVA TABLE FOR LINEAR REGRESSION WITH VALUES**

Source	Degrees of Freedom	Sum of Squares	Mean Square	F	p-value
Model	1	29.58	29.58	215.72	<0.0001
Error	662	90.78	0.14		
Total	663	120.36			

© Cengage Learning, 2012.

CONCLUSION: This *p*-value is small; there is evidence that the ratio is large or that a significant amount of the total variability is explained by the model (tap water consumption) significant.

- The model's ability to explain enough of the variability in hemoglobin changes implies a linear relationship between tap water consumption and hemoglobin change, *change* = α + β(tap water consumption) + ε, where ε follows a normal distribution with a mean of 0 and a variance of σ^2. Therefore, the linear relationship between the explanatory (*x*) variable and the response (*y*) variable is quantified by the slope (β).

- If there is no linear relationship, then the slope (β) would be 0 and the model would be Hemoglobin change = $\alpha + 0 + \varepsilon$. When the slope is 0, the scatterplot of the response and explanatory variable is just a horizontal, random scatter of datapoints (Figure 3-10a).
- For a positive linear relationship, the slope (β) is positive, and the model is *Change* = $\alpha + \beta$(tap water consumption) + ε. When the slope is positive, the scatterplot of the response and explanatory variable displays a positive correlation (Figure 3-10b).
- If the linear relationship is negative, then the slope (β) is negative, and the model is *Change* = $\alpha - \beta$(tap water consumption) + ε. When the slope is negative, the scatterplot of the response and explanatory variable displays a negative correlation (Figure 3-10c).

Therefore, the hypothesis of the variability explained by the model translates to a hypothesis about the linear relationship between the response and explanatory variable or a hypothesis about the slope (β).

RESEARCH HYPOTHESIS: Tap water consumption and hemoglobin change are linearly related: $\beta \neq 0$.

NULL HYPOTHESIS: Tap water consumption and hemoglobin change are not linearly related: $\beta = 0$.

The *F*-statistic from the ANOVA (Table 3-6) was 215.72. Using an *F*-distribution with numerator degrees of freedom equal to 1 and denominator degrees of freedom equal to 662, the *p*-value was obtained ($p < 0.001$).

CONCLUSION: Since this *p*-value is small, there is evidence that the ratio is large or that the variability explained by the model is large enough to suggest that tap water consumption and hemoglobin change are linearly related. Because this *p*-value is small, the null hypothesis indicating that the true slope is 0 can be rejected. Hence, there is sufficient evidence to reject the null hypothesis of no linear relationship, tap water consumption and hemoglobin are linearly related.

Figure 3-10 Examples of slopes.
© *Cengage Learning, 2012.*

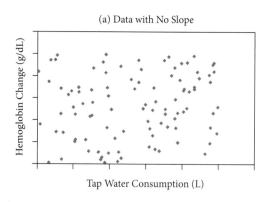

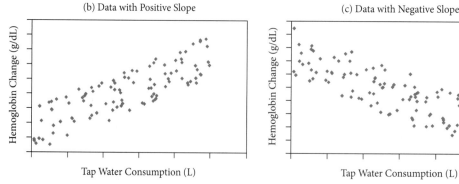

Although the ANOVA table helped to provide an answer to the question of whether a linear relationship existed between the response variable and the explanatory variable, specific questions about the slope and the strength of the linear relationship remain. Because the ANOVA resulted in an F-statistic that was significant (the p-value was small), the specific slope associated with the explanatory variable can be investigated further. However, if an ANOVA results in an F-statistic that is not significant (the p-value is large), there is no evidence of a linear relationship, that is, that the true slope could be 0. When this happens, the data do not support further investigation of the specific properties of the slope.

Estimates for the intercept and slope are obtained using least squares regression. ANOVA and least squares regression are related since least squares regression obtains the line (estimates of the intercept and slope) by minimizing the sum of the squared errors (SSE). While inferences regarding the model (ANOVA) are an important step in the analysis, a linear regression analysis is usually implemented to better understand the relationship of the response and an explanatory variable, and the properties of the specific slope rather than the overall effect of the model are of greater interest. Therefore, reports of the linear regression results typically focus on the estimates and inferences related to the slope. However, in this introductory example there is only one variable in the model, so statistical tests for the variability explained by the model and the specific slope are the same.

Specific Hypothesis Test for Slope

RESEARCH QUESTION:
Is exposure to herbicides (measured by tap water consumption) in drinking water associated with hemoglobin changes?

Once the ANOVA has been performed, two pieces of information are obtained: (1) whether there is evidence of a linear relationship and further investigation of the slope is warranted and (2) an estimate of the common variance (mean squared error). The goal of this study is to better understand the relationship between herbicides exposure and hemoglobin changes in pregnant women. While the overall question of whether there is a linear relationship is important, investigators are specifically interested in how tap water consumption is related to hemoglobin changes.

After establishing that there is a linear relationship between hemoglobin change and tap water consumption, the specific slope associated with tap water consumption can be investigated. A positive slope suggests that increases in tap water consumption are related to increases in hemoglobin change, whereas a negative slope would suggest that increases in tap water consumption are related to smaller hemoglobin changes. A slope of zero would suggest no linear relationship.

RESEARCH HYPOTHESIS: The true slope (β) is not 0. There is a linear relationship between the response and the explanatory variable.

NULL HYPOTHESIS: The true slope (β) is 0. There is no linear relationship between the response and the explanatory variable.

Using the data from pregnant women who consume tap water ($n = 664$), the least squares regression results in estimates for the intercept and the slope (Table 3-7).

TABLE 3-7 **LEAST SQUARES REGRESSION RESULTS**

	Estimate	Standard Error	Test Statistic	*p*-value
Intercept	2.647316	0.0525200	50.41	<0.001
Tap Water Consumption	0.002241	0.0001526	14.69	<0.001

© Cengage Learning, 2012.

Application of Formula

Test statistic for the slope $(t) = \dfrac{b}{\text{Standard error}}$

b = The estimate of the slope

Standard error = The standard error is a function of the mean square error.

What you need to test for nonzero slope:

1. *An estimate of the slope:* $b = 0.002241$.
2. *The standard error:* Take the square root of the MSE divided by the total (corrected) sum of squares for x. The standard error associated with the slope is 0.0001526.

To calculate the test statistic (t): Divide the slope estimate (1) by the standard error (2): $0.002241 \div 0.0001526 = 14.7$. The test statistic follows a t-distribution with degrees of freedom equal to the degrees of freedom of the mean squared error (DF = 662). The test statistic (14.7) is quite large. Therefore, the percentage of test statistics that are even farther away from the null parameter than the test statistic (the p-value) will be small. The hypothesis test for the slope in this example results in a p-value < 0.0001.

CONCLUSION: The p-value (<0.0001) is small; so this test statistic is considered rare and would not be expected if $\beta = 0$. This is sufficient evidence to reject the null hypothesis. Because the hypothesis of a zero slope is rejected, there is evidence that tap water consumption and hemoglobin change have a linear relationship.

The estimated slope of 0.0022 is quite small. So it may seem odd that this estimate of the slope provides evidence *against* the null hypothesis that the true slope is 0. Consider more than the point estimate; the standard error and the units for the explanatory variable play an important role as well. Although the estimate of the slope is very close to 0, the standard error is even smaller (0.0001526). Whenever the standard error is small, the test statistic resulting from taking the estimate divided by the standard error is going to be large. Also, the units of the explanatory variable impact the interpretation; the slope describes the change in the response for every 1 unit increase in the explanatory variable. The tap water consumption is measured over the course of 36 weeks in liters (L), and a pregnant women should be drinking about 2 L of water a day. Therefore, part of the reason the estimate of the slope is not very large is that the unit increase in tap water consumption is not very large. Because of the linear relationship between tap water and hemoglobin change, the estimate can be modified for larger increases in tap water consumption. For example, a 10-L increase in the tap water consumption would increase the observed hemoglobin change by 0.022 g/dL, and a 100-L increase in tap water consumption over the pregnancy would increase the observed hemoglobin change by 0.22 g/dL. Hence, just because an estimate seems close to 0, the units and the standard error have to be considered to determine the existence and strength of the linear relationship.

It may seem redundant to consider the specific slope after the overall F-test already answered the question of whether there is evidence of a linear relationship. In fact, the hypotheses for the overall test and for the specific test were exactly the same. Furthermore, the two tests result in the same test statistic; the t-statistic obtained in the specific test is simply the square root of the F-statistic found in the overall test. The reason is that, in the case of simple linear regression, where there is only one explanatory variable, the model is the same as looking at only one explanatory variable, and the overall test for the model and the specific test for the slope are the same. However, when multiple explanatory variables are included in the model, this is no longer the case.

Specific Confidence Interval for Slope

The hypothesis tests indicate a linear relationship between tap water consumption and hemoglobin change, investigators are often more interested in estimating the slope than stating whether a relationship exists. Specifically, the point estimate for the slope ($b = 0.002$) indicates that on average, for every 1L increase in tap water consumption, a change of 0.002 g/dL is observed. The point estimate of 0.002 indicates the slope for this sample, but to use this point estimate in estimating the true population slope, confidence intervals are needed.

Confidence intervals are based on the idea of sampling distributions and the fact that not all samples result in the same statistic. Although, it is unlikely that another sample of 664 pregnant women would have the same relationship between tap water consumption and the hemoglobin change, the statistics (estimates of the slopes) from these different samples should all pile up fairly close to the parameter (the true slope β), resulting in the sampling distribution of the slope. The sampling distribution is a t-distribution with the same degrees of freedom as the mean squared error and can be used to obtain confidence intervals.

Application of Formula

C% confidence interval for the mean: $b \pm t^* \times SE$

b = The slope obtained from the sample data

C = The confidence level for a C% confidence interval

t^* = The number of standard deviations from the center of the sampling distribution

SE = The standard error of the slope

What you need to calculate the confidence interval:

1. *The sample mean or the point estimate of the slope:* $b = 3.5$ g/dL.
2. *The standard error:* The standard error of the slope (found by using the mean squared error) is 0.0001526.
3. *The confidence level:* C% is typically 95%, but 90% and 99% are also common.
4. *The number of standard deviations from the center of the sampling distribution:* This depends on C% (3) and the sampling distribution. Because the mean square error is used to calculate the standard error, the degrees of freedom of the mean square error is used to define the t-distribution. In this case, where the sampling distribution is a t-distribution with 662 degrees of freedom, the t^* for a 90% confidence interval is 1.65, the t^* for a 95% confidence interval is 1.96, and the t^* for a 99% confidence interval is 2.58. Therefore, confidence intervals can be calculated as

90% confidence interval: $b \pm (1.65 \times SE)$

95% confidence interval: $b \pm (1.96 \times SE)$

99% confidence interval: $b \pm (2.58 \times SE)$

To calculate the 95% confidence interval: The number of standard errors from the slope is $1.96 \times (0.0001526) = 0.0003$ and is also known as the margin of error. Adding and subtracting the margin of error from the point estimate results in the 95% confidence interval for the true slope, $[0.0022 - 0.0003, 0.0022 + 0.0003]$, or $[0.0019, 0.0025]$.

Because 95% of the confidence intervals cover the true slope, the interval provides a range of plausible values for the true slope. A slope of 0 is not in this range, and the interval estimate suggests that the true slope is larger than 0. Hence, tap water consumption and the hemoglobin change have a positive linear relationship.

This confidence interval provides an estimate of the slope associated with a 1-L change in tap water consumption. As previously discussed, this is a pretty small increase in tap water consumption. Finding the confidence interval for a different increment of change in the regressor may be of interest. For example, suppose it was of interest to estimate the slope associated with a 10-L increase in tap water consumption. The 95% confidence interval for this increase is simply the 95% confidence interval for a 1-L increase multiplied by 10 [0.019, 0.025].

Prediction Equation

Because the slope was found to be statistically significant (different from 0), the estimate can be used in the equation of line $\hat{y} = a + bx$ or $\widehat{change} = a + b \times$ tap water consumption. Therefore, the equation of the line that best fits the data (Figure 3-11) is $\widehat{change} = 2.647 + 0.0022 \times$ tap water consumption. This line can now be used to "predict" the hemoglobin change if a certain amount of tap water is consumed. For example, if a pregnant woman consumes 250 L of tap water, then the predicted amount of hemoglobin change is 3.2 g/dL. On the other hand, a pregnant woman who drinks only 100 L of tap water has a predicted hemoglobin change of 2.9 g/dL. The range of tap water consumption values in this study is 88–604 L. These values are used in finding the regression line, $\widehat{change} = 2.647 + 0.0022 \times$ tap water consumption. The regression line is appropriate only for predicting values in the range used to create it. For example, using the equation to find the change of hemoglobin for a pregnant woman who consumes 1800 L of tap water in 36 weeks results in a hemoglobin change of 6.6 g/dL. This value is too large a change to be reasonable. However, this result should not be surprising because 1800 L is three times the amount of the most tap water consumed in the study. To avoid unreasonable predictions, possible explanatory values must be limited to ones similar to those used to find the regression line.

Diagnostics

Statistical models are functions that define how the explanatory variable can explain changes in the response variable. Models provide a way for investigators to understand how the data might have been produced. Therefore, a model is helpful only if it is appropriate for the data or if the data fit well. To determine whether a linear regression

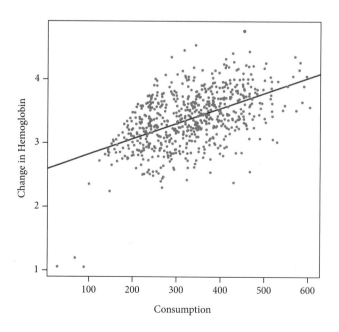

Figure 3-11 Example of the fit of the regression line. © *Cengage Learning, 2012.*

is the most appropriate model, check the assumptions. The assumptions of a linear regression model are predominantly assumptions about the errors. The assumptions for this model are as follows:

1. *The subjects are independent:* The hemoglobin change for one pregnant woman has nothing to do with the hemoglobin change for another pregnant woman. If the subjects are independent, then the errors are independent as well. The distance between one point and the line has nothing to do with the distance between another point and the line.
2. *The errors come from a normal distribution* that has
   a. A mean of 0
   b. A constant variance (represented as σ^2)

Assumptions on these error terms can be checked by considering the residuals.

In a regression model statement, the errors (ε) represent the random variation about the line because it is unlikely that all observations will fall exactly on the line. Once the regression line is found, some of the observed points will be above the line and some below it. The distance between the observed points and the lines are the observed errors from the model, or *residuals.*

For example, in the tap water consumption study, one of the pregnant women had a tap water consumption of 298.85 L. Her hemoglobin change was 2.85 g/dL. The regression line obtained from the tap water consumption sample ($n = 664$) was $\widehat{change} = 2.647 + 0.0022 \times$ tap water consumption. Using this line, a pregnant woman who consumes 298.85 L of tap water in 36 weeks should have a hemoglobin change of 3.30 g/dL. The actual hemoglobin change of 2.85 g/dL is a point that occurred below the regression line because it is below the 3.30 g/dL value. The 2.85 g/dL is the actual observed value of the response variable (y), and the 3.30 g/dL is the response that would be predicted by the line ($\hat{y}$). The difference between these two points is the error, or residual, for this pregnant woman: $y - \hat{y} = change - \widehat{change} = 2.85 - 3.30 = -0.45$.

Thus each pregnant woman in the sample has an actual response and a response predicted by the equation line. The differences between these two values (for each woman) are the residuals. Based on the assumptions of the linear regression model,

- The mean of all of these residuals should be 0.
- The histogram of all these residuals should be symmetric and bell-shaped (normal distribution).
- The residuals should be uncorrelated and have a constant variance (or a variance that does not depend on the explanatory variable).

When the response variable and the explanatory variable have a linear relationship, the variability in the response can be partially explained by the changes in the explanatory variable. The hope of any regression analysis is that the explanatory variable does an excellent job of explaining why one subject's response is different from another's. If it does, then the only reason the observed points do not fall exactly on the regression line ($y = a + bx$) is random variation. Further, there will be no leftover pattern, no further trend in the response; nothing else can help to explain the variability in the response because the only variability left is random. The distances between the observed outcomes (y) and the regression line ($\hat{y} = a + bx$) are called residuals because they represent the "leftover," or residual, information that cannot otherwise be explained.

Therefore, if the linear model ($y = \alpha + \beta x + \varepsilon$) is appropriate, then the plot of the residuals (the difference between the line and the actual response) versus the predicted value from the line ($\hat{y}$) will:

- Have no pattern.
- Be centered around 0 (there should not be more points above the line than below it).

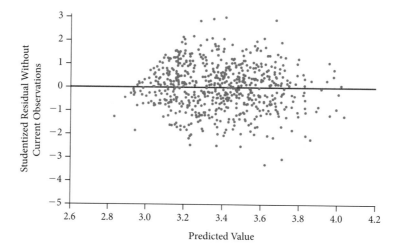

Figure 3-12 Plot of residual versus predicted change. © Cengage Learning, 2012.

- Have constant variance (the residuals should be just as scattered for small values of the explanatory variable as for large values of it).
- Not be correlated (one error has nothing to do with another error).

The plot of the residuals versus the predicted change from the 664 pregnant women in the tap water consumption study appear to be randomly and evenly distributed around a residual (or difference) of 0 (Figure 3-12).

The residuals represent the errors between the actual response (y) and the response predicted from the regression line ($\hat{y}$). The assumptions of the linear regression model are assumptions about the errors (ε). Therefore, to determine whether there are violations, a plot of the residuals versus the predicted response is often used. The predicted response is just $\hat{y} = a + bx$. So the patterns in the plot of the residuals versus the predicted responses ($a + bx$) is essentially the same as the patterns observed in the residuals versus x. If gross violations of the model assumptions are found, then adjustments to the linear model must be made. The adjustment depends on the violation found.

The differences between the observed and predicted response variables are known as raw residuals. There are actually additional types of residuals, which provide different types of information. The residuals presented in Figure 3-12 and the sections that follow are *studentized residuals*, or residuals that have been divided by the estimated standard deviation. This standardizing of the residuals allows for checking the assumptions of the regression model and also helps to identify potential outliers in the data.

Violations to Constant Variance

Constant variance means that the response (hemoglobin change) follows the regression line equally well for different values of the explanatory variable. *Nonconstant variance* occurs when, for example, the hemoglobin change follows the regression line quite well for small values of tap water consumption but does worse for larger values. When this is the case, the result is that the residuals for small values of tap water consumption are all fairly similar and have a small amount of variability, but the larger values of tap water consumption have residuals that are very different and that demonstrate a larger amount of variability. If a scatterplot of the residuals versus explanatory variable (x) exhibits a fan shape, the assumption of constant variance has been violated. A fan shape results when the variability of the residuals is different depending on the value of the explanatory variable (Figure 3-13).

One way to lessen the fan shape in the residuals is to stabilize the variance by transforming the response variable. Some common transformations include the natural log and the square root. In the example, to fix the violation observed in Figure 3-13, one solution is to take the natural log (ln) of the hemoglobin change and use this as the response variable. The new model would be $\ln(y) = \alpha + \beta x + \varepsilon$.

Figure 3-13 Plot of residuals with a violation of constant variance.
© *Cengage Learning, 2012.*

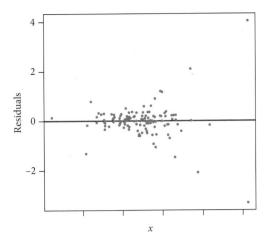

Violations of Normality

The best way to verify whether the assumption of normality has been violated is to investigate plots of the errors. A histogram of the residuals provides an indication of whether the distribution of the residuals is skewed and not normally distributed. A skewed distribution is possible when the data contain **outliers**, which are points that lie outside the pattern of the other datapoints. An outlier can be an extreme point with respect to the explanatory variable, to the response variable, or to both. If an outlier is suspected, run the regression analysis with and without the suspicious datapoint. Although removing datapoints from the analysis is never desirable, seeing what the analysis would be when outliers are removed can be helpful. If the datapoint is truly an anomaly, there may be some justification for preferring the regression analysis without this point.

Consider an example of a scatterplot with an obvious outlier in Figure 3-14:

- This outlier (Figure 3-14a) has a much larger value for the explanatory variable than any of the other datapoints.
- The histogram of the residuals is somewhat normal, but the outlier clearly creates a tail; so the distribution is more skewed to the left than a normal distribution would be (Figure 3-14b).
- The residuals can also be helpful in identifying potential outliers. Because an outlier is a point that does not follow the pattern of the other points, it does not follow the linear pattern. In other words, the outlier is not as close to the line as other points. Therefore, the residual for that point (the distance between the point and the line) is larger in magnitude than that of the other residuals (Figure 3-14c).

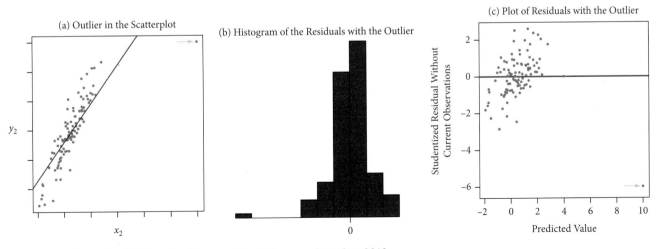

Figure 3-14 Example of a dataset with an outlier. © *Cengage Learning, 2012.*

Figure 3-15 Example of a dataset with influence points.
© *Cengage Learning, 2012.*

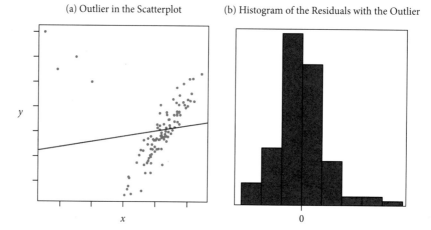

(a) Outlier in the Scatterplot   (b) Histogram of the Residuals with the Outlier

Another type of extreme point that may impact the normality assumption are **influence points**, which are points with extreme explanatory values. They are particularly troublesome because the least squares regression line is created by minimizing the squared errors (the distances between the line and the points). If a point influences the regression line by pulling it away from the other datapoints and closer to itself, the resulting regression line may not be as accurate as it could be in describing the linear relationship between the explanatory and response variables. When the least squares regression is performed with these points removed, the regression line can be considerably different.

An influential point can alter the relationship (and the least squares regression line) between the response and explanatory variables. In Figure 3-15a, the four points in the upper left-hand corner of the scatterplot are pulling the regression line from a positive slope to a more negative slope, which results in a flattening of the line. The regression line without the influence points is $\hat{y} = 2.99 + 1.92x$, and the p-value for the slope is less than 0.0001. The regression equation for the data with the influence points is $\hat{y} = 4.15 + 0.3x$. Furthermore, the p-value for the slope is larger than 0.05, indicating that there is no longer evidence that the slope is not 0 (no linear relationship). Again, the result of these extreme points is to skew the distribution of the residuals so that the histogram no longer resembles a normal distribution (Figure 3-15b).

In addition to extreme points, violations to the normality assumption can occur when the distribution of the response variable is non-normal (Figure 3-16).

Figure 3-16 Response variable is non-normal.
© *Cengage Learning, 2012.*

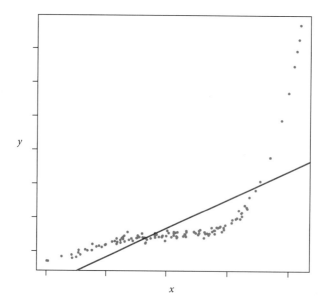

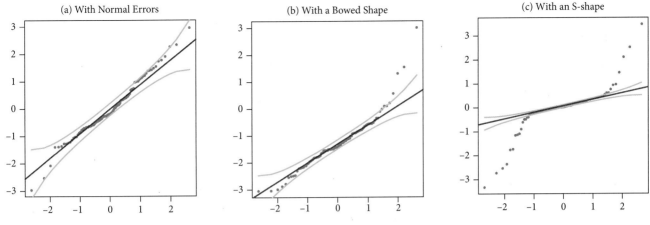

Figure 3-17 Examples of Q-Q plots. © *Cengage Learning, 2012.*

An additional way to identify whether the normality assumption has been violated is to consider normal probability plots. The *normal probability* (or *Q-Q*) *plot* is a plot of the error distribution and the plot of a normal distribution with the same mean and variance as the errors. A normal probability plot is sometimes referred to as a normal Q-Q plot because quantiles from the error and the true normal distribution are plotted on the vertical and horizontal axes, respectively.

- If the error distribution is normal, then the two plots should match up along a diagonal line (Figure 3-17a).
- If, however, there are too many large errors in one direction and the error distribution is skewed, then the plot bows out from the diagonal line, suggesting that the normality of the errors is violated (Figure 3-17b).
- The normal probability plot can also take on an S-shape when the normality assumption is violated (Figure 3-17c). This occurs with either too many or too few errors in either direction.

Violations of Linearity

Simple linear regression is, by definition, the process of using a line to summarize the relationship between the response and explanatory variables. If a line does a poor job of describing that relationship, then the assumption of linearity has been violated. The assumption of linearity can be checked simply by viewing the scatterplot of the response and the explanatory variables to see whether it demonstrates a linear pattern. If it does, then the points should line up fairly well along the line. If, however, the relationship is not linear, then a line may do a poor job of explaining the relationship between the explanatory and response variables (Figure 3-16).

When this occurs, transformations of the explanatory variable may be necessary. Typical transformations include the natural log and the square root so that the model becomes $y = \alpha + \beta \ln(x) + \varepsilon$ or $y = \alpha + \beta \sqrt{x} + \varepsilon$, respectively.

Polynomial Regression

Even when the plot of the explanatory and the response variable appear to be fairly linear, leftover patterns may be evident in the plot of the residuals, which should have no pattern. A leftover pattern indicates that more in the unexplained variability can be explained by additions to the model. As an example. The plot of the response versus the explanatory variable appears fairly linear (Figure 3-18a). However, the plot of the residuals versus the explanatory variable clearly indicate that a curve is evident (Figure 3-18b). In the residual plot of Figure 3-18b, a pattern obviously remains in the residuals; the points are not randomly scattered. In particular, the errors are larger for small and large values of the explanatory variable but small for the middle explanatory values. The result is a leftover pattern in the residuals that can be explained by a parabola (a U-shaped curve). However, by squaring the explanatory variable and adding it to the model, it is

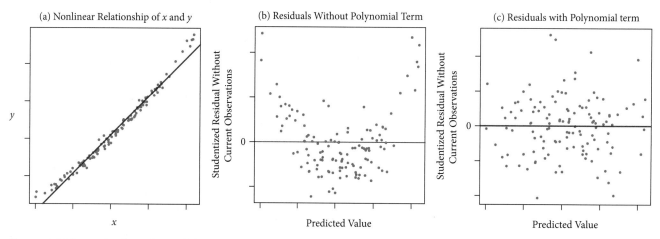

(a) Nonlinear Relationship of x and y (b) Residuals Without Polynomial Term   (c) Residuals with Polynomial term

Figure 3-18 Examples for polynomial regression. © *Cengage Learning, 2012.*

possible to account for the parabola (curve) that is left over in the residuals. The model (a quadratic regression) with the squared term is $y = \alpha + \beta_1 x + \beta_2 x^2 + \varepsilon$. The residual plot of residuals versus the predicted response ($a + b_1 x_1 + b_2 x_1^2$) now reveals no remaining patterns (Figure 3-18c).

Adding a squared (quadratic) term, may not eliminate all of the curve pattern still in the residuals. When there is still a curve leftover in the residuals, adding a cubic (x^3) term or other higher-powered terms may be needed.

Violations of Independence

Most statistical software packages have tests that can help determine whether the independence assumption has been violated. However, as long as the explanatory variable is measured on independent subjects and the observations are independent the residuals should be independent as well.

Implementing Regression Diagnostics

Assumptions may be investigated without performing statistical tests. In fact, most diagnosing of the model assumptions involves the use of plots. In general, a linear regression analysis needs to include a scatterplot of the two variables, a scatterplot of the residuals, and plots assessing the normality of the residuals.

- Consider the scatterplot of the response variable y versus the explanatory variable x. Is the plot fairly linear? Would it make sense to draw a line between the points? Is a transformation needed to make the relationship linear?
- A plot of the residuals versus the predicted response should be randomly scattered around 0. Is fanning apparent suggesting non-constant variance? A violation may suggest that the response variable should be transformed.
- Plots of the residuals versus the explanatory variable can also indicate if polynomial regression is needed. If the plot of the residuals are not randomly distributed about 0 but demonstrate a leftover curve, higher-order terms may need to be added to the model.
- Histograms and probability plots of the residuals assess normality of the residuals. A histogram of the residuals should resemble the normal distribution and be centered at 0, and a probability plot should look like a diagonal line.

If violations are found in any of these plots, then transformations to the response variable may be necessary. If these fixes do not address the violation of linearity, then an alternative to linear regression should be considered.

Keep in mind that it is always necessary to check and recheck for violations of the linear regression model assumptions. Furthermore, significance tests (overall F-tests and specific t-tests of slopes) should also be revisited. Changes to the variables involved in the model are likely to effect more than just a single plot. If a transformation of the response is made, then do not forget to re-plot the newly transformed variables. Likewise, if a higher-order term is added to the regression model, do not forget to re-check the residuals. The final regression equation should be fully vetted for possible violations of the statistical model assumptions.

Planning a Correlation Study

A correlation or simple linear regression study generally involves only one sample of subjects. The goal is to obtain two continuous measurements on each subject. The research question involves trying to understand how these two continuous variables are related. To plan a correlation study, a sample size must be selected so that either a correlation can be precisely estimated or a decision can be made about a hypothesized correlation coefficient.

When the goal is simply to estimate a correlation coefficient, a one-sided confidence interval is typically planned. Using sample size calculation software, investigators can estimate the number of subjects needed to estimate the correlation coefficient with a certain amount of precision, provided they have a confidence level, a guess of the correlation coefficient, and the upper or lower limit on the correlation. For example, suppose that the goal is to plan a study where the expected correlation coefficient is 0.6 and that the investigator wants to be able to estimate the correlation with a lower limit of 0.50. Using a 95% one-sided confidence interval, the investigator would need 134 subjects. If the investigator had been interested in a negative correlation of 0.6, then the limit of -0.50 would be an upper limit and would still require 134 subjects. The sample size is dependent on the size of the correlation as well as the upper/lower bound. A study trying to detect a small correlation (e.g., 0.20) requires a larger sample; a 95% one-sided confidence interval would require 262 subjects for a lower limit of 0.10. Likewise, decreasing the distance between the limit and the proposed correlation also increases the sample size. Assuming the same correlation of 0.20, a 95% confidence interval would require 1020 subjects for a lower limit of 0.15.

When the goal of the study is to perform a hypothesis test, sample size estimation involves the relationship of power and type 1 error (discussed in Chapter 1). Furthermore, the sample size depends on how big a difference the test needs to detect. This requires stating a null correlation and an alternative correlation. Generally, studies are planned with 80–90% power and significance levels (probability of a type 1 error) of 0.05. Observational, exploratory studies where a type 1 error is not as critical can handle larger significance levels ($\alpha = 0.1$).

Once decisions are made on power and the probability of a type 1 error, the only other decision is the effect size. In a one-sample study involving correlation, the effect size involves the difference between the null and alternative correlations. For example, suppose the goal is to determine whether a correlation exists between two continuous variables. The null hypothesis might be that the true correlation is 0. If an investigator wanted to plan a study so that a correlation of 0.25 could be detected with 90% power (assuming a two-sided significance level of 0.05), then a sample size of 165 subjects is needed (Table 3-8).

TABLE 3-8 **EXAMPLES OF SAMPLE SIZES FOR A CORRELATION STUDY (TESTING)**

Null Hypothesis	Detectable Correlation	Sample Size Estimates	
		Power = 80%	Power = 90%
$\rho = 0$	0.1	783	1047
	0.25	124	165
	0.5	30	38
$\rho = 0.5$	0.35	652	871
	0.5	94	125
	0.75	19	24

Assuming a two-sided significance level of 0.05.

© Cengage Learning, 2012.

Suppose that the explanatory variable of water consumption is not the only variable suspected of impacting the hemoglobin change. In this study, the primary outcome of interest is the hemoglobin change. Many times the change is dependent on where the subjects started; so investigating the change without considering the initial value can be misleading. In this example, the pregnant women have differing week 9 hemoglobin values; some women have values in a normal range, and some were already anemic at week 9 (baseline). This is an issue when investigating the hemoglobin change since pregnant women who were already anemic (low hemoglobin measures) at baseline may not experience much change in the hemoglobin measures over the course of the pregnancy because their values started out low. Likewise, women with high hemoglobin measures at baseline might experience a large hemoglobin change simply because their starting values were so high. For example, one pregnant woman might experience only a 1.0 g/dL hemoglobin change, while another experiences a 2.5 g/dL hemoglobin change. If the first pregnant woman had a baseline hemoglobin value of 9.1 g/dL and the second pregnant woman had a baseline hemoglobin of 13.1 g/dL, the baseline values could partially explain why the hemoglobin changes were different for the two women. To investigate the relationship of water consumption and hemoglobin changes, an additional variable (the baseline hemoglobin) should also be considered. When multiple variables might explain differences in the response variable, *multiple linear regression* can be used.

The underlying concepts of a multiple linear regression are very similar to those of simple linear regression. The main difference is the number of explanatory variables. Simple linear regression involves only one explanatory variable, but multiple linear regression involves multiple variables that can help explain differences in the response. Often, the multiple variables in the multiple linear regression are referred to as **regressors**. A regressor is any variable that appears on the right hand side of the model equation or any variable that is associated with a slope in a linear regression model. In order to explain the principles for a multiple linear regression and to make analogies to simple linear regression, multiple linear regression is first discussed with only two regressors (tap water consumption and baseline hemoglobin), but the concepts can be extended to any number of regressors.

Given two regressors, the associations of both variables with the response should be examined for correlations, and scatterplots again provide a simple description of the relationships.

- The estimated correlation between tap water consumption and hemoglobin change is still positive and fairly strong ($r = 0.50$, $p < 0.0001$) (Figure 3-19).
- The estimated correlation between hemoglobin change and baseline hemoglobin is still negative and pretty weak ($r = -0.04$, $p = 0.2850$) (Figure 3-20).

The datapoints in the scatterplot in Figure 3-20 do not exhibit a linear relationship, which is supported by the small correlation estimate. The correlation between the hemoglobin change and baseline hemoglobin is not significantly different from 0, indicating no linear relationship between the baseline and change values ($r = -0.04$, $p = 0.2849$). However, considering two-variable relationships (water consumption and hemoglobin change, baseline hemoglobin and hemoglobin change) separately does not provide a complete picture. Both of these regressors are expected to impact the hemoglobin change, and it does not suffice to consider them one at a time. Moreover, considering the bivariate relationships of tap water consumption with hemoglobin change and baseline hemoglobin with hemoglobin change ignores the potential relationship between tap water consumption and baseline hemoglobin (and how both variables together have a relationship on the hemoglobin change).

Figure 3-19 Scatterplot of tap water consumption and hemoglobin change.
© Cengage Learning, 2012.

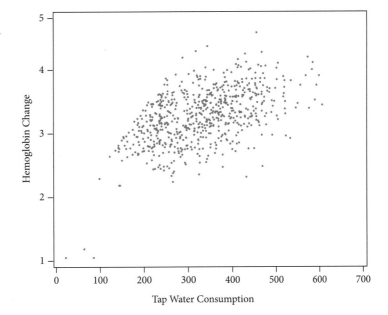

Figure 3-20 Scatterplot of baseline hemoglobin and hemoglobin change.
© Cengage Learning, 2012.

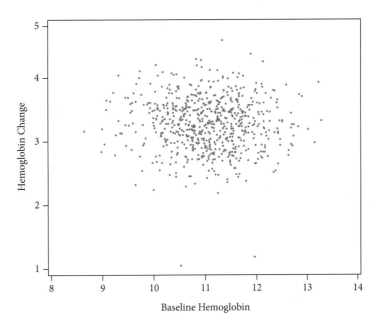

Instead of three two-dimensional plots with only a vertical (y-axis) and horizontal (x-axis), a three-dimensional scatterplot may provide a better representation of the relationship of the three variables (Figure 3-21). There are no longer two axes (y-axis and x-axis) but three axes (y-axis, x_1-axis, and x_2-axis). Hence, each point no longer represents a pair of continuous measurements (x, y), but three values (y, x_1, and x_2), or (Hemoglobin Change, Tap Water Consumption, Baseline Hemoglobin).

Although the three-dimensional scatterplot is somewhat different than the scatterplot used in simple linear regression, the goal is the same: Is there a "line" that best fits these data? The major difference is that the line is replaced by a plane or flat surface (Figure 3-22). Even though the picture is a little different with three variables than with two variables, the purpose is the same: Find the plane that best fits the data by minimizing the error between the plane and the observed points. In simple linear regression, least squares regression was used to identify the best line, and, in multiple linear regression, least squares regression is also used to find the best plane.

Figure 3-21 Three-dimensional scatterplot.
© *Cengage Learning, 2012.*

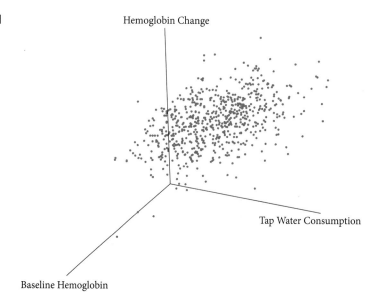

Figure 3-22 Three-dimensional scatterplot with fitted plane.
© *Cengage Learning, 2012.*

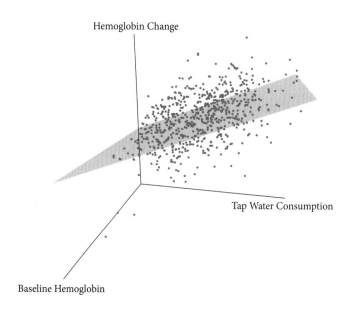

The Model (Two Regressors)

With a response and two regressors, the goal is still to understand the relationship among the three variables. In particular, why do the hemoglobin changes differ among pregnant women? Could the different hemoglobin changes values be attributed to differing tap water consumption values, to different baseline hemoglobin values, or to both? Understanding the relationship of tap water consumption, baseline hemoglobin, and hemoglobin change helps answer the research question of whether exposure to herbicides impacted hemoglobin changes. Statistical models can again be used to help understand relationships in the data and how the data could have been produced.

In simple linear regression, a line is used to model how the response variable relates to the explanatory variable. With more than one regressor, a linear relationship is still observed, and the response is associated to the regressors by a linear model:

$$\alpha + \beta_1 x_1 + \beta_2 x_2$$

where x_1 represents tap water consumption and x_2 represents baseline hemoglobin.

Like simple linear regression, the response and the regressor are related to each other using a linear combination of the variables plus an error term to account for random variation about the line:

$$y = \alpha + \beta x + \beta_2 x_2 + \varepsilon$$

where the ε comes from a normal distribution with mean 0 and constant variance. The intercept is denoted as α, and the slopes by βs.

- If the response and a regressor have a positive association, the slope is positive.
- If the response and a regressor have a negative association, the slope is negative.
- If the response and a regressor are not associated, then the slope is 0.

In the case of multiple linear regression, there are now multiple regressors and multiple slopes.

Because the model describes the population, the intercept and the slopes in the model are parameters (α, β_1, β_2) and are represented by Greek symbols. The errors (ε) are also represented by a Greek symbol. Because the data are not expected to arise exactly from this plane, the errors represent the random variation that might occur in the real data. The random variations are assumed to come from a normal distribution with a mean of 0 and a constant variance (σ^2).

In summary, given a response and two regressors, the linear relationship between these two variables can be modeled as $y = \alpha + \beta_1 x_1 + \beta_2 x_2 + \varepsilon$. The assumptions for this model are the same as in simple linear regression:

1. *The subjects are independent.* The hemoglobin change in one pregnant woman has nothing to do with the hemoglobin change in another pregnant woman. If the subjects are independent, then the errors are independent as well. The distance between one point and the line has nothing to do with the distance between another point and the line.
2. *The errors come from a normal distribution* that has
   a. A mean of 0
   b. A constant variance (represented as σ^2)

Getting the Intercept and Slopes

Even though the scatterplot has changed from two dimensions (tap water consumption, hemoglobin change) to three dimensions (tap water consumption, baseline hemoglobin, hemoglobin change), the relationship is still linear. The line in two-dimensional space, however, becomes a plane in three dimensions (or three variables). Any plane could be fit through the data, but only one plane fits the data so that the errors (the distance between the plane and the points) are minimized.

The plane that best fits the data is obtained by finding estimates of the intercept (α) and the slopes (β_1 and β_2) so that the resulting plane ($\hat{y} = a + b_1 x_1 + b_2 x_2$) minimizes the difference between the points and the plane. Like simple linear regression, the plane that results is the one that minimizes the squared distance between the points and the plane. Therefore the regression method is still called least squares regression.

Therefore, using the data, the true intercept and the true slopes in the model ($y = \alpha + \beta_1 x_1 + \beta_2 x_2 + \varepsilon$) are estimated by least squares regression resulting in $\hat{y} = a + b_1 x_1 + b_2 x_2$, the prediction equation. The prediction equation contains no Greek symbols because this equation for the plane is found using sample data. The intercept a and the slopes b_1 and b_2 are statistics, not parameters. The y wears a hat because it is not the response observed in the data, but the response that would result from the plane. The formula ($\hat{y} = a + b_1 x_1 + b_2 x_2$) is the equation for the plane that best fits the data, not the statistical model, so it contains no ε, or errors. Furthermore, both of the regressors are involved in the estimation of the slopes and intercept; so particular values of all regressors (x_1 and x_2) are needed to predict a response ($\hat{y}$).

The ANOVA Table (Two Regressors)

Just like in the simple linear regression, the ANOVA and the overall *F*-test can be used to analyze the variability of the response or to explain why one pregnant woman has a different hemoglobin change than another pregnant woman. The ANOVA is used to divide the variability observed in the responses into the variability that is attributable to the model and the variability that is just error. With multiple variables, the model now represents the set of multiple regressors as a group.

In an ANOVA analysis, the goal is to divide the variability of the response into the variability that can be explained by the set of regressors (the model) and the variability that cannot be explained (error). The difference between the ANOVA table with one regressor (Table 3-5) versus the ANOVA table with two regressors (Table 3-9) is that the model now represents multiple variables (tap water consumption and baseline hemoglobin) instead of just one (tap water consumption).

TABLE 3-9 **ANOVA TABLE (TWO REGRESSORS)**

Source	Degrees of Freedom	Sum of Squares	Mean Square	F
Model	Number of explanatory variables	SSM	$MSM = \dfrac{SSM}{Model\ DF}$	$\dfrac{MSM}{MSE}$
Error	(Total DF − Model DF)	SSE	$MSE = \dfrac{SSE}{Within\ DF}$	
Total	Number of observations − 1	SST		

© Cengage Learning, 2012.

In Table 3-9:

- The total sum of squares (SST) of the response is still the sum of the model sum of squares (SSM) and the error sum of squares (SSE).
- The total sum of squares and its degrees of freedom (DF) for the two regressor model versus simple linear regression are exactly the same; there has been no change to the left side of the statistical model (the response variable), and SST still describes the total variability in the response.
- The model sum of squares, on the other hand, has changed and is larger because an additional regressor was added to the model; more variables are explaining the differences in the response.
- Accordingly, the error sum of squares, on the other hand, is now smaller than in the one-regressor model. In simple linear regression, the model consisted of only one variable (tap water consumption), leaving some unexplained variability in the response. The unexplained variability is represented by the error sum of squares. In the ANOVA table with two regressors in the model, some of the unexplained variability in the error sum of squares is now explained by adding another regressor (baseline hemoglobin).
- The degrees of freedom have also changed. The degrees of freedom for the model sum of squares is increased by 1 because of the additional regressor in the model. Consequently, the degrees of freedom for the error sum of squares has to be reduced by 1.
- The mean square model and mean square error are still found by dividing the sum of squares model and sum of squares error by their respective degrees of freedom.
- The *F*-statistic is still the mean square model divided by the mean square error.

The purpose of the ANOVA is still to answer the question: Is there a linear relationship between the response and regressors? Just as in simple linear regression, the sources of variability are split. If the variability seen in the response variable can be explained by the model, then an association between the response and at least one of the regressors is established. A linear relationship between the response and the regressors helps to explain the variability in the response. In other words, two response values appear at different places on the y-axis (hemoglobin change) because, in part, the two responses have different corresponding regressor values on the x_1-axis (tap water consumption) and x_2-axis (baseline hemoglobin). For example, if one woman had higher hemoglobin changes than another woman, the difference between the hemoglobin changes might be explained by larger tap water consumption and/or a higher baseline hemoglobin. The explained variability represents the variability in the response that can be explained by the variables in the model. However, the tap water consumption and baseline hemoglobin (regressors the model) do not completely explain why one pregnant woman has a different hemoglobin change than another pregnant woman does; some variability remains in the response variable (hemoglobin change) that cannot be explained by tap water consumption and baseline hemoglobin.

In any regression analysis, the goal is to explain as much of the variability in the response as possible so that there is little unexplained variability. Therefore, regressors that can explain much of the variability in the response are considered to have strong linear relationships with the response variable. If a lot of variability remains unexplained or is attributed to error, then the model (the set of regressors) does not do an adequate job of explaining the variations in the response values, and the regressors do not exhibit much of a linear relationship with the response.

The ANOVA table can provide information on how well the model explains changes in the response. Ideally, the model explains much of the variation in the response, and very little is left over for the errors. In other words, a good model is able to explain a large proportion of the variability in the response.

Just as in simple linear regression, the R^2 value is obtained by dividing the model sum of squares by the total sum of squares. It represents the proportion of the total variability explained by the model. The maximum R^2 is 1, or 100%. An $R^2 = 0.9$ indicates that the model was able to explain 90% of the variability in the response variable. An $R^2 = 0.01$, on the other hand, indicates that the model does a poor job because only 1% of the total variability can be explained by the model. Visually, as the area covered by the two circles (the model) in Figure 3-23 increases, so does the proportion of the square (total sum of squares) covered, i.e. R^2 increases. Unlike simple linear regression, the square root of R^2 is no longer the correlation between x and y. Now that there are two regressors in the model, the R^2 is calculated using both regressors (x_1 and x_2).

Figure 3-23 Visualization of R^2 (two regressors).
© *Cengage Learning, 2012.*

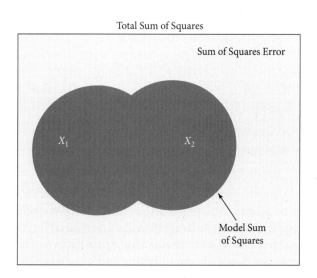

Overall Hypothesis Test

Although the ANOVA table provides a mechanism for partitioning the variability that comes from the response, the question is still whether the variability attributable to the model (measured by the mean square model) is large enough when compared to the error variability (measured by the mean square error) to claim that a linear relationship exists. The variability attributed to the model and the error is compared by considering the ratio of the mean squared model and the mean squared error. If the mean squared error is small compared to the model, then the ratio will be large. If the mean squared error is large compared to the model, then the ratio is small. The ratio can be used to determine whether the variability due to the model is large enough to claim that the regressor(s) are linearly related to the response.

The ratio has a sampling distribution that follows an F-distribution, just as it did in simple linear regression. However, with two regressors, the numerator degrees of freedom from the mean square model is 2 (the total number of regressors in the model), and the denominator degrees of freedom from the mean squared error 661 ($661 = 663 - 2$). Therefore, using the F-distribution with 2 and 661 degrees of freedom, the F-statistic can be used to test the hypothesis of a linear relationship between the regressors (x_1 and x_2) and the response (y).

RESEARCH HYPOTHESIS: Tap water consumption or baseline hemoglobin is linearly related to hemoglobin change.

NULL HYPOTHESIS: Tap water consumption and baseline hemoglobin are not linearly related to hemoglobin change.

The hypotheses with multiple regressors are the same as simple linear regression in that the hypotheses involve testing for a linear relationship. Multiple linear regression hypotheses differ, however, from simple linear regression because multiple variables are considered at one time. The research hypothesis is that tap water consumption [water] or baseline hemoglobin [hgb] is linearly related to hemoglobin change [change]. To enable investigators to reject the null hypothesis, the data have to support a linear relationship with the response and at least one of the regressors; both regressors do not have to be linearly related to the response.

A linear relationship between the hemoglobin change and the regressors (tap water consumption and baseline hemoglobin) is modeled as

$$\text{Change} = \alpha + \beta_1 (\text{water}) + \beta_2(\text{hgb9}) + \varepsilon$$

where ε follow a normal distribution with a mean of 0 and a variance of σ^2. Therefore, the hypothesis of the linear relationship between the response and regressors becomes a hypothesis about the slopes (β_1 and β_2).

RESEARCH HYPOTHESIS: *At least one* of the true slopes is not 0 ($\beta_1 \neq 0$ or $\beta_2 \neq 0$). There is a linear relationship between the response and *at least one* of the regressors.

NULL HYPOTHESIS: The true slopes (β_1 and β_2) are both 0. There is no linear relationship between the response and the regressors.

Using the ANOVA table (Table 3-10), a ratio of mean square model and mean square error results in $F = 109.55$. Is this ratio (F-statistic) large enough to claim that the model variability is larger than the error variability? In other words, is it large enough to claim that a linear relationship exists between hemoglobin change and at least one regressor (tap water consumption and/or baseline hemoglobin)?

$$\text{Test statistic } (F) = \frac{\text{Mean square model}}{\text{Mean square error}}$$

What you need to calculate the test statistic:

1. *The mean square:* MSM = 14.98.
2. *The mean square error:* MSE = 0.14.
3. *The degrees of freedom:*
   a. MSM, DF = the number of explanatory variables = 2
   b. MSE, DF = 661

To calculate the test statistic (F): The ratio is MSM (1) divided by MSE (2): $14.98 \div 0.14 = 109.55$.
Using an *F*-distribution with numerator degrees of freedom of 2 and denominator degrees of freedom of 661, the percentage of ratios observed with this sample that are farther from the ratio is less than 0.01% (p-value < 0.0001).

TABLE 3-10 **ANOVA TABLE RESULTS**

Source	Degrees of Freedom	Sum of Squares	Mean Square	F	p-value
Model	2	29.96	14.98	109.55	<0.0001
Within (error)	661	90.40	0.14		
Total	663	120.36			

© Cengage Learning, 2012.

Point to Ponder

The ideal R^2 is close to 1. The complexity of some research questions may impact how much variability can be explained by the model. How does the type of data impact the interpretation of the R^2?

CONCLUSION: Because this p-value is small, there is evidence that the ratio is large or that the variability attributable to the model is large enough to suggest a linear relationship. In other words, there is sufficient evidence to reject the null hypothesis that there is no linear relationship between the hemoglobin change, tap water consumption, and baseline hemoglobin.

The relationship between the response and the regressors is further confirmed by the $R^2 = \text{SSM} \div \text{SST} = 29.96 \div 120.36$, indicating that 24.9% of the variability in the hemoglobin changes can be explained by the model.

The objective of this analysis is to determine whether the hemoglobin change is linearly related to either tap water consumption or baseline hemoglobin. Of the two regressors, the model mean square does not provide information for each independently; it provides only how much variability is explained by the model with both regressors combined. Both regressors could have a linear relationship with the response and do a good job of explaining the variability in the response. In contrast, it may be that only tap water consumption helps to explain the variability in the hemoglobin change, and baseline hemoglobin might not help at all; or, perhaps the baseline hemoglobin explains the variability in the hemoglobin change, and tap water consumption does not contribute. Because the *F*-statistic involves the mean square model, the conclusions have to involve the model, not the individual regressors. This was not an issue in simple linear regression because there was only one regressor; testing for how well the model explained the variability in the response was the same as testing the individual regressor.

A statistically significant p-value associated with the overall *F*-test simply indicates that a linear relationship exists somewhere. It could be with one or both of each of the regressors, but it does not indicate which regressor contributes significantly or the direction of the association. To investigate the impact of each of the regressors, specific hypothesis testing needs to performed and specific confidence intervals need to be constructed. However, these more specific investigations of the contribution of each regressor can be performed only *after* a linear relationship has been determined to exist between at least one of the regressors and the response. If the ANOVA results in an F-statistic that is not significant (the p-value is large), then the null hypothesis cannot be rejected; there is no evidence of a linear relationship. If there is no evidence of a linear relationship, then there is no reason to continue searching for the contribution of the individual regressors.

Adjusted Sum of Squares and Partial Correlations (Two Regressors)

Although the ANOVA table has helped to determine whether a linear relationship exists between the response variable and the regressors, how these regressors individually contribute to understanding the variability in the response is still unknown. In multiple linear regression, considering the effect of just one regressor is not sufficient; the impact of the other regressors must be considered as well.

The sum of squares model (SSM) from the ANOVA table is produced when the response is regressed on both the x_1 and x_2 simultaneously. The model sum of squares still represents the variability in the response that can be explained by x_1 and x_2, but having more than one regressor in the model allows for more interpretations. In fact, the model sum of squares can be thought of as the sum of the squares related to x_1 and the sum of squares related to x_2. However, x_1 and x_2 are not likely to be independent; the explanations they provide may overlap. Because of this overlap, the sum of squares model is not simply the sum of squares for x_1 plus the sum of squares for x_2. To avoid overcounting the overlap between x_1 and x_2, the sum of squares model can be partitioned into the separate contributions of the two regressors in one of two ways:

1. The sum of squares for x_1 + the sum of squares for x_2 that remains after considering x_1 (Figure 3-24)
2. The sum of squares for x_2 + the sum of squares for x_1 that remains after considering x_2 (Figure 3-25)

If the individual contribution of each regressor is considered, so that the overlap is ignored, the sum of these individual contributions does not add up to the model sum of squares; the overlap is missing (Figure 3-26). After the removal of any overlapping contribution, the individual contribution of each regressor is known as the *adjusted sum of squares*: the contribution to the model sum of squares that only that regressor independently contributes. The adjusted sum of squares is found by assuming that all the other regressors have already been included in the model. The nonoverlapping regions represent the adjusted sum of squares for the two regressors in the model.

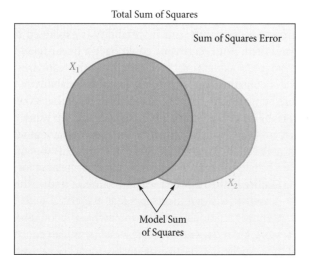

Figure 3-24 Proportion of total variability explained by the regressors (x_1, then x_2).
© *Cengage Learning, 2012.*

Total Sum of Squares

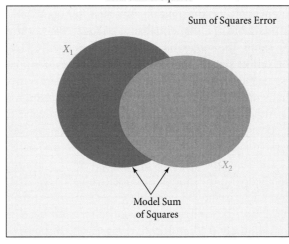

Figure 3-25 Proportion of total variability explained by the regressors (x_2, then x_1).
© *Cengage Learning, 2012.*

Total Sum of Squares

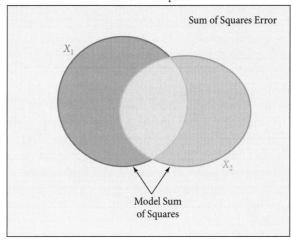

Figure 3-26 Proportion of total variability explained independently by the regressors.
© *Cengage Learning, 2012.*

Instead of considering the impact of a regressor after all other regressors have been included, it is also possible to consider the contribution of a regressor by considering them sequentially, where the order they are entered into the model matters. By considering regressors sequentially, the additional amount of variability explained as each regressor is added can be quantified. For example, in the simple linear regression, only x_1 (tap water consumption) was a regressor in the model. The sum of squares model and the sum of squares contribution of x_1 were exactly the same. However, when x_2 (baseline hemoglobin) is included in the model, more of the variability in the response (hemoglobin change) is explained. The sum of squares model becomes the contribution of the tap water consumption variable (x_1) plus the contribution of baseline hemoglobin variable (x_2) that had not already been accounted for by the tap water consumption. The so-called *sequential sum of squares* provides the sum of squares model contribution as variables are sequentially added in the model.

The order in which variables are considered in the model matters in the sequential sum of squares. The complete contribution of the first variable entered into the model is used for understanding the variability in the response. The next variable included in the model is credited only for the contribution to the sum of squares not already accounted for by the previous regressor. Hence, the sequential sums of squares can be summed to provide the model sum of squares. Because order matters, the sequential sum of squares can differ depending on the order in which variables are entered into the model. If x_1 is entered first, then the whole contribution of x_1 is used, and only the additional contribution of x_2 is used (Figure 3-24). However, if x_2 is entered first, then the whole contribution of x_2 is used, and only the additional contribution of x_1 is used (Figure 3-25).

Hence, the sequential sum of squares for the *last regressor* included in the model represents only its contribution after all other regressors have been considered. So, for that last variable, the sequential sum of squares and the adjusted sum of squares are really the same. The sequential sum of squares for the *first regressor* included in the model is the sum of squares that would result if there were no other variables. For this reason, the sequential sum of squares for the first regressor is the same as the model sum of squares that would result if only a simple linear regression were performed.

Although the circle figures (Figures 3-24 through 3-26) present a conceptual description of adjusted and sequential sums of squares, consider actual values in the example involving hemoglobin change, tap water consumption, and baseline hemoglobin (Table 3-11).

The SSM (model sums of squares) for this example is 30.0, the sums of squares associated with the model. Because two variables are in the model (tap water consumption and baseline hemoglobin), these are the sums of square associated with the two variables. The sequential sums of squares for baseline hemoglobin and tap water consumption are 0.40 and 29.6, respectively. Because baseline hemoglobin is first in the model, the 0.40 represents the sum of squares associated with baseline hemoglobin, without tap water consumption in the model. The sequential sum of squares for the tap water consumption is assigned the remaining part of the model sums of squares not accounted for by the baseline hemoglobin. Therefore, the two sequential sums of squares can be added (0.40 + 29.6) to get the model sums of squares (30.0).

The *adjusted sum of squares*, on the other hand, represents the sums of squares associated with each variable controlling for the other. For example, the adjusted sums of squares for the tap water consumption variable is the same as the sequential sum of squares because tap water consumption was the last variable included in the model. The adjusted sums of squares for baseline hemoglobin and tap water consumption no longer add up to the model sums of squares (0.40 + 29.8 ≠ 30.0) because each piece assumes that the other variable is already in the model.

Sequential sums of squares and adjusted sums of squares are helpful in multiple linear regression because the regressors are considered simultaneously. Considering each regressor individually would defeat the purpose of a multiple linear regression. Sequential sums of squares are often used when trying to determine whether adding an additional regressor will contribute significantly to the model sum of squares. In public health, the adjusted sum of squares, which describe the individual contribution of a regressor after all other regressors have been considered, is commonly used. In fact, the adjusted sum of squares correspond to the statistics (partial correlations and slopes) most often used to describe the individual regressor.

TABLE 3-11 **EXAMPLE OF ADJUSTED AND SEQUENTIAL SUMS OF SQUARES**

Analysis of Variance					
Source	DF	Sum of Squares	Mean Square	F-Value	Pr > F
Model	2	29.96318	14.98159	109.55	<0.0001
Error	661	90.39943	0.13676		
Corrected Total	663	120.36262			

Results of Regression Analysis						
Variable	Parameter Estimate	Standard Error	t-Value	Pr > |t|	Sequential SS	Adjusted SS
Intercept	2.27635	0.22826	9.97	<0.0001	7627.41798	13.60153
water	0.00229	0.00015539	14.75	<0.0001	29.58182	29.75529
hgb9	0.03202	0.01917	1.67	0.0954	0.38136	0.38136

© Cengage Learning, 2012.

In a multiple linear regression with two regressors, a datapoint consists of three variables (x_1, x_2, and y). In this example, a datapoint would include three values, one for tap water consumption, baseline hemoglobin, and hemoglobin change. Clearly, from the discussion of model sum of squares, the impact of x_1 on y cannot be adequately described without considering the impact of x_2 on y. The three variables are connected; describing the relationship of a regressor and the response one at a time would be an incomplete explanation. Simple two-variable correlations do not capture this multiple-variable relationship, so describing how x_1 and y are correlated in the presence of x_2 or to consider the association of x_2 and y after accounting for the effect of x_1 is now an important numerical summary. These correlations are known as *partial correlations*.

Given two regressors (x_1 and x_2) and one response variable (y), the correlation between the response (y) and one of the regressors (x_1) while accounting for the other regressor (x_2) is known as a *partial correlation*, and this statistic is represented as $r_{y \cdot x_1 | x_2}$. Likewise, the correlation between the response (y) and one of the regressors (x_2) while accounting for the other regressor (x_1) is also known as a partial correlation and this statistic is represented as $r_{y \cdot x_2 | x_1}$. A partial correlation coefficient shares the same properties as a correlation coefficient (r). A partial correlation coefficient is between -1 and 1, which represent the strongest negative or positive association between the response and one of the regressors while accounting for the other regressor.

In simple linear regression, the R^2 represented the proportion of the variability in the response that was explained by the explanatory variable or the single regressor. In addition, squaring the correlation coefficient that resulted between the response and the regressor also provided R^2. Given the additional regressor, R^2 is no longer simply the square of the correlation coefficients. However, each partial regression coefficient can be squared to obtain the proportion of variability in the response explained by the regressor while accounting for the additional regressor (Table 3-12). Specifically, $(r_{y \cdot x_2 | x_1})^2$ measures the proportion of the variation in y explained by x_2 that has not already been explained by x_1. Similarly, $(r_{y \cdot x_1 | x_2})^2$ measures the proportion of the variation in y explained by x_1 that has not already been explained by x_2. Hence, adding tap water consumption as a regressor explains 0.248 (24.8%) of the total variability left unexplained by baseline hemoglobin alone. Likewise, adding baseline hemoglobin as a regressor explains only 0.004 (0.4%) of the total variability left unexplained by tap water consumption alone.

The R^2 for the whole model (all the regressors) is $R^2 = 1 - [1 - (r_{y \cdot x_1})^2] (1 - (r_{y \cdot x_2 | x_1})^2]$. In other words, R^2 is the area covered by the circles and does not over-count the overlap. The partial correlations ($r_{y \cdot x_2 | x_1}$ and $r_{y \cdot x_1 | x_2}$) are calculated from sample data and are statistics. These partial correlations are useful when estimating the true partial correlations of the population ($\rho_{y \cdot x_2 | x_1}$ and $\rho_{y \cdot x_1 | x_2}$).

Often of interest is testing whether these partial correlations are equal to 0. A 0 partial correlation is similar to a 0 correlation. If the partial correlation is 0, for example if $\rho_{y \cdot x_2 | x_1}$ is 0, then there is no linear relationship between y and x_2 after taking x_1 into account. The statistical test for whether the partial correlation ($\rho_{y \cdot x_2 | x_1}$) is 0 turns out to be the exact same statistical test that tests whether β_2 is 0. Likewise the statistical test for whether the partial correlation $\rho_{y \cdot x_1 | x_2}$ is 0 turns out to be the very same statistical test for whether β_1 is 0.

TABLE 3-12 **EXAMPLE OF PARTIAL CORRELATIONS**

Variable	Parameter Estimate	Standard Error	t-Value	Pr > |t|	Partial Correlation Estimates
Intercept	2.27635	0.22826	9.97	<0.0001	
hgb9	0.03202	0.01917	1.67	0.0954	0.00420
water	0.00229	0.00015539	14.75	<0.0001	0.24764

© Cengage Learning, 2012.

Specific Hypothesis Tests for Slopes (Two Regressors)

In a multiple linear regression, the model connects multiple regressors to a single response, and a datapoint is comprised of all three variables (x_1, x_2, and y). All three of these variables are used in the least squares regression simultaneously; so all three variables (x_1, x_2, and y) are used to obtain estimates of the slopes (b_1 and b_2) and intercept a. The slope for each regressor is found assuming that all the regressors are in the model ($y = \alpha + \beta_1 x_1 + \beta_2 x_2 + \varepsilon$) or that all the datapoints are made of three values (x_1, x_2, and y). Hence, each slope can be thought of as being adjusted for the other regressors in the model. Consequently, the hypotheses for individual slopes have to reflect that other regressors are in the model. For this reason, these slopes are discussed as being adjusted for all other variables in the model (i.e., all other regressors).

RESEARCH HYPOTHESIS: The true slope $\beta_1 \neq 0$ and $\beta_2 \neq 0$. After including x_2 in the model, there is a linear relationship between the response and the x_1.

NULL HYPOTHESIS: The true slope $\beta_1 = 0$ and $\beta_2 \neq 0$. After including x_2 in the model, there is no linear relationship between the response and the x_1.

RESEARCH HYPOTHESIS: The true slope $\beta_2 \neq 0$ and $\beta_1 \neq 0$. After including x_1 in the model, there is a linear relationship between the response and the x_2.

NULL HYPOTHESIS: The true slope $\beta_2 = 0$ and $\beta_1 \neq 0$. After including x_1 in the model, there is no linear relationship between the response and the x_2.

The estimate of the slope obtained from the least squares regression can be used to determine whether there is sufficient evidence against the null hypothesis, assuming the other regressor is in the model. Using the data from pregnant women who consume tap water ($n = 664$), the least squares regression results in estimates for the intercept and the slope (Table 3-13).

Application of Formula

$$\text{Test statistic for the slope } (t) = \frac{b_j}{\text{Standard error}}$$

b_j = The estimate of the slope associated with x_j

Standard error = A function of the MSE

What you need to test for nonzero slope:

1. *An estimate of the slope:* $b_1 = 0.002292$.
2. *The standard error:* 0.0001554.

To calculate the test statistic (t): Divide the slope estimate (1) by the standard error (2): $0.002292 \div 0.0001554 = 14.8$. The test statistic follows a t-distribution with degrees of freedom equal to the degrees of freedom of the mean squared error (DF = 661). This test statistic is quite large, 14.8. Therefore, the proportion of test statistics that are even farther away from the null parameter than the test statistic (the p-value) will be small. The hypothesis test for the slope in this example results in a p-value < 0.0001.

TABLE 3-13 **LEAST SQUARES REGRESSION RESULTS**

	Estimate	Standard Error	Test Statistic	p-value
Intercept	2.276348	0.228259	9.97	<0.001
Tap water consumption	0.002292	0.0001554	14.75	<0.001
Baseline hemoglobin	0.032018	0.0191739	1.67	0.0954

© Cengage Learning, 2012.

CONCLUSION: The p-value that results for the slope associated with tap water consumption is small ($p < 0.0001$). This is sufficient evidence to reject the null hypothesis that the slope is 0 when baseline hemoglobin is in the model; there is evidence that tap water consumption and hemoglobin change have a linear relationship, after controlling for baseline hemoglobin. On the other hand, the slope for baseline hemoglobin is not significantly different from 0 (p-value = 0.0954), when tap water consumption is in the model. Therefore, there is not enough evidence to reject the null hypothesis that the slope for baseline hemoglobin is 0 when tap water consumption is in the model.

Although the p-value associated with baseline hemoglobin is not smaller than 0.05, it is not large, either. In fact, it is smaller than 0.10. More importantly, the investigator wants to describe the relationship of tap water consumption and hemoglobin change, controlling for the baseline hemoglobin. Therefore, baseline hemoglobin is kept in the model. Keeping the baseline hemoglobin in the model is useful because now the relationship between tap water consumption and hemoglobin change has been adjusted for any differences between the subjects with respect to the baseline hemoglobin.

In a multiple linear regression, whenever a variable is included in the model, it explains some of the variability in the response. Each variable contributes something to the model sum of squares. Unless the regressors are completely independent, some of their contributions will overlap. A regressor is considered to be significant when it contributes significantly to the model sum of squares or when it does a good job of explaining the variability in the response, when the overlap of the other variables are removed. Likewise, the specific hypothesis test for the slope results in a small p-value when the regressor independently explains variability sufficient amount of variability in the response. Given multiple regressors, a single regressor has to be able to contribute a sufficient amount of explanation on its own, excluding the contribution that overlaps with other regressors (Figure 3-27).

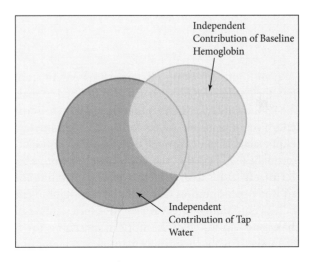

Independent
Contribution of Baseline
Hemoglobin

Independent
Contribution of Tap
Water

Figure 3-27 Visualization of adjusting for other variables.
© *Cengage Learning, 2012.*

Specific Confidence Intervals for Slopes (Two Regressors)

Hypothesis tests indicate a linear relationship between tap water consumption and hemoglobin change, even in the presence of baseline hemoglobin. Specifically, the point estimate for the slope ($b_1 = 0.002$), controlling for baseline hemoglobin, indicates that a change of 0.002 g/dL is expected for every 1-L increase in tap water consumption for this sample, but to estimate the true slope (β_1), confidence intervals are used.

Application of Formula

C% confidence interval for the slope: $b_j \pm t^* \times SE$

b_j = The slope obtained from the sample data

C = The confidence level for a C% confidence interval

t^* = The number of standard deviations from the center of the sampling distribution

SE = The standard error for the slope

What you need to calculate the confidence interval:

1. *The point estimate of the slope:* $b = 0.002$ g/dL.
2. *The standard error:* 0.0001554.
3. *The confidence level:* C% is typically 95%, but 90% and 99% are also common.
4. *The number of standard deviations from the center of the sampling distribution:* This depends on C% (3) and the sampling distribution. Because the mean square error is used to calculate the standard error, the degrees of freedom of the mean square error are used to define the t-distribution. In this case, where the sampling distribution is a t-distribution with 661 degrees of freedom, the t^* for a 90% confidence interval is 1.65, the t^* for a 95% confidence interval is 1.97, and the t^* for a 99% confidence interval is 2.59. Therefore, confidence intervals can be calculated as

90% confidence interval: $b \pm (1.65 \times SE)$

95% confidence interval: $b \pm (1.96 \times SE)$

99% confidence interval: $b \pm (2.58 \times SE)$

To calculate the 95% confidence interval: The number of standard errors from the slope is $1.96 \times 0.0001554 = 0.0003$ and is also known as the *margin of error*. Adding and subtracting the margin of error from the point estimate results in the 95% confidence interval for the true slope, $[0.0022 - 0.0003, 0.0022 + 0.0003]$, or $[0.0019, 0.0025]$.

In addition to making a better estimate than a point estimate of the true parameter (β_1), the confidence interval can also be used to make inferences about the parameter. The 95% confidence interval that was obtained from these data $[0.0019, 0.0025]$ represents a set of plausible values for the true parameter, the slope. Because 0 is not in the set of plausible values provided by the 95% confidence interval, the true parameter (β_1) cannot be 0. In fact, the true slope must be positive because the interval covers a parameter that is larger than 0. Hence, after controlling for baseline hemoglobin, increasing tap water consumption increases the hemoglobin change.

This confidence interval provides an estimate of the slope associated with a 1-L change in tap water consumption, adjusting for baseline hemoglobin. As already discussed, such a small increment as 1 L may not be of interest when investigating the relationship between tap water consumption and hemoglobin change. In simple linear regression, the confidence interval is simply multiplied by the number of units needed for an interesting increment. The same can be done in multiple linear regression. The confidence interval for a 10-L increase is simply the confidence interval for a 1-L increase multiplied by 10 [0.019, 0.025]. Therefore, the adjusted hemoglobin change is 0.23 (95% CI: 0.019, 0.025) for every 10-L increase in tap water consumption.

Prediction Equation

Using the estimates from Table 3-13, the equation of the plane $\hat{y} = a + b_1 x_1 + b_2 x_2$, or $\widehat{change} = a + b_1$ (water) $+ b_2$ (hgb9). Therefore, the equation of the plane that best fits the data is $\widehat{change} = 2.2764 + 0.0023$ (water) $+ 0.0202$ (hgb9). This can now be used to "predict" the hemoglobin change if a certain amount of tap water is consumed and a particular hemoglobin is observed at baseline. However, in public health research, it may be of lesser interest to use this regression for prediction and of greater interest to explore the interpretation of the estimates.

More Than Two Regressors

In public health, it is often of interest to investigate the relationship of two variables while controlling for the effect of others. In this example, even after adjusting for the baseline hemoglobin, the hemoglobin change increases 0.023 g/dL for every 10 L increase in tap water consumed ($p < 0.0001$). Because baseline hemoglobin is included in the model, the estimate for the slope associated with tap water consumption has been adjusted for baseline hemoglobin or the part of the variability in the hemoglobin change that is explained by both tap water consumption and baseline hemoglobin has been removed.

However, a study is not likely to result in only one response and one or two regressors. Public health problems are complicated, and the outcome is probably going to depend on more than one variable. Furthermore, studies are expensive to conduct, and collecting data on only one response and one explanatory variable is inefficient. Therefore, nearly all studies measure several variables on each subject. The concepts presented for a regression model with two regressors ($y = \alpha + \beta_1 x_1 + \beta_2 x_2 + \varepsilon$) are analogous for a regression model with multiple (k) regressors ($y = \alpha + \beta_1 x_1 + \beta_2 x_2 + \beta_3 x_3 + \beta_4 x_4 + \cdots + \beta_k x_k + \varepsilon$). The two-regressor model was introduced first because visualizing the two-regressor model (three-dimensional plot) is possible; four-dimensional, five-dimensional, or k-dimensional plots cannot be visualized. Also, it is simpler to discuss the impact of two regressors on the response and introduce the concepts of sequential and adjusted sums of squares, partial correlations, and adjusted slopes. Adding more regressors adds to the relationships that must be considered and to the complexity of the model. There are more sequential and adjusted sums of squares, more partial correlations, and more adjusted slopes. Although the calculations for obtaining these have the same foundation, performing the calculations becomes more complicated. Software to implement a multiple linear regression is highly recommended.

Regressors Do Not Have to Be Continuous

When thinking of a linear regression, some tend to think that all the variables have to be continuous or ordinal. This is due in part to the interpretation of the slopes; as the regressor increases by 1 unit, the change in the response is the slope. However, multiple linear regression is more flexible than this. In fact, all that is required is that the *response* comes from an approximately normal distribution. The regressors can actually be any kind of variable: continuous, ordinal, nominal, dichotomous. Although the interpretations of the slopes corresponding to these different types of variables may be different, each type of variable is allowed to be considered in the model.

The general interpretation of the slope is that, as the regressor increases by 1 unit, the response changes by the slope. As long as the regressor is a variable type where order makes sense (continuous or ordinal), this interpretation holds. However, when the regressor is nominal, then the phrase "increasing the regressor by 1 unit" does not make sense because the categories of the nominal variable can be reordered and a different conclusion will result. For a dichotomous variable, the order of the levels of the variable does not matter because there are only two levels. So, for a dichotomous variable, the interpretation can still be that, as the regressor increases by 1 unit, the response changes by the slope. However, think about what this means: Because there is only one possible 1-unit increase, the change in the outcome for a 1-unit increase in the dichotomous regressor is the same as the difference between the two categories. Therefore, for a dichotomous variable, the slope can be interpreted as the average difference in the response between the two levels. So the slope can be easily interpreted when the regressor is continuous, ordinal, or dichotomous.

What can be done for nominal variables with more than two levels? The definition of the slope does not change, so the variable has to be transformed so that the interpretation of the slope is reasonable. Therefore, nominal variables are included in the multiple regression as a set of dichotomous variables. As an example, consider a nominal variable like marital status (never married, married, divorced/separated, widowed). These levels have no order. If dichotomous variables for married or not, divorced/separated or not, and widowed or not were included in the regression, then the slopes could just be interpreted as they would for any dichotomous variable. Notice that never married is not included in this set of dichotomous variables. The reason is that, if the married variable is 0, and the divorced/separated variable is 0, and the widowed variable is 0, then the participant must be "never married". As a rule, if a nominal variable has C categories, then only $C - 1$ dichotomous variables are needed. Because the never married level is not included in the regression, it becomes the reference.

- The interpretation of the slope for married is the average difference in hemoglobin change for married compared to never married
- The interpretation of the slope for divorced/separated is the average difference in hemoglobin change for divorced/separated compared to married.
- The interpretation of the slope for widowed is the average difference in hemoglobin change for widowed compared to married.

When a categorical variable is converted into multiple dichotomous variables, they are known as **dummy variables**.

A dummy variable only takes on values of only 0 or 1. The slope associated with a dummy variable can be interpreted as the mean change in the response between two groups. When a categorical variable is converted to dummy variables, the slope associated with each dummy variable is interpreted as the mean change in the response between a group and a reference. The reference group is the group that was not converted to a dummy variable and that was not included in the model. Even though studies in public health commonly use "never married" as a comparison or reference group, an investigator may want to use a different reference, such as divorced/separated. To use divorced/separated as the reference, dummy variables are created for married, never married, and widowed, and divorced/separated is not included in the model.

Dummy variables are generally used in the regression model when a variable is categorical. For this reason, a linear regression that includes categorical variable(s) is referred to as dummy variable regression. When a multiple linear regression, involves dummy variable regressors, the slopes associated with the dummy variables provide **adjusted means**. For example, consider a regression that includes a dummy variable for smoking prior to pregnancy [psmoke]. A value of 0 indicates no smoking prior to pregnancy and a value of 1 indicates smoking prior to pregnancy. The regression model that also includes tap water consumption [water] and baseline hemoglobin [hgb9] would be:

$$\text{Change} = \alpha + \beta_1(\text{water}) + \beta_2(\text{hgb9}) + \beta_3(\text{psmoke}) + \varepsilon$$

where ε is independent and comes from a normal distribution with 0 mean and constant variance. For women who smoked prior to pregnancy, the value of the dummy variable for smoking prior to pregnancy is 1. Therefore, the model for these women who smoked prior to pregnancy is:

$$\text{Change} = \alpha + \beta_1(\text{water}) + \beta_2(\text{hgb9}) + \beta_3(1) + \varepsilon$$

or

$$\text{Change} = \alpha + \beta_1(\text{water}) + \beta_2(\text{hgb9}) + \beta_3 + \varepsilon.$$

The β_3 is just a constant, so the intercept is really $\alpha + \beta_3$. For women who did not smoke prior to pregnancy, the dummy variable for smoking prior to pregnancy is 0. Therefore, the model for these women is:

$$\text{Change} = \alpha + \beta_1(\text{water}) + \beta_2(\text{hgb9}) + \beta_3(0) + \varepsilon$$

or

$$\text{Change} = \alpha + \beta_1(\text{water}) + \beta_2(\text{hgb9}) + \varepsilon$$

For the nonsmokers, the intercept is simply α. Therefore, when prior smoking is included in the model, the result is essentially two parallel regression lines separated by β_3.

Recall that any slope in a multiple linear regression is adjusted for all other variables in the model. Therefore, the beta associated with a dummy variable becomes the shift or the average difference in the response between the two groups, adjusting for all the other variables in the model (Figure 3-28). For this reason, the slope associated with the dummy variable can be interpreted as the adjusted mean difference. Figure 3-28 shows that β simply represents the difference between the two groups, making the interpretation of β a mean difference. The "adjusted" part occurs when the model includes other variables and that the estimate of the slope is obtained by simultaneously considering the other variables. Hence, the adjusted mean difference represents the average difference in the response variable, after the other variables in the model have been considered.

Often investigators treat ordinal variables as nominal variables. This is because the "1-unit increase" interpretation is generally not applicable to ordinal variables in public health, i.e. the jumps between units are not equal. For example, the educational attainment variable in this study has three levels (less than high school, high school/GED, and more than high school). Technically, this variable has an order to it and can be considered an ordinal variable. If this ordinal educational attainment variable [ed] is added to the regression model with tap water consumption [water] and baseline hemoglobin [hgb9], the model is:

$$\text{Change} = \alpha + \beta_1(\text{water}) + \beta_2(\text{hgb9}) + \beta_3(\text{ed}) + \varepsilon$$

where ε is independent and comes from a normal distribution with 0 mean and constant variance. The slope (β_3) represents the hemoglobin change for a 1-unit increase in education, controlling for all other variables in the model. A 1-unit

Figure 3-28 Example of dummy variable regression.
© *Cengage Learning, 2012.*

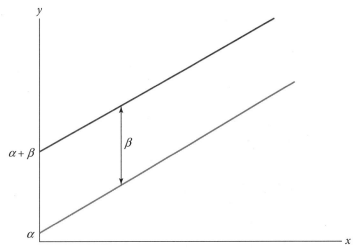

increase here describes the increase from less than high school to high school/GED or the increase from high school/GED to more than high school. The slope implies that a 1-unit increase represents the same-size increase regardless of whether the increase is from less than high school to high school/GED or from high school/GED to more than high school. This may not be the case and it may be more appropriate to treat the educational attainment variable as a categorical variable without order (nominal variable). This means that educational attainment is included in the regression model by using dummy variables. Because educational attainment has three levels, two dummy variables are required. If high school is made the reference, dummy variables for less than high school and for GED/high school should be added to the regression model.

- The dummy variable lessHS takes on a value of 1 if the pregnant woman attained less than a high school degree and 0 otherwise.
- The dummy variable GEDHS takes on a value of 1 if the pregnant woman attained a GED or high school degree and 0 otherwise.
- If lessHS = 0 and GEDHS = 0, the subject must have obtained more than a high school degree.

The model becomes:

$$\text{Change} = \alpha + \beta_1(\text{water}) + \beta_2(\text{hgb9}) + \beta_3(\text{lessHS}) + \beta_4(\text{GEDHS}) + \varepsilon$$

The adjusted mean difference in hemoglobin change for those with less than high school compared to those with more than high school is β_3. The adjusted mean difference in hemoglobin change for those with GED/high school compared to those with more than a high school degree is β_4. The result of including educational attainment as two dummy variables is three parallel regression planes: one for those with less than high school (lessHS = 1 and GEDHS = 0); one for those with high school/GED (lessHS = 0 and GEDHS = 1); one for those with more than high school (lessHS = 0 and GEDHS = 0).

Interpreting the Results of a Multiple Linear Regression

RESEARCH QUESTION:
How is the hemoglobin change related to tap water consumption, baseline hemoglobin, and maternal factors (education, age, and smoking status prior to pregnancy)?

Suppose a multiple linear regression is conducted using the hemoglobin change as the response variable. In addition to tap water consumption and baseline hemoglobin, it is of interest to determine how other factors (baseline hemoglobin [hgb9], prenatal care [prenatal], mother's education [ed], mother's age [age], and mother's smoking status prior to pregnancy [psmoke]) are related to the hemoglobin change.

The multiple linear regression model for this research question is

$$\text{Change} = \alpha + \beta_1(\text{water}) + \beta_2(\text{hgb9}) + \beta_3(\text{prenatal}) + \beta_4(\text{ed0}) + \beta_5(\text{ed1}) + \beta_6(\text{age}) + \beta_7(\text{psmoke}) + \varepsilon$$

where ε is independent and comes from a normal distribution with mean of 0 and constant variance. Using statistical software, the following output results from implementing this multiple linear regression (Table 3-14).

The overall test results in an F-statistic of 72.69 with a small p-value ($p < 0.0001$). Therefore, there is sufficient evidence to reject the global null hypothesis and to continue on to investigate which variables are related to hemoglobin change. The R^2 for this model is very good for observational studies, indicating that 44% of the variability in hemoglobin change can be explained by the variables in the model. With the exception of age and baseline hemoglobin, all of the variables in the multiple linear regression are significant ($p < 0.05$). In other words, the slopes associated with the variables (except for age and baseline hemoglobin) are statistically different from 0. Typically, the results of a multiple linear regression are presented in a table with the estimates, confidence intervals, and p-values (or asterisks to denote $p < 0.05$). A footnote regarding the R^2 may also be included (Table 3-15).

TABLE 3-14 RESULTS OF A MULTIPLE LINEAR REGRESSION

Dependent Variable: Change					
Analysis of Variance					
Source	DF	Sum of Squares	Mean Square	F-Value	Pr > F
Model	7	52.5759875	7.5108554	72.69	<0.0001
Error	656	67.7866303	0.1033333		
Corrected total	663	120.3626178			

R^2 0.436813

Results of the Regression Analysis				
	Parameter Estimate	Standard Error	t-Value	Pr > $|t|$
Intercept	2.392035992	0.29389949	8.14	<0.0001
water	0.001464796	0.00014651	10.00	<0.0001
hgb9	0.031447506	0.01675783	1.88	0.0610
prenatal 0	0.222763409	0.02599150	8.57	<0.0001
prenatal 1	0.000000000	.	.	.
psmoke 0	−0.170357816	0.02821071	−6.04	<0.0001
psmoke 1	0.000000000	.	.	.
age	−0.006481127	0.00789389	−0.82	0.4119
ed 0	0.485434784	0.05275459	9.20	<0.0001
ed 1	0.248138089	0.05146066	4.82	<0.0001
ed 2	0.000000000	.	0.01	

© Cengage Learning, 2012.

TABLE 3-15 TABLE OF REGRESSION RESULTS

	Parameter Estimate	95% CI	p-value
Intercept	2.39	(1.82, 2.97)	<0.0001
Tap water consumption (10 L)	0.015	(0.012, 0.018)	<0.0001
Baseline Hgb (g/dL)	0.03	(0, 0.06)	0.0610
Age (years)	−0.01	(−0.02, 0.01)	0.4119
Adequate prenatal care			
Yes	−0.22	(−0.27, −0.17)	<0.0001
No	Ref	—	
Prior smoking			
No	−0.17	(−0.23, −0.12)	<0.0001
Yes	Ref	—	
Educational attainment			
Less HS	0.49	(0.38, 0.59)	<0.0001
HS/GED	0.25	(0.15, 0.35)	<0.0001
More than HS	Ref	—	

R^2 for the model is 0.4368.

© Cengage Learning, 2012.

The results of the regression analysis can be interpreted like the simple linear regression analysis; there are just more slopes to investigate. Unlike a simple linear regression, however, these estimates represent adjusted estimates because all of the estimates were obtained using all the variables in the model. Therefore, interpretations for specific variables need to mention that the relationship between the response and the regressor has been adjusted for the other variables in the model.

The estimate for tap water consumption obtained for the multiple linear regression is again quite small ($\hat{\beta} = 0.0015$, SE $= 0.00015$). Part of the reason is the fact that a 1-L change in tap water consumption is not a very big change; so the small increment would not be expected to have much of an impact on hemoglobin change. As in simple linear regression, counting in 10 L instead of 1 L may be a more appropriate increment. Therefore, Table 3-15 includes the slope estimate associated with a 10-L increase.

CONCLUSION: The overall model did a fairly good job at explaining differences in hemoglobin changes among pregnant women ($R^2 = 0.44$). A positive linear relationship was found for hemoglobin change and tap water consumption ($p < 0.0001$). For every 10-L increase in tap water consumption, it is estimated that the hemoglobin change will increase by 0.015 g/dL (95% CI: 0.012, 0.018), controlling for all other variables in the model. Although not statistically significant ($p = 0.0610$), an expected positive association was observed between baseline hemoglobin and hemoglobin change, suggesting that pregnant women with larger baseline values tend to have larger observed hemoglobin changes. Education, prenatal care, and prior smoking were also found to be related to hemoglobin changes, even after controlling for the other variables in the model. Specifically, a dose-response relationship was observed with education, indicating that greater educational attainment results in smaller hemoglobin changes; the adjusted mean difference in hemoglobin changes for less-HS compared to greater-than-HS attainment is 0.49 g/dL ($p < 0.0001$) and for HS/GED compared to greater-than-HS degree is 0.25 g/dL ($p < 0.0001$). Finally, when compared to smokers prior to pregnancy, nonsmokers have a 0.17 g/dL ($p < 0.0001$) lower adjusted mean difference in hemoglobin change.

Confounding

Some regressors are included in the regression model not because they are particularly interesting, but because they might interrupt the relationship between response and explanatory variables. Including these variables in the model allows the investigator to control or adjust for their effects. Variables that are not of primary importance but that are collected and included in the model because they could potentially influence the relationship between the response and explanatory variables are called **confounding variables**.

A variable is a confounding variable (also known as a *confounder*) when it is suspected of impacting the relationship between the explanatory and response variables. Public health data often result from observational studies, in which the investigator may not have control over who is exposed, who gets the intervention, or who has a particular value on an explanatory variable of interest. In such cases, other factors may be involved in explaining why a subject has a particular outcome and a particular value for the explanatory variable. These other factors—confounders—may alter the relationship between the response and the explanatory variable and may prevent the investigator from making accurate conclusions.

The premise of any regression analysis is that the explanatory variable(s) explain the changes in the response variable. However, confounding variables can cause a regression analysis to suggest misleading results. For example, suppose it is known that women who do not receive prenatal care are likely to drink more tap water. Additionally, it is known that women who do not receive prenatal care are more likely to experience greater decreases in hemoglobin over the course of the pregnancy. Therefore, the

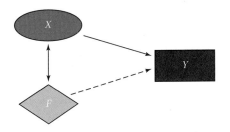

Figure 3-29 Diagram of relationship of explanatory, response, and confounding variables.
© *Cengage Learning, 2012.*

Legend: X = exposure to herbicides through drinking water
F = prenatal care
Y = change in hemoglobin

amount of prenatal care is related to both hemoglobin change and tap water consumption, making the amount of prenatal care a potential confounding variable. The amount of prenatal care that a woman receives becomes a confounding variable because it is unclear whether the hemoglobin changes are due to drinking more tap water or to the lack of prenatal care. In Figure 3-29, although prenatal care (F) is not a variable of primary interest in explaining the relationship between exposure to herbicides through drinking water (X) and hemoglobin changes (Y), F must be considered because it impacts the relationship of the explanatory and response variables.

Confounding is a common problem in public health studies because the studies are generally observational and involve the comparison of groups. In this example, although the goal may be to compare maternal outcomes based on exposure to herbicides in the water, the investigator may not have the choice of deciding who is exposed. Ideally, an investigator allows random chance to choose the exposed and unexposed groups. By randomly assigning the groups, the groups end up being fairly similar. This means that the same confounding variables that impact the exposed also impact the unexposed. When comparisons are made between randomly assigned groups, the impacts of the confounding cancel out so that only the relationship between the response and explanatory variables remain. In public health, however, investigators do not always have the luxury of random assignment to exposure groups. In fact, many times public health questions involve comparisons where assigning participants to groups is unethical. Examples are exposure to violence, smoking, lead paint, and even herbicides. Randomly assigning some children to be exposed to lead paint in order to compare developmental outcomes would be unethical. Similarly, assigning individuals to smoke cigarettes in order to examine differences in health outcomes would be unacceptable.

In this study, exposure to herbicides in drinking water entails the potential for harm, and randomly assigning pregnant women to be exposed to herbicides or not would be unethical. Therefore, investigating the impacts of herbicides in the water depends on how much tap water the pregnant woman decides to drink on her own. Because the pregnant women get to decide their levels of exposure to herbicides in the water, the impact of tap water consumption on hemoglobin changes may be confounded by other variables related to the choice of drinking water. In such cases, researchers must control for potential confounding variables to investigate relationships between the exposure and response variables. One way to adjust for potential confounders is to use regression models. Therefore, although the research questions may simply be a comparison between groups (Chapter 2), more complicated analyses are required because of confounding.

Analysis of Covariance and Adjusted Means

The principles of multiple linear regression can be used to control for potential confounding variables. Because the estimates that result from a multiple linear regression are adjusted for everything else in the model, including confounders in the model implies that the estimates associated with the exposure variables have been adjusted for the effects of the confounders. Many times an exposure variable is a categorical variable, the levels of the variable are the levels of exposure, and the research question involves comparing the outcome among those levels. The group exposure variable is included in the regression model as a dummy variable(s), and when dummy and continuous regressors are mixed, the multiple linear regression is often referred to as *analysis of covariance (ANCOVA)*. Analysis of covariance can be thought of as the combination of an ANOVA and a multiple linear regression with continuous or ordinal regressors. Therefore, ANCOVA is often used when the research question involves the comparison of group means, but it is necessary to account for potential confounding variables.

Although a research question may involve simply the comparison of means, either through a two-sample *t*-test or a one-way ANOVA (Chapter 2), the presence of confounding may prevent this simple analysis. Group means that do not take confounding into consideration are referred to as *unadjusted means*, and means resulting from regressions or ANCOVAs are called *adjusted means*. In any multiple linear regression, the parameters (βs) associated with the explanatory variable provide a description of the relationship of the explanatory variable to the response variable while controlling for other variables in the model. When the explanatory variable is a dummy variable(s), the parameter is really a mean difference. Therefore, when the other variables in the model are confounders, the parameters (βs) associated with dummy exposure variables are still the true mean difference between exposure levels, but the mean differences have been adjusted for the confounders.

For example, in Chapter 2 the goal was to use the water consumption groups to determine whether a relationship existed between exposure to herbicides and hemoglobin change. In this example, the water consumption group is really the explanatory variable. Ideally, a comparison of hemoglobin changes among the three water consumption groups would provide an answer to the research question of whether herbicides have an adverse effect on maternal hemoglobin outcomes. In Chapter 2, this comparison was performed using a one-way ANOVA, and the groups were determined to be different with respect to hemoglobin change. However, this analysis was too simplistic. The groups were not assigned by random chance but were based on the type of water the participant chose to consume during pregnancy. A simple comparison among these three groups is not possible, however, because the pregnant women in these three groups differ on other variables that may impact hemoglobin changes.

Table 3-16 shows that the groups are different with respect to baseline hemoglobin, income, prenatal care, mother's education, mother's age, and mother's smoking status. For this sample, women who consumed only tap water had lower baseline hemoglobin, lower incomes, and lower high school graduation rates. Furthermore, they also had higher percentages reporting prepregnancy smoking and the lowest percentages receiving adequate prenatal care. Investigators may reasonably assume that baseline hemoglobin, income, education, prenatal care, and smoking may all impact how the hemoglobin changes during pregnancy. Determining whether a variable is a confounder often depends on the literature and/or the investigator's knowledge about the variables. However, according to the definition of a confounder (a variable that is related to both the response and the explanatory variable), it is possible to investigate the data to determine whether a variable is a potential confounder. Table 3-16 identifies variables that may be related to group membership; so it remains to determine whether these variables are also related to the response, the hemoglobin change. For continuous confounding variables, correlations between the outcome and the potential confounder can be investigated, while the mean of the response can be compared for different levels of a categorical confounding variable (Table 3-17).

All of these potential confounding variables exhibited a relationship with hemoglobin change, suggesting that these variables should be used to adjust the mean hemoglobin change for the three exposure groups. Even though weight gain does not appear to be related to the exposure group or the hemoglobin change in this example, weight gain is often considered a confounder when investigating maternal outcomes during pregnancy. So baseline hemoglobin [hgb9], income [inc], prenatal care [prenatal], parity [parity] mother's education [ed], mother's age [age], mother's smoking status [psmoke], and weight gain [wtgain] are potential confounders. Hence, it is unclear whether the

RESEARCH QUESTION:
Do differences exist in the hemoglobin change for women who are exposed to herbicides (tap water only), marginal exposure to herbicides (both tap and bottled water), and no exposure (bottled water only), controlling for potential confounders?

TABLE 3-16 CHARACTERISTICS OF THE THREE WATER CONSUMPTION GROUPS

	Tap Only (N =)	Bottled Only (N =)	Both (N =)
Age (years)	*n = 270*	*n = 315*	*n = 394*
Mean (SD)	25.03 (1.907)	27.11 (1.467)	25.00 (1.336)
Median (min, max)	25.1 (18.9, 30.7)	27.1 (22.9, 31.0)	25.0 (21.3, 28.9)
Income ($10K)	*n = 270*	*n = 312*	*n = 393*
Mean (SD)	3.75 (1.434)	4.06 (1.775)	3.92 (1.702)
Median (min, max)	3.3 (2.2, 10.9)	3.5 (2.2, 12.2)	3.5 (2.2, 11.8)
Weight Gain (lb)	*n = 270*	*n = 315*	*n = 394*
Mean (SD)	41.60 (4.106)	42.01 (4.152)	41.95 (3.937)
Median (min, max)	41.5 (29.5, 56.4)	42.1 (30.0, 51.7)	42.0 (30.5, 52.9)
Adequate Prenatal Care			
No	175 (64.8%)	52 (16.5%)	167 (42.4%)
Yes	95 (35.2%)	263 (83.5%)	227 (57.6%)
Smoked Prior to Pregnancy			
No	183 (67.8%)	261 (82.9%)	297 (75.4%)
Yes	87 (32.2%)	54 (17.1%)	97 (24.6%)
Education			
Less HS	149 (55.2%)	46 (14.6%)	141 (35.8%)
HS/GED	111 (41.1%)	238 (75.6%)	218 (55.3%)
College +	10 (3.7%)	31 (9.8%)	35 (8.9%)
Number of Previous Births (parity)			
None	45 (16.7%)	48 (15.2%)	57 (14.5%)
One	137 (50.7%)	167 (53.0%)	211 (53.6%)
Two	78 (28.9%)	92 (29.2%)	115 (29.2%)
Three or more	10 (3.7%)	8 (2.5%)	11 (2.8%)

© Cengage Learning, 2012.

differences observed in the hemoglobin changes between the three groups in the ANOVA (Chapter 2) were due to the consumption of tap water exposed to herbicides or due to the characteristics of the groups. To address the relationship between herbicide exposure and hemoglobin changes, adjustments for these confounders need to be made, and they can be made using ANCOVA.

The ANCOVA is not really different from any other multiple linear regression. The discussion of partitioning the variability, overall F-tests, partial correlations, and specific inferences for slopes all remain the same. The difference is really in the focus of the analysis. The goal is simply to determine whether there are differences in the responses for different groups, controlling for confounding variables. In this example, the water consumption variable is *group* and has three levels (1 = tap only, 2 = bottled only, and 3 = both tap and bottled). Using the bottled-only group as the reference, the two remaining categories are tap-only and both. Therefore, the model includes two βs for the water consumption groups, and these βs represent the true mean difference in hemoglobin change between tap-only and bottled-only and between both and bottled-only,

TABLE 3-17 **THE RELATIONSHIP OF HEMOGLOBIN CHANGE AND POTENTIAL CONFOUNDERS**

	Hemoglobin Change		
	N	Mean	Std Dev
Level of Prenatal			
0	394	3.38297599	0.55755192
1	585	2.66294448	0.74986808
Level of Psmoke			
0	741	2.85958095	0.76875326
1	238	3.24271251	0.67768708
Level of Ed			
0	336	3.42181931	0.54749191
1	567	2.73918574	0.75039195
2	76	2.47191391	0.69406695
Level of Parity			
0	150	2.67920797	0.74493677
1	515	2.88996418	0.75126285
2	285	3.16910409	0.74649307
3	29	3.35543597	0.60571737
Pearson Correlation Coefficients Prob > |r| under H0: Rho = 0			
hgb9			
r		−0.19182	
p-value		<0.0001	
n		979	
age			
r		−0.46205	
p-value		<0.0001	
n		979	
inc			
r		−0.10737	
p-value		0.0008	
n		975	

© Cengage Learning, 2012.

controlling for all other variables in the model. Because the parameters (βs) are really adjusted mean differences, the primary focus of the analysis is to estimate these parameters and to determine whether these differences are significantly different from 0. Mean differences that are 0 suggest that the means of the two groups are the same. Therefore the ANCOVA model is as follows:

$$\text{Change} = \alpha + \beta_1(\text{group1}) + \beta_2(\text{group3}) + \beta_3(\text{hgb9}) + \beta_4(\text{prenatal}) + \beta_5(\text{ed0})$$
$$+ \beta_6(\text{ed1}) + \beta_7(\text{age}) + \beta_8(\text{psmoke}) + \beta_9(\text{parity0}) + \beta_{10}(\text{parity1})$$
$$+ \beta_{11}(\text{parity2}) + \beta_{12}(\text{inc}) + \beta_{13}(\text{wtgain}) + \varepsilon$$

where ε are independent and come from a normal distribution with mean of 0 and constant variance.

RESEARCH HYPOTHESIS: The true mean difference (β_1) is not 0, after including all the other variables in the model (this implies that all the other βs $\neq$ 0 too).

NULL HYPOTHESIS: The true mean difference (β_1) is 0, after including all the other variables in the model (this implies that all the other βs $\neq$ 0).

RESEARCH HYPOTHESIS: The true mean difference (β_2) is not 0, after including all the other variables in the model (this implies that all the other βs $\neq$ 0 too).

NULL HYPOTHESIS: The true mean difference (β_2) is 0, after including all the other variables in the model (this implies that all the other βs $\neq$ 0).

By means of statistical software, the results from the ANCOVA can be used to test these hypotheses and to investigate the comparison of herbicide exposure means while controlling for confounding variables (Table 3-18). It is clear from the adjusted sums of squares associated with the group effect that there is a significant ($p < 0.0001$) association with water consumption type (tap-only, bottle-only, and both) and hemoglobin change, after controlling for potential confounders. Specifically, the estimate $(\hat{\beta}_1)$ associated with the mean difference in hemoglobin change between tap-only and bottle-only is 1.11 (SE = 0.033), and the combination compared to bottle-only has an estimate of $\hat{\beta}_2 = 1.14$ with an SE = 0.027, controlling for the potential confounding variables. Most of the results of the ANCOVA analysis have significant p-values ($p < 0.05$). However, the variables of income, weight gain, age, and baseline hemoglobin are not significant. If these variables are removed from the analysis, the parameter estimates no longer represent adjusted means where these variables have been controlled for. If the literature suggests that these are important confounders, including them (or a subset of them) in the model might be useful even though the p-values are not statistically significant. Again, the goal of this analysis is to get better estimates for the water consumption groups, adjusting for confounding variables. Therefore, many times the results of the ANCOVA are presented in a table where the adjusted means are emphasized, and the confounding variables included in the model are noted (Table 3-19), in addition to a description of the adjusted means in a table, a plot of the means, as described in Chapter 2, may also be helpful (Figure 3-30).

In a table like Table 3-19, confidence interval or standard errors are generally presented instead of p-values. The reason is that the goal in these types of studies is to estimate the adjusted means, and, given multiple groups, presenting the p-values for the multiple comparisons can become distracting. However, p-values for comparing the three groups can be easily obtained (tap-only versus bottled-only ($p < 0.0001$); both versus bottled-only ($p < 0.0001$); tap-only versus both ($p = 0.3767$). Notice that the comparison of tap-only versus both is not statistically significant, suggesting that these two groups have similar average hemoglobin changes, controlling for all other variables in the model.

The estimates obtained from the ANCOVA for tap-only and both were $\hat{\beta}_1 = 1.11$ ($p < 0.0001$) and $\hat{\beta}_2 = 1.14$ ($p < 0.0001$), respectively. To demonstrate that these estimate the adjusted mean difference, consider the adjusted means for tap-only and bottled-only, 3.375 and 2.262. The difference between these two adjusted means is $3.375 - 2.262 = 1.112$, which is $\hat{\beta}_1$. Likewise, the difference between the adjusted means for both types and bottled-only is $3.398 - 2.262 = 1.136$, or $\hat{\beta}_2$. Therefore, the research question can be addressed by making inferences about the adjusted slopes or the adjusted means.

CONCLUSION: Even after controlling for potential confounding variables, the hemoglobin change is smaller in pregnant women who drank only bottled water when compared to those that drank only tap water ($\hat{\beta}_1 = 1.11, p < 0.0001$) or drank a combination of tap and bottled water ($\hat{\beta}_2 = 1.14, p < 0.0001$). Because these p-values are small ($p < 0.0001$), the null hypothesis suggesting no difference between these two groups can be rejected. Furthermore, the adjusted means for tap-only and both water types are similar ($p = 0.3767$). This further supports the association with drinking herbicide exposed water and hemoglobin change.

TABLE 3-18 COMPARISON OF HERBICIDE EXPOSURE WHILE CONTROLLING CONFOUNDING VARIABLES

Dependent Variable: Change					
Source	DF	Sum of Squares	Mean Square	F-Value	Pr > F
Model	13	472.1973408	36.3228724	402.50	<0.0001
Error	961	86.7240868	0.0902436		
Corrected total	974	558.9214276			

R^2 0.844837

Source	DF	Type III SS	Mean Square	F-Value	Pr > F
group	2	161.2204959	80.6102480	893.25	<0.0001
hgb	1	0.0034293	0.0034293	0.04	0.8455
prenatal	1	17.7437852	17.7437852	196.62	<0.0001
psmoke	1	8.4126929	8.4126929	93.22	<0.0001
age	1	0.0004578	0.0004578	0.01	0.9432
wtgain	1	0.0108880	0.0108880	0.12	0.7284
ed	2	24.1242339	12.0621170	133.66	<0.0001
inc	1	0.0450163	0.0450163	0.50	0.4802
parity	3	26.6100698	8.8700233	98.29	<.0001

Results of Regression Analysis					
	Level	Parameter Estimate	Standard Error	t-Value	Pr > |t|
intercept		3.368175970	0.25990822	12.96	<0.0001
group	1	1.112610511	0.03321077	33.50	<0.0001
group	3	1.135577090	0.02746793	41.34	<0.0001
group	2	0.000000000	.	.	.
hgb9		0.002725492	0.01398144	0.19	0.8455
prenatal	0	0.298293607	0.02127301	14.02	<0.0001
prenatal	1	0.000000000	.	.	.
psmoke	0	−0.219163153	0.02269908	−9.66	<0.0001
psmoke	1	0.000000000	.	.	.
age		−0.000444017	0.00623394	−0.07	0.9432
wtgain		−0.000830831	0.00239192	−0.35	0.7284
ed	0	0.561739523	0.03915003	14.35	<.0001
ed	1	0.251598172	0.04171527	6.03	<0.0001
ed	2	0.000000000	.	.	.
inc		0.000000543	0.00000077	0.71	0.4802
parity	0	−0.618276112	0.06110421	−10.12	<0.0001
parity	1	−0.382049202	0.05749977	−6.64	<0.0001
parity	2	−0.143942217	0.05868328	−2.45	0.0143
parity	3	0.000000000	.	.	.

TABLE 3-19 ADJUSTED AND UNADJUSTED MEANS OF HEMOGLOBIN CHANGE

Water Consumption Group	Unadjusted Means (95% CI)	Adjusted* Means (95% CI)
Tap-only (n = 270)	3.49 (3.42, 3.52)	3.38 (3.32, 3.43)
Both tap and bottled (n = 393)	3.34 (3.30, 3.38)	3.40 (3.35, 3.44)
Bottled-only (n = 312)	2.04 (1.99, 2.09)	2.26 (2.21, 2.32)

*Adjusted for baseline hemoglobin, age, weight gain, income, education, parity, prior smoking status, and prenatal care.

© Cengage Learning, 2012.

Figure 3-30 Plot of adjusted means.
© *Cengage Learning, 2012.*

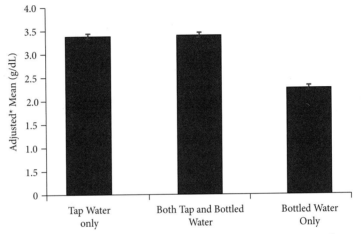

*Adjusted for baseline hemoglobin, age, weight gain, income, education, parity, prior smoking status, and prenatal care.

Error bars represent 95% confidence intervals,

Cause Versus Association

Regardless of whether the explanatory variable is continuous, ordinal, categorical, or dichotomous, the discussion of the relationship between explanatory and response variables has been very carefully worded. Explanatory variables were defined as variables that explain a change in a response. Another way of thinking of explanatory variables is that changes in an explanatory variable cause a change in the response. Many times regression models are employed because investigators want to understand the cause-and-effect relationship of explanatory and response variables. However, the word "cause" has been purposely omitted from the discussion of explanatory and response variables. Words like "association" and "relationship" have been used instead—words that are not as strong in meaning as cause—because of confounding variables. The presence of confounding variables has the potential to change the relationship of explanatory and response variables. Therefore, although tap water consumption and hemoglobin change appear to have a relationship, stating that increased tap water consumption *causes* a greater hemoglobin change is not appropriate. Even when a multiple linear regression is performed and confounding variables are included, a significant slope cannot be interpreted as the explanatory and response variables having a cause-and-effect relationship. The reason is that using a regression adjusts only for the confounding variables that have been measured. As long as the subjects have control over the amount of exposure or the group they belong to, unmeasured confounders may impact the relationship between the explanatory and response variables. For this reason, when dealing with observational studies where confounding may be present, the term "association" is preferred, and care must be taken not to overinterpret the results of the regression.

Diagnostics

The assumptions of a simple linear regression model, ANOVA, multiple linear regression model, or ANCOVA are always the same; the model assumptions are predominantly assumptions about the errors. The assumptions for the model are as follows:

1. *The subjects are independent.* The hemoglobin change in one pregnant woman has nothing to do with the hemoglobin change in another pregnant woman. If the subjects are independent, then the errors are independent as well.
2. *The errors come from a normal distribution* that has the following:
   a. A mean of 0
   b. A constant variance (represented as σ^2)

These assumptions can be checked by considering the residuals. The same strategies that were presented for investigating the diagnostics with one regressor in simple linear regression can be used to assess violations with multiple regressors.

With the additional regressors involved in multiple linear regression and ANCOVA, however, an additional assumption is needed: that the regressors are not highly correlated. Recall that the estimates of the regression equation are obtained by simultaneously regressing all the regressors on the response. If any of the regressors are highly correlated, then the estimates become unstable and inferences (statistical tests and confidence intervals) become unreliable. If the regressors are highly correlated, the regressors are *co-linear,* and the regression is said to suffer from **multicollinearity**.

If any two regressors are highly correlated, the correlation between the two regressors is close to -1 or 1, then the two regressors are considered to be co-linear. If any two regressors are co-linear, then the two regressors are essentially trying to explain the same variation in the response. In other words, when the highly correlated regressors are included in the model, there is significant overlap in the contribution to the sum of squares model (Figure 3-31).

Multicollinearity is problematic because the goal of a regression is to use the regressors to help explain the variability in responses. Although one of these regressors may help to explain a significant portion of the variability in the response (y), if multiple regressors explaining the same aspect of the response variable are included in the regression, then the part that is explained by the regressors individually is minimal (Figure 3-31). When two collinear regressors are included in the model, the least squares regression results in slope estimates for these regressors that are often similar

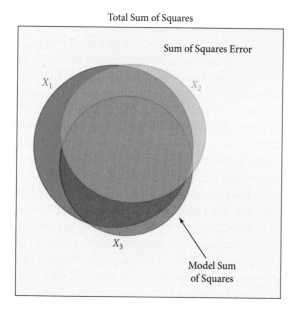

Figure 3-31 Visual example of multicollinearity.
© *Cengage Learning, 2012.*

and large but with opposite signs (one is positive and one is negative). They appear to "cancel out" each other's effects. In addition and even more problematic for statistical tests and confidence intervals, the standard errors of these estimates are inflated. Having large standard errors can result in hypothesis tests indicating that the slopes are not significantly different from 0 when they really are.

Although the circles representing the collinear regressors are large (Figure 3-31), they overlap so much that the individual contribution of the regressors ends up being quite small. Because the hypothesis test for the slopes involves testing for the individual contribution of the regressor (after all other regressors have been accounted for), the individual contribution appears to be quite small. Hence, the overall F-test that determines whether the regressors explain the variability in the response could be significant (small p-value) because the area covered by the circles is large. However, the individual tests on the regressors could be insignificant (large p-value) because the individual slices of the circles with no overlap are quite small. One of the solutions to dealing with multicollinearity is to remove regressors until all of the regressors in the model are not highly correlated.

Variable Selection

One of the most difficult tasks in completing a multiple linear regression analysis is deciding which variables to include. Including too many variables, can result in biased estimates with inflated standard errors while including too few variables can overlook important relationships. If performing a primary data analysis, the problem is a little more straightforward because the data are collected to answer a particular question. However, if performing a secondary data analysis, the problem can be considerably more complicated.

There are two main reasons for performing a regression analysis: (1) forecasting or prediction and (2) covariate-adjustment (adjusting for confounders). The strategies employed in variable selection depend on the purpose.

Forecasting or Prediction

When forecasting is the primary goal of the regression analysis, the research question usually involves trying to predict an outcome based on values from explanatory variables. Choosing an appropriate set of explanatory variables is very important because the variables need to do a good job of explaining changes in the outcome. So the model-fit measures (R^2, for example) are particularly important. If the regression model does not fit the data, then the resulting prediction equation will not do a very good job of forecasting outcomes. In addition, outliers and influence points must be considered because they may alter the regression estimates. Furthermore, the assumptions of the regression analysis must be rigorously tested because the model is being used to predict outcomes.

A good strategy for performing a regression analysis for forecasting or prediction is to follow the strategies for regression diagnostics. Plotting the data provides a good first step to identifying variables that may be related to the outcome, as well as the opportunity to visually assess whether transformations may be warranted. Once plots have been created and reviewed, a set of potential variables can be identified. Some of these variables may be measuring the same thing; so the set of potential variables can be further reduced by removing variables that demonstrate multicollinearity. With this set of variables, a regression can be performed, the assumptions of the model checked, and potential outlier/influence points identified. Making appropriate corrections here can eliminate the need for certain variables or transformations. In evaluating the regression output, some variables may not really contribute to the prediction of the outcome. Diagnostic tools for model fit can again be used in deciding whether these variables should be in the model. Generally, this involves removing and adding variables one at a time to determine whether the removal or addition has an impact on the model fit.

Most statistical software packages have options for variable selection. Common procedures include forward, backward, and stepwise selection. However, relying solely on automated model selection strategies—including forward, backward, and stepwise selection—should generally be avoided. These methods may do a poor job because they cannot incorporate prior knowledge or the investigator's perspective. This is less of an issue when using regression methods for prediction/forecasting than when using regression models for adjusting for confounders.

Covariate-Adjustment

When adjustment for covariates or confounders is the primary goal of the regression analysis, the emphasis is on the interpretation of the regression coefficients (the slopes). The research question usually involves trying to compare two (or more) groups, and data are generally obtained from an observational study where these groups are defined by something other than random chance. To get a better estimate of the differences between groups, variables are included in the model that impact group assignment and the outcome of interest. Unlike regression analyses where prediction is the primary goal, the selection of variables has much more to do with published literature and an understanding of the groups/outcome. Although good model fit is important, the rationale for selecting a variable is based more on the context of the problem and less on statistical justification. The assumptions of the regression model should still be evaluated so that the most appropriate regression analysis is used. Remember that providing good estimates are the goal, and good estimates rely on using an appropriate model.

The first step to variable selection is to consult the literature. Identify variables that were used in other analyses and include them as potential covariates. A next step is to provide descriptive statistics (either through simple statistical tests or simple regressions). Variables that impact the outcome and the group assignment should be considered candidates in the regression analysis. A larger cutoff than 0.05 can be used to determine whether variables are potential candidates for the regression analysis (e.g., 0.2–0.3). If the p-value cutoff is stringent (e.g., $p < 0.05$), important variables may be omitted. However, when trying to determine whether a variable has an impact, do not focus entirely on the p-value; consider the statistics too.

In addition to these steps, implement strategies for regression diagnostics. In general, a complete regression analysis should include the following:

- Plots of the data (scatteplots of y versus x, as well as mean plots, box-and-whisker plots, and histograms)
- Descriptive statistics and simple statistical tests (simple linear regression, ANOVA, and chi-square tests)
- Checks for multicollinearity
- Investigation of outliers/influence points
- Check of model assumptions (verify the residuals are normally distributed and randomly scattered around 0 with constant variance)

Plotting the data provides a visual method for identifying variables that may be important, as well as the opportunity to visually assess whether transformations may be warranted. Once the literature has been consulted, simple tests have been performed, and plots have been created and reviewed, a set of potential variables can be identified. Some of these variables may be measuring the same thing; so the set of potential variables can be further reduced by removing variables that demonstrate multicollinearity. With this set of variables, a regression can be performed, the assumptions of the model can be checked, and potential outlier/influence points can be identified. Although outlier and influence points are generally not omitted, these points may cause issues in the regression estimates. In evaluating the regression output, some variables may not really contribute to understanding changes in the outcome. However, be careful in eliminating variables. If a variable is removed from the model, the estimates will no longer be adjusted for that variable. A decision must be made as to whether having that variable involved in the covariate-adjustment is important. Diagnostic tools for model fit should also be used to determine whether these variables should be in the model, but keep in mind that in public health research the reason for including the variables is typically not based on statistical rationale. Hence, relying on automated model selection strategies (forward, backward, and/or stepwise) has little justification in this setting.

Planning a Multiple Regression Study

There are many reasons to conduct a linear regression when multiple variables are involved. In general, the goal is to explain the variability in the outcome or to compare groups while controlling for other variables. When a study is planned that will involve multiple explanatory variables, estimating the sample size really depends on how much variability the explanatory variables can explain (measured by the size of the R^2). One option for estimating sample sizes in a multiple linear regression is to determine the sample size necessary to test whether the R^2 is equal to 0. For example, given five explanatory variables, a sample of 72 subjects will have at least 90% power to detect an R^2 of 0.2, assuming a two-sided significance level of 0.05. As the number of explanatory variables increases, so does the sample size (Figure 3-32)

Often, however, the goal of the multiple linear regression is simply to adjust for a confounder. In public health, research questions often involve simple comparisons of means but require more complicated analyses due to the adjustment for confounders. Although the analyses often require the ultimate use of a multiple linear regression or ANCOVA, studies comparing group means are generally planned using the sample size estimates for simple comparisons (presented in Chapter 2).

Figure 3-32 Examples of sample sizes for multiple linear regression.
© *Cengage Learning, 2012.*

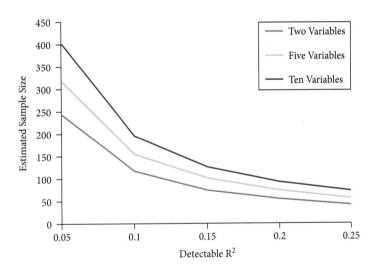

SUMMARY

This chapter began with an environmental health problem: groundwater impacted by an herbicide, atrazine. As in the public health application, the data presented in this chapter involved investigating maternal health outcomes for women exposed to water that had been affected by herbicides. The research question involved two continuous outcomes: hemoglobin change and tap water consumption. Specifically, it was of interest to investigate how the hemoglobin change during pregnancy is altered by the amount of tap water (exposed to herbicides) consumed.

Research questions involving clinical outcomes often result in continuous data, the level of detail is limited only by how precisely the instrument measures. Hence, graphical and numerical summaries are particularly important with continuous outcomes because they provide a mechanism for understanding and interpreting the data. When there are multiple continuous variables of interest, scatterplots and correlation estimates become even more important when trying to make sense of the collected data.

The most common analyses associated with continuous outcomes were explained in this chapter. Specifically, methods were presented for investigating associations with multiple variables. The use of regression techniques to predict an outcome or simply adjust for confounding was also discussed. Considerable detail was given to topics such as simple linear regression because the fundamental concepts can be modified and applied to many different types of regression models. One modification of the simple linear regression was discussed in this chapter: multiple linear regression. Regression models with multiple regressors are often used in analyzing public health data because this is one method for controlling for confounding variables. Further modifications can be made to multiple linear regression to account for outcomes that are not continuous. Because not every research question results in a continuous outcome, generalizing these methods to handle different types of outcome variables will be a component of the remaining chapters.

SUMMARY OF CHAPTER CONCEPTS

RESEARCH QUESTION	GRAPHICAL DESCRIPTIONS	NUMERICAL DESCRIPTIONS	STATISTICAL METHOD
Is there a linear relationship between two variables?	Scatterplot	Correlation	
Is there a linear relationship between a response and independent variable?	Scatterplot	Correlation slope	Simple linear regression
Is there a linear relationship between explanatory variables and the response variable?	Scatterplots	Correlations slopes	Multiple linear regression
Is there a difference between the groups, controlling for other variables?	Mean plots Scatterplots	Unadjusted and adjusted means (SE) Slopes (adjusted mean differences)	ANCOVA

KEY TERMS

association

explanatory variable

response variable

outlier

influence points

regressor

dummy variable

adjusted mean

confounding variables

multicolinearity

PRACTICE WITH DATA

1. DESCRIBING THE DATA

a. Provide descriptive statistics for the correlation between tap water consumption, hemoglobin change, and weight gain.

b. Use a scatterplot to display the relationship between tap water consumption and weight gain. What does the plot show?

2. SIMPLE LINEAR REGRESSION

a. Perform a linear regression to investigate the relationship between tap water consumption and weight gain. Provide the ANOVA table. What can you conclude?

b. Estimate (using a 95% confidence interval) the true slope associated with tap water consumption. Interpret.

c. Provide a plot of the studentized residuals. Use the plot to investigate the model assumptions. Are there any violations of the model assumptions? If so, suggest recommendations for addressing these violations.

d. Use the studentized residuals and create a normal probability (Q-Q) plot. What can you conclude?

3. MULTIPLE LINEAR REGRESSION

a. What is the model for the multiple linear regression when weight gain is a dependent variable and the explanatory variables are hemoglobin change, tap water consumption, and age. Be sure to define all symbols and model assumptions.

b. Provide the global null and research hypotheses (defining all symbols) for investigating the relationship of hemoglobin change, tap water consumption, and age on weight gain.

c. Perform a multiple linear regression for the model described in part (a). Write up the results of the regression. Be sure to include a discussion of diagnostics and variable selection.

4. ANALYSIS OF COVARIANCE

a. Provide the null and research hypotheses (defining all symbols) for investigating the difference in mean weight gain for the two water consumption groups (tap-only and bottled-only), controlling for potential confounders. Potential confounders include education, parity, previous smoking.

b. Create a table providing the unadjusted and adjusted means. What can you conclude?

PRACTICE WITH CONCEPTS

1. Consider the following research questions/study scenarios. For each study, discuss the most appropriate methods for describing the data (graphically and numerically). What statistical method would be *most* appropriate for addressing the research questions? Be sure to provide a justification of the statistical method. Provide the appropriate regression model and statistical test when appropriate.

a. A study was performed to determine the differences in pain experienced by children with sickle cell disease (SCD) in inpatient and outpatient settings. Pain intensity (visual analog scale) was the primary outcome of interest, but potential confounders include age and physical activity.

b. Elderly subjects are participating in a trial to investigate the benefits of strength training. One of the outcomes is to investigate the expression levels of inflammatory biomarkers, a continuous variable. Is there a relationship between post-training expression levels and the intensity of the training (a continuous variable).

c. A workplace wellness program was instituted to improve employee health outcomes as related to obesity and cardiovascular health. Blood lipid levels were measured on employees prior to the implementation of the wellness program and five years later. Changes in blood lipid levels were the outcome of interest. Participants in the program were offered weekly health education meetings and time off for exercise. Data on the number of health education meetings attended, weight loss, and waist circumference were collected prior to and five years after the implementation of the wellness program. Is compliance with the program (measured by the number of meetings attended), weight loss, and changes in waist circumference related to changes in triglycerides?

d. Exposure to arsenic in drinking water during pregnancy may have an impact on infant outcomes. Infants born to mothers residing in two cities, one with arsenic concentrations in the drinking water and one without, are compared to investigate whether arsenic exposure is associated with smaller head circumferences. However, the two cities are different with respect to income, prenatal care, parity, and iron supplementation.

2. *Poor cardiorespiratory fitness predicts cardiovascular disease (CVD) risk. Low serum vitamin D level is also associated with an increased prevalence of CVD risk factors and all-cause mortality. Whether low serum vitamin D level independently predicts cardiorespiratory fitness in healthy adults without CVD is not known. The aim of this study was to determine the relationship between serum 25-hydroxy vitamin D [25(OH)D] concentration and cardiorespiratory fitness in healthy adults.* (Ardenstani et al., 2010)
   a. When investigating the relationship between aerobic exercise capacity (as measured by VO2max, a continuous variable) and serum concentration of vitamin D, the authors of this study report a Pearson correlation coefficient estimate of $r = 0.23$ with a p-value < 0.01. Interpret.
   b. Consider the outcome of serum concentration vitamin D and the predictor cardiorespiratory fitness. Provide a definition of confounding variables in the context of this study, and provide some examples of potential confounders.
   c. The authors indicate that a multiple linear regression was used to adjust for potential confounders. Explain how using multiple linear regression controls for confounding (conceptually).

3. *Maternal smoking during pregnancy can result in both pregnancy complications and reduced size of the fetus and neonate. Among women who smoke, genetic susceptibility to tobacco smoke also is a likely causative factor in adverse pregnancy outcomes. A prospective cohort study was conducted among 460 pregnant women who delivered live singletons in Sapporo, Japan, from 2002 to 2005. Multiple linear regression models were used to estimate associations of maternal smoking and polymorphisms in two genes encoding N-nitrosamine-metabolizing enzymes—NQO1 and CYP2E1—with birth size.* (Sasaki et al., 2008)
   a. Why was the use of multiple linear regression appropriate?
   b. Based on the results provided in the following table, what conclusions can be drawn about the relationship between smoking status and gene type with birth weight? Be sure to include a discussion of statistical inference in your conclusion.

	Parameter Estimate* (SE)	p-value
Maternal smoking during pregnancy		
Nonsmoker	Reference	—
Former Smoker	−31 (40)	0.443
Current Smoker	−148 (42)	<0.001
NQO1 genotype		
Pro/Ser + Ser/Ser	Reference	—
Pre/pro	−9 (32)	0.781
CYP2E1 genotype		
c1/c2 +c2/c2	Reference	—
c1/c1	−73 (32)	0.023

Source: Adapted from Table 2 (Sasaki et al.).

*Adjusted for maternal age, height, weight before pregnancy, weight gain during pregnancy, alcohol consumption during pregnancy, parity, infant gender, gestational age, and household income.

© Cengage Learning, 2012.

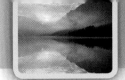
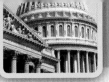
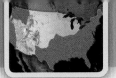
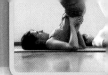

CHAPTER 4

categorical data comparisons and associations

When the possible values of a variable represent categories, data are referred to as *categorical*. Generally, categorical variables have a limited number of levels, or categories, and only these levels or categories occur; no values between categories are observed. Because of the gaps between the levels of a categorical variable, categorical data are considered to be discrete. Categorical data come in three forms:

- *Dichotomous—only two levels*: Dichotomous data are very common in public health problems: disease (yes/no), exposure (yes/no), or screening test (positive/negative).

- *Nominal—multiple levels without order*: Nominal variables are also quite common in public health. Many demographic variables are considered nominal variables: race, marital status, or type of housing.

- *Ordinal—multiple levels with order*: Severity of disease (mild, moderate, severe), a pain scale (0–10), or rankings are examples of ordinal variables. These are categorical variables whose categories have a natural ordering. Ordinal variables were also discussed in Chapter 2 (nonparametric methods). Analyses of these variables depend on whether the ordering is taken into account or not.

Categorical outcomes are the most common type of data collected in public health; many public health research questions naturally result in categorical outcomes. Any yes/no response, disease status, or health indicator is a categorical variable. Even when a continuous variable is of interest, these variables often have natural breaks or cutoffs that allow them to easily be treated as categorical variables.

For example, body mass index (BMI) is a continuous variable, but often the BMI measures are grouped into underweight, normal, overweight, and obese. Hence, whether collected with categories or later categorized, categorical data are prevalent in public health applications.

This chapter will focus on the common statistical methods for comparing categorical outcomes and investigating associations between categorical variables.

LEARNING OBJECTIVES

How do I describe categorical data?

Identify, create, and present appropriate descriptive statistics and figures specific for categorical data.

How do I make comparisons?

Identify appropriate statistical tests for making comparisons.

Understand when to use exact tests versus approximations.

Interpret the results of the statistical tests.

How do I investigate associations?

Identify, create, and present the appropriate measures of associations.

Utilize statistical inference to provide accurate interpretations.

What method do I use?

Identify the most appropriate method for the data.

Public Health Application

Malaria represents about 1.4% of the global burden of disease [1] and in Africa, it is the primary cause of disease burden as measured by Disability Adjusted Life Years (DALY) lost of 10.8% [2,3]. The continent bears over 90% of the global burden of about 2.7 million deaths attributable to malaria; and houses over 300 million people who suffer from this disease yearly, the worst hit being young children and pregnant women [2-4].

More than three quarter of global malaria deaths occur in under-five children living in malarious countries in sub-Saharan Africa (SSA) [5], where 25% of all childhood mortality below the age of five (about 800,000 young children [6]) is attributable to malaria [2]. Of those children who survive cerebral malaria, a severe form of the disease, more than 15% suffer neurological deficits [4,7], which include weakness, spasticity, blindness, speech problems and epilepsy. Where such children are poorly managed and do not have access to specialized educational facilities, these deficits may interfere with future learning and development [5].

About 30–40% of all fevers seen in health centres in Africa are due to malaria with huge seasonal variability between rainy and dry seasons. At the end of the dry season, it is less than 10% and more than 80% as the rainy season winds up [8].

In Nigeria, malaria is the leading cause of under-five mortality contributing 33% of all childhood deaths and 25% infant mortality. As a child will typically be sick of malaria between 3–4 times in one year, the disease is a major cause of absenteeism in school-aged children, thus impeding their educational and social development [5] and subsequently robbing the country of its future human resources.

(Korenromp, E.L., Miller, J., Cibulskis, R.E., Kabir, C.M., Alnwick D., Dye C. (2003). *Monitoring mosquito net coverage for malaria control in Africa: possession vs. use by children under 5 years.* Tropical Medicine & International Health, *8(8), 693–703. http://www.ncbi.nlm.nih.gov/pubmed/12869090)*

Data Description

To investigate the factors related to insecticide-treated net use, a cross-sectional study was conducted. In the study, a survey was given to the head of the household in a tropical region where malaria is a public health problem. Households were surveyed by using in-person interviews.

Households ($n = 1876$) in a tropical region owning an insecticide-treated net (ITN) were sampled and asked whether the ITN had been used the previous night. The head of the household was provided a questionnaire that included age of the head of household, a measure of household wealth, the miles to the nearest healthcare facility, whether the household was located in a rural or urban area, the family size in the household, and whether there was a child younger than 5 years old residing in the household. The type of roof for the household was also recorded (thatched, corrugated metal, or other). The measure of wealth was recorded as a 4-level ordinal variable: lowest 25%, next lowest, next highest, and highest 25%. The distance to the nearest healthcare facility was categorized into three levels: within 15 miles, between 15 and 50 miles, and greater than 50 miles. All questionnaires were completed with an interviewer and were conducted during the rainy season.

The primary goal of this study is to understand the factors associated with using insecticide-treated nets. The primary outcome is whether an ITN was used on the previous night.

DESCRIBING THE DATA

Because categorical data have a limited number of categories (or levels), describing the data means summarizing the possible categories and the number of subjects in particular categories. The most common numerical summaries are counts, proportions, and percentages. Graphically, pie charts and bar graphs are often used to describe categorical data.

This study involves several types of categorical data. The use of insecticide-treated nets is a dichotomous variable because it only has two levels: yes or no. The type of roof, which has three levels or categories, is another type of categorical variable, a nominal variable. Because this variable has no particular order (thatched, corrugated metal, and other), the ordering of the categories does not matter. The wealth and distance to a healthcare facility variables were also collected as categorical variables, except the categories do have an order. A wealth ranking of next-to-high is higher than a wealth ranking of next-to-low. Likewise, a family within 15 miles of a healthcare facility is closer than a family that has to travel more than 50 miles to a facility. Wealth and distance to healthcare are considered ordinal variables.

Graphical Summaries: Bar Graphs and Pie Charts

Bar graphs (introduced in Chapter 1) are often used as graphical representations of nominal and ordinal variables, where the heights of the bars indicate the number of percentage of subjects within a category. When the categorical variable is ordinal, the horizontal axis has a defined order because the order of the categories has meaning (Figure 4-1). Nominal data, on the other hand, do not have a specified order, and the horizontal axis of the bar graph can be ordered in any way but are most often ordered according to the heights of the bars (Figure 4-2).

Figure 4-1 Bar graph of wealth index.
© *Cengage Learning, 2012.*

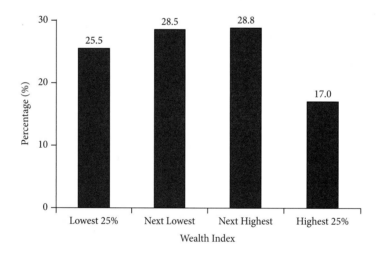

Figure 4-2 Bar graph of roof type.
© *Cengage Learning, 2012.*

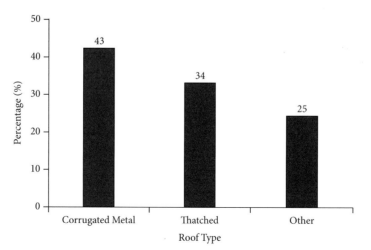

Pie charts (introduced in Chapter 1) can also be used to graphically describe categorical variables. However, because pie charts provide a description of how the parts relate to the whole, they are found less often in published works (Figure 4-3). Pie charts, however, may be very helpful in describing data for presentations where numerical summaries are harder to present.

Although dichotomous data, with only two categories to describe, can be described using either pie charts or bar graphs, the graphical summaries result in fairly simplistic pictures (Figure 4-4). Furthermore, these graphical summaries may be somewhat uninformative because there are only two categories. When the variable is dichotomous, once the number or proportion of subjects in one category is known, the remaining number or proportion of subjects automatically belongs to the other category.

However, when comparisons are of interest, combining the dichotomous variable with other variables in a bar graph can be very informative (Figure 4-5). For example, a description of the wealth according to insecticide-treated net use allows a visual comparison of net use differences for the wealth categories. In this example, the greatest differences in net use occur at the lowest and highest levels of the wealth index.

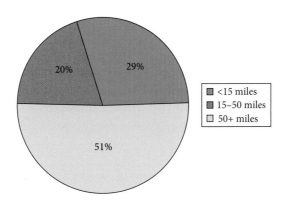

Figure 4-3 Pie chart of distance to healthcare.
© *Cengage Learning, 2012.*

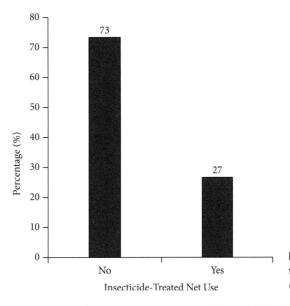

Figure 4-4 Bar graph of insecticide-treated net use.
© *Cengage Learning, 2012.*

Figure 4-5 Bar graph of wealth index by insecticide-treated net use.
© Cengage Learning, 2012.

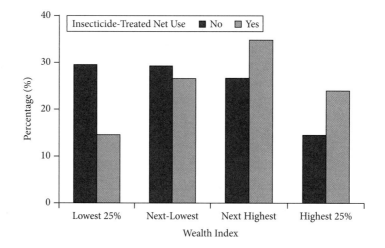

Numerical Summaries: Prevalence, Risk, and Odds

Numerical summaries provide an additional way to describe categorical data. Numerical summaries for categorical variables (introduced in Chapter 1) include counts (number of subjects in a category), proportions (number of subjects in a category out of the total number of subjects), and percentages (proportions multiplied by 100). Counts, percentages, and proportions can all be used in creating graphical descriptions of categorical data. However, the proportion serves as the building block for other useful numerical summaries (prevalence rates, risks, and odds). The proportion represents the fraction of the population with a particular characteristic or category. The population proportion is represented by p. Using a sample, the population proportion p is estimated by the sample proportion $\hat{p}$. The sample proportion, a statistic, is the fraction of the sample with a particular characteristic or category.

Application of Formula: SAMPLE PROPORTION

$$\hat{p} = \frac{\sum_{i=1}^{n} x_i}{n}$$

$x_i = 0$ or 1; Subjects with characteristic (success) are assigned a 1 and 0 otherwise

$n = $ The total number of subjects

What you need to calculate the proportion:

1. *Category count:* The number of subjects with the characteristic (success). In this example, 500 are using ITNs (assigned a 1) and 1376 are not (assigned a 0). Therefore, $\sum_{i}^{n} x_i = 500$.

2. *Total number of subjects:* The study includes 1876 households, $n = 1876$.

To calculate the proportion: Divide (1) by (2) = $500 \div 1876 = 0.27$, so $\hat{p} = 0.27$.

For the sample percentage, the sample proportion is multiplied by 100, $0.27 \times 100 = 27\%$.

The primary numerical summary in categorical data is the proportion. However, the proportion can be used in different ways to describe the data. In particular, prevalence rates, risks, and odds are all numerical summaries that involve proportions.

A **prevalence rate** is a proportion that describes a population at a specific point in time. It provides a summary of the proportion of subjects with a particular characteristic at the time data were collected. In this example, data were collected using a cross-sectional study, where households were surveyed at one point in time.

Therefore, the proportions represent prevalence rates. If the sample proportion of households using insecticide-treated nets is 0.27, then the estimated prevalence insecticide-treated net use is 0.27.

Risks are also proportions. However, risks are reserved for prospective studies. Statements referring to risk assume that data collection began when the subjects were *disease-free* or before the outcome of interest occurred. If data had been collected prospectively, households might have been identified before the start of the rainy season or when the ITN was first purchased and then followed to see how certain factors influenced net usage, and the proportion could be described as a risk.

Both prevalence rates and risks are proportions and are calculated in the same way. The difference between them is the interpretation, which depends on how the data are collected. Prevalence rates are used when collecting data at one point in time (cross-sectional); risks are used when data are collected prospectively. An additional numerical summary, the odds, is more versatile. It can be used in any type of study, irrespective of how the data were collected. However, odds are not proportions. Proportions are used to create the odds.

Application of Formula: SAMPLE ODDS

$$\text{Estimate of odds} = \frac{\hat{p}}{1 - \hat{p}}$$

$\hat{p}$ = The proportion of subjects in the sample with a particular characteristic (success)

$1 - \hat{p}$ = The proportion of subjects in a sample *without* a particular characteristic (failure)

What you need to estimate the odds:

1. *The estimated proportion of successes, $\hat{p}$:* In this example, this is the proportion of subjects using insecticide-treated nets: $\hat{p} = 500 \div 1876 = 0.27$.
2. *The estimated proportion of failures, $1 - \hat{p}$:* In this example, this is the proportion of subjects not using an insecticide-treated net: $1 - (1) = 1 - 0.27 = 0.73$ or $1376 \div 1876 = 0.73$.

To calculate the estimated odds: Divide (1) by (2) = 0.27/0.73 = 0.37. Therefore, the estimated odds of using an insecticide-treated net is 0.37.

The **odds** are obviously different from a simple proportion. In fact, a proportion must be between 0 and 1, but odds can be any number greater than or equal to 0.

- When the odds are less than 1, the chance of failure $(1 - p)$ is greater than the chance of success (p).
- When the odds are greater than 1, the chance of success (p) is greater than the chance of failure $(1 - p)$.
- When the odds are 1, then the chance of success (p) is the same as the chance of failure $(1 - p)$, which happens only when $p = 0.5$.

In this case, the estimated odds are 0.37; so in this sample, households are more likely not to use insecticide-treated nets than to use them.

Choosing the appropriate numerical summary depends on how the data were collected, that is, the study design. Three primary types of studies [prospective (cohort), retrospective (case-control), and cross-sectional] were described in Chapter 1.

- In a *prospective study*, groups of interest (cohorts) are specified at the start of the study. The cohorts are followed to see whether the outcome of interest develops. The data collection starts at the beginning of the study and continues as subjects are followed throughout the study.

- In a *case-control study*, the outcome is known, and data that have already been collected are reviewed to determine whether any characteristics impacted the development of the outcome (whether a subject is a case or a control). Data collection occurs before the study starts, and groups are defined based on data that have already been collected.
- In a *cross-sectional study*, the outcome and other variables are collected at a particular point in time and the results represent a cross-section of time. The data collected in this study are an example of a cross-sectional study because surveys were given to households and information about the households and net use were collected at one point in time.

The type of study design dictates the type of numerical summary (Table 4-1).

TABLE 4-1 **STUDY DESIGNS**

Study Design	Pros	Cons	Numerical Summary
Prospective	Data collection begins with study enrollment for all subjects.	May require significant resources	Risk Odds
Retrospective	Because data collection occurs in the past, it is easier to collect data on subjects.	Potential for missing data May increase bias	Odds
Cross-sectional	Obtaining data on subjects at only one point in time is easier.	Only one point in time can be summarized May increase bias	Prevalence Odds

© Cengage Learning, 2012.

ONE-GROUP STUDIES WITH A DICHOTOMOUS OUTCOME

Many times it may only be feasible to collect data on a single group. For example, when investigators are trying to understand the utilization of insecticide-treated nets, practical constraints might force them to collect data only on those using insecticide-treated nets, to focus on only one tribe or region, or to collect data only on those coming to a particular clinic. When data collection is constrained so that data are collected on only one group, investigators may still have research questions that involve comparisons. However, if data are collected on only one group, the investigators do not have a control or comparator group available for comparison. When a one-sample study is conducted because an independent comparator group is not practical, results collected from other studies (historical controls) can be used to make comparisons and inferences. Historical controls are estimates of the true parameter based on data from another study, perhaps from a different time period, a different region, different population, or a different exposure.

This study, for example, includes only households surveyed during the rainy season. It may be of interest to compare the proportion of those who use insecticide-treated nets during the rainy season to those who use nets in the dry season. Suppose a study investigating net use in the dry season reported that 20% of households used insecticide-treated nets. The proportion of households using ITNs in the dry season represents the historical control.

RESEARCH QUESTION:
Is the season (rainy or dry) associated with the utilization of insecticide-treated nets?

One-Sample Proportion: Hypothesis Test

Although the observed proportion ($\hat{p} = 0.27$) of net use found in this study is different from the historical control, the sample proportion ($\hat{p} = 0.27$) may be specific to this sample of 1876 households. Is the proportion found in this sample of households different enough from the historical control to conclude that the rate of net use in the rainy season is truly different from the rate in dry seasons? Hypothesis testing can help.

> **RESEARCH HYPOTHESIS:** The true proportion (*p*) in the rainy season is not 0.20.

> **NULL HYPOTHESIS:** The true proportion (*p*) in the rainy season is 0.20.

Point to Ponder

There are several symbols for representing a proportion: p, p_0, and $\hat{p}$. Why are different symbols necessary? How do they represent different proportions?

The hypothesis test assumes that the true parameter (the true proportion of households using an insecticide-treated net during the rainy season) is 0.20. In other words, the historical control serves as the null parameter ($p_0 = 0.20$). The data from this sample ($n = 1876$) provide a statistic (an estimate of the proportion: $\hat{p} = 0.27$). Would this statistic be expected if the true parameter really was the null parameter ($p_0 = 0.20$)?

In Chapters 1 and 2, the sampling distribution of the mean was described. When the sample size is large and the proportion is not too small, the sampling distribution of the proportion is similar to the sampling distribution of the mean. In fact, it is normally distributed (Figure 4-6). This means that if the proportions of net use were obtained from many samples of 1876 households, the distribution of all the sample proportions of net use would be normally distributed. Because the normal distribution is used to determine whether there is enough evidence against the null hypothesis, this hypothesis test is referred to as a one-sample *z*-test for a proportion.

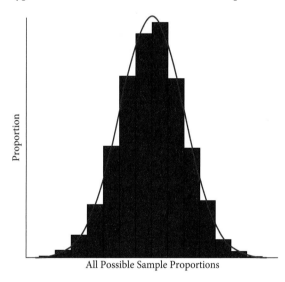

All Possible Sample Proportions

Figure 4-6 Sampling distribution for the proportion (large-sample approximation).
© *Cengage Learning, 2012.*

Application of Formula: ONE-SAMPLE *z*-TEST

Test statistic $(z) = \dfrac{\hat{p} - p_0}{\sqrt{\dfrac{p_0(1 - p_0)}{n}}}$

$\hat{p}$ = The proportion of subjects in the sample with a particular characteristic (success)

p_0 = The proportion of successes proposed by the null hypothesis (null parameter)

$\sqrt{\dfrac{\hat{p} - p_0}{n}}$ = The standard error when the null hypothesis is true

What you need for a one-sample *z*-test for a proportion:

1. *The difference between the sample proportion and the null parameter:* $\hat{p} - p_0 = 0.27 - 0.20 = 0.07$

2. *The standard error under the null:* The standard error involves the null proportion of successes (p_0) and failures ($1 - p_0$)

   a. Multiply the null proportions of successes and failures: $p_0 \times (1 - p_0) = 0.2 \times 0.8 = 0.16$

continues

continued

  b. The variance under the null: Divide (a) by the sample size ($n = 1876$) $= 0.16 \div 1876 = 0.0000853$.
  c. The standard error under the null: Take the square root of (b): $\sqrt{0.000085} = 0.0092$.

To calculate the test statistic (z) for the one-sample z-test: Divide (1) divided by (2): $0.07 \div 0.0092 = 7.6$.

Using a normally distributed sampling distribution, this test statistic would be considered rare. As a general rule, test statistics that are bigger than 3 or smaller than -3 are considered to be far enough away from the center of the sampling distribution to be defined as rare. When the test statistic is rare, the null hypothesis can be rejected.

The proportion of statistics that are even farther away from the center than the observed test statistic (*p*-value) can be obtained by means of statistical tables or a statistical software package. This one-sample *z*-test results in a *p*-value of <0.0001 (Table 4-2).

TABLE 4-2 **RESULTS OF A ONE-SAMPLE z-TEST OF A PROPORTION**

Test of H_0: Proportion (p) = 0.2	
ASE under H_0	0.0092
Z	7.2034
One-sided Pr $>$ Z	<0.0001
Two-sided Pr $>$ |Z|	<0.0001
Sample size = 1876	

© Cengage Learning, 2012.

CONCLUSION: Because the *p*-value is small ($p < 0.0001$), the test statistic would be considered rare if the null hypothesis were true. Hence, there is sufficient evidence ($p < 0.0001$) to reject the null hypothesis. The proportion of insecticide-treated net use in the rainy season is not 0.20.

One-Sample Proportion: Confidence Intervals

Although the one-sample hypothesis test is helpful for determining whether the true proportion is equal to some value, it does not provide an estimate for the true proportion. Based on the one-sample hypothesis test, there is evidence that the true proportion of households using nets in the rainy season is not 0.20. However, to estimate the true proportion, confidence intervals can help.

Because the sample size in this example is somewhat large and the rate of net use is not too small, the normal distribution can also be used to help create confidence intervals. Like the hypothesis test, confidence intervals are also based on the idea that not all samples will result in the same statistic (sampling variability). Another sample of 1876 households is not likely to result in 500 ($\hat{p} = 0.27$) households using insecticide-treated nets. The estimate of $\hat{p} = 0.27$ is a point estimate and describes only this sample; a better estimate of the true proportion can be found with an interval estimate or a confidence interval. Confidence intervals are calculated using the idea that, if many more samples of 1876 households were selected, the statistics (estimates of the proportions of net use) would all pile up fairly close to the true parameter (the true proportion of net use *p*), resulting in a sampling distribution that is normally distributed and centered at the true parameter. In contrast to the one-sample hypothesis test, where the null parameter is assumed to be the center of the sampling distribution, confidence intervals are calculated with the assumption that most of the statistics will be within a certain distance of the true parameter (*p*).

Before interval estimates can be found, however, an estimate of the variability is needed. For dichotomous variables, the variance is easily calculated from the sample proportion and the sample size.

$$\text{Standard error} = \sqrt{\frac{\hat{p} \times (1 - \hat{p})}{n}}$$

n = The sample size

$\hat{p}$ = The proportion of subjects in the sample with the characteristic (success)

What you need to calculate the standard error:

1. *The sample proportion of successes:* $\hat{p} = \frac{500}{1876} = 0.27$. In this example, a success is using an ITN.
2. *The sample proportion of failures:* $1 - (1)$ or $1 - \hat{p} = 1 - 0.27 = 0.73$. In this example, a failure is not using an ITN.
3. *The sample size:* $n = 1876$.
4. *The numerator:* (1) multiplied by (2): $\hat{p}(1 - \hat{p}) = 0.27 \times 0.73 = 0.1971$.
5. *The sample variance:* Divide (4) by (3): $0.1971 \div 1876 = 0.000105$.

To calculate the standard error: Take the square root of (5): $\sqrt{0.000105} = 0.01$.

$C\%$ confidence interval for the proportion: $\hat{p} \pm z^* \times SE$

$\hat{p}$ = The sample proportion

C = The confidence level for a $C\%$ confidence interval

z^* = The number of standard deviations from the center of the sampling distribution

SE = The standard error of the proportion

What you need to calculate the confidence interval:

1. *The sample proportion (point estimate):* $\hat{p} = 0.27$.
2. *The standard error:* $\sqrt{0.000105} = 0.01$.
3. *The confidence level:* $C\%$ is typically 95%, but 90% and 99% are also common.
4. *The number of standard deviations from the center of the sampling distribution:* This depends on $C\%$ (3) and the sampling distribution. So, when the sampling distribution is a normal distribution, the z^* for a 90% confidence interval is 1.65, the z^* for a 95% confidence interval is 1.96, and the z^* for a 99% confidence interval is 2.58. Therefore, confidence intervals can be calculated as

90% confidence interval: $\hat{p} \pm (1.65 \times \text{standard error})$

95% confidence interval: $\hat{p} \pm (1.96 \times \text{standard error})$

99% confidence interval: $\hat{p} \pm (2.58 \times \text{standard error})$.

To calculate the 95% confidence interval: The number of standard errors from the center (margin of error) is $1.96 \times 0.01 = 0.0196$. Adding and subtracting the margin of error to and from the point estimate results in the 95% confidence interval, $[0.27 - 1.96 \times 0.01; 0.27 + 1.96 \times 0.01]$, or $[0.25, 0.29]$.

Because 95% of all confidence intervals cover the true proportion, this interval represents a set of plausible values for the true proportion of net use. Because the proportion of 0.20 is not covered by this interval, 0.20 is not a plausible value for the true proportion of net use in the rainy season. Furthermore, because the confidence interval provides an estimate, and the interval estimate suggests that the proportion of net use in the rainy season is actually greater than reported use in the dry season.

Planning a One-Sample Study

Planning a study with the appropriate number of subjects depends on the research question (or the outcome) and on the purpose of the study. When the outcome is dichotomous, the research question typically involves a proportion. Depending on the research question, the purpose of the study could be to estimate the proportion or actually to test that the proportion is different from a historical control.

Unlike sample size estimation, there are fewer unknowns when dealing with proportions and the outcome is continuous (see Chapter 2). In particular, estimating the variance is much easier. When a dichotomous outcome is measured on a sample, the outcome comes from the binomial distribution. In the binomial distribution, the variance is a function of the proportion. If the proportion is known (or can be reasonably guessed), a reasonable estimate of the variance is obtainable. Because most studies focus on the parameter of interest (the proportion), finding a measure of variability is fairly easy.

Planning for Estimating a Proportion

When the outcome is dichotomous (only two levels), the goal is often to estimate a proportion. When the objective of the study is estimation, sample size calculations are based on the calculation of confidence intervals. To determine the sample size, an investigator needs:

- A guess of the proportion
- The amount of precision

Luckily, the worst-case scenario (the largest sample size needed) when guessing the proportion occurs when the proportion is 0.50 or the percentage is 50%. Therefore, even when investigators have no idea what to use to estimate the percentage, the best solution is to potentially overestimate the sample size and use 50%.

Estimation generally involves creating an interval estimate, and precision is determined by the width of the interval. A smaller interval means that the proportion can be estimated with greater precision. The width of the interval is usually decided by the investigator. If an investigator wants to estimate the percentage, for example, within 3%, then the width of the interval is ±3%. Estimating a proportion within ±3−5% is common. A larger width (less precision) requires fewer subjects. However, care must be taken when making a width too large. If the width of the interval is 20%, the proportion is estimated within ±20%—a pretty large range. In fact, it is so large that it may not be helpful in providing an estimate of the true proportion of net use.

Table 4-3 provides a summary of how the sample size estimate changes with increased proportion estimates and increased precision (smaller width). For example, assuming a percentage of 50% and a two-sided 95% confidence interval, a sample size of 385 subjects will allow for the estimation of the proportion within ±5%, but a sample size of 1068 is needed to estimate the true percentage within 3%.

Planning for Making Comparisons with a Proportion

When the goal of the study is making a comparison by using hypothesis tests, sample size estimation involves the relationship of effect size, power, and type 1 error. In a one-sample test for a proportion, the effect size is determined by considering the difference between the null parameter and some other alternative parameter (a parameter that might be found if the research hypothesis were true).

TABLE 4-3 SAMPLE SIZE ESTIMATES (95% CONFIDENCE INTERVAL OF A PROPORTION)

Proposed Sample Size	Estimate of the Proportion	Width of the Interval
897	0.3	
1025	0.4	0.03
1068	0.5	
323	0.3	
369	0.4	0.05
385	0.5	

Sample size estimates are based on a two-sided 95% confidence interval.

© Cengage Learning, 2012.

Power and type 1 error were discussed in Chapter 1. A sample size is found by planning a study so that the null hypothesis can be rejected when it should be rejected (high power) while keeping the chance of rejecting the null hypothesis when it should not be (type 1 error) low. Usually potential power values are 80–90%. Furthermore, the possible values of the significance level (probability of a type 1 error) range from 0.01 to 0.1. Observational, exploratory studies, where a type 1 error is not as critical, can handle larger significance levels ($\alpha = 0.1$). However, most studies are planned with a two-sided significance level of 0.05. If the study is very concerned with making a type 1 error, a lower significance level is used ($\alpha = 0.01$).

Table 4-4 provides a summary of how the sample size estimates change with different power and null and alternative proportions. When the difference between the null and alternative proportions increases, the sample size decreases. The sample size

TABLE 4-4 SAMPLE SIZE ESTIMATES (TESTING WITH A PROPORTION)

Proposed Sample Size	Null Proportion	Alternative Proportion	Power
171	0.25	0.15	
742	0.25	0.20	
214	0.25	0.35	90
36	0.25	0.50	
113	0.50	0.35	
1047	0.50	0.45	
259	0.50	0.60	90
38	0.50	0.75	
133	0.25	0.15	
563	0.25	0.20	
157	0.25	0.35	80
26	0.25	0.50	
85	0.50	0.35	
783	0.50	0.45	
194	0.50	0.60	80
29	0.50	0.75	

Assumes a two-sided significance level of 0.05.

© Cengage Learning, 2012.

estimates also decrease as the power decreases. For example, when the sample size is 214 subjects, the one-sample test of proportion (using the normal approximation) would have 90% power to detect a difference in proportions between 0.25 and 0.35, assuming a two-sided significance level of 0.05, but would only need 157 subjects for 80% power.

One-Sample Proportion: Exact Methods

The hypothesis tests and confidence intervals provided so far used the normal approximation because the sample size was relatively large and the proportion was not too small.

- In *hypothesis testing*, this means that $n \times p_0 \times (1 - p_0)$ must be greater than or equal to 10 to use the normal distribution (i.e., to use the z-test).
- For *confidence intervals*, this means that $n \times \hat{p}$ and $n \times 1 - (\hat{p})$ must be greater than or equal to 5 to use the normal distribution, that is, $z = 1.96$ for a 95% confidence interval.

Very possibly, however, studies arise when the sample size is not large enough and/or the proportion is too small. In such cases, using the normal approximation to make statistical inferences with a dichotomous outcome is no longer appropriate.

The outcome in this example is whether an insecticide-treated net was used the previous night; this is a dichotomous variable with only two options (yes/no). Asking each household whether a net was used represents a sample of 1876 trials where a success is defined as using a net. Recall from Chapter 1 that the distribution of the successes in these trials is the binomial distribution. Luckily, when the normal distribution cannot be assumed, hypothesis tests and confidence intervals can be calculated using the properties of the binomial distribution. A hypothesis test that cannot use the normal approximation and that must use the binomial distribution is referred to as an *exact test*.

For example, suppose each household was also asked whether the household had had a death due to malaria during the rainy season; and 5 households out of 1876 experienced a death: $\hat{p} = \frac{5}{1876} = 0.003$. If the investigators already know that the malaria mortality proportion during the dry season is 0.001 (historical control), is the mortality proportion for the rainy season different from the dry season?

Although the sample size is still large, this is a very small mortality rate. Therefore, hypothesis tests and confidence intervals that rely on the normal distribution can no longer be used. The exact binomial test and confidence intervals will have to help in answering the research question.

RESEARCH QUESTION: Is the proportion of deaths due to malaria associated with the season (rainy or dry)?

RESEARCH HYPOTHESIS: The true proportion of households with malaria deaths in the rainy season is not 0.001.

NULL HYPOTHESIS: The true proportion of households with malaria deaths in the rainy season is 0.001.

These hypotheses are structured like the hypotheses used when the normal approximation is appropriate; the event proportions are just much smaller. The main difference between using the normal approximation (one-sample z-test) and the exact method is that in the exact method the p-value is obtained directly from the binomial distribution.

Public Health Professional

Application of Formula: EXACT TEST

How do I get the p-value for an exact test?

Determine whether the observed proportion in the sample ($\hat{p}$) is less than or equal to the null parameter (p_0).

a. If the observed proportion ($\hat{p}$) is less than or equal to the null proportion (p_0), then the binomial distribution can be used to find the probability of getting even fewer successes than what was observed. This calculation can be somewhat complicated, but any statistical software package will provide the probability. In fact, several online probability calculators can compute the probability by using the number of successes, the sample size, and the p_0.

b. If the observed proportion ($\hat{p}$) is greater than or equal to the null proportion (p_0), then the binomial distribution can be used to find the probability of getting at least as many successes as what was observed. This calculation can be somewhat complicated, but any statistical software package or online probability calculator can supply the probability.

To calculate the p-value: If the test is a one-tailed test, the research hypothesis refers to the proportion being either larger or smaller. The p-value is then simply the value found in (a) or (b). If it is a two-tailed test, the p-value is two times the probability found in (a) or (b). The probability is doubled because the research hypothesis refers to the proportion being different, the proportion could be larger or smaller. If the result of doubling the probability is a value greater than 1, the p-value is just 1.

In this example, 5 households experienced a malaria-related death; so $\hat{p} = 0.003$. Because 0.003 is larger than 0.001, the p-value has to be found using the method described in (b). Using a binomial distribution with a sample size of 1876 and a probability of success of $p_0 = 0.001$, the probability of observing 5 or more (i.e., at least 5) malaria deaths is 0.0421. Therefore, the p-value for this hypothesis test is $2 \times 0.0421 = 0.0841$.

The p-value for this hypothesis test is 0.0841 and can be found using any statistical software package (Table 4-5).

TABLE 4-5 **RESULTS OF THE ONE-SAMPLE BINOMIAL EXACT TEST**

Test of H_0: Proportion (p) = 0.001	
One-sided Pr >= P	0.0421
Two-sided = 2 × One-sided	0.0841
Sample size = 1876	

© Cengage Learning, 2012.

CONCLUSION: The p-value that results from the exact test is 0.0841. This value is not statistically significant at the 0.05 level ($\alpha = 0.05$). Therefore, there is not enough evidence to reject the null hypothesis. However, this p-value is not large; some might even call this p-value marginally significant. Although not significant at the 0.05 level, a rate of malaria higher than 0.001 was observed in the rainy season ($p = 0.0841$).

Point to Ponder
The hypothesis test in this example resulted in a two-tailed test because the research hypothesis indicated that the rate in the rainy season was different (higher or lower). If the research hypothesis had been that a higher rate of malaria was expected in the rainy season, then there would have been enough evidence to reject the null hypothesis (rate is less than or equal to 0.001) at the 0.05 significance level because the one-tailed p-value is 0.0421.

Sometimes *p*-values can be troublesome because they indicate only whether the null hypothesis can be rejected. Having a confidence interval, an interval estimate of the true proportion, may be more helpful. However, if the normal approximation is not appropriate for performing a hypothesis test, then it is also not appropriate for the calculation of an interval estimate. Exact methods using the binomial distribution can also be used to get an interval estimate for the true proportion. Exact confidence intervals can be obtained from statistical software and online calculators (Table 4-6)

TABLE 4-6 **EXAMPLE OF EXACT CONFIDENCE INTERVAL FOR A PROPORTION**

Binomial Proportion for Malaria = 1	
Proportion Estimate	0.0027
Exact Confidence Limits	
95% lower confidence limit	(0.0009, 0.0062)
90% upper confidence limit	(0.0011, 0.0056)

© Cengage Learning, 2012.

Hence, the exact 95% confidence interval for the proportion of household with a malaria death during the rainy season is [0.0009, 0.0062]. This represents a set of plausible values for the true proportion. Although most of the interval is larger than the historical control, the dry season proportion (0.001) would be covered by this interval. Therefore, based on the 95% confidence interval, the rainy season proportion of malaria deaths could be the same as 0.001. If less confidence is used, the 90% confidence interval indicates that the rate of malaria deaths is larger than 0.001.

MULTIPLE-GROUP STUDIES

Many studies in public health are conducted to compare proportions between groups, where the group is a categorical variable. Therefore, multiple-group studies that investigate categorical outcomes involve two variables: the outcome and the categorical group variable. If a study involves collecting data on multiple groups, comparisons can be made directly among the categories of the group variable (historical controls are not used). Generally, when comparing more than one group, one of the groups (one of the categories) serves as the control group.

For example, in this study, households without children under the age of 5 have been known to use insecticide-treated nets less often (Noor, 2009). Therefore, the variable for whether the household has children under 5 represents the group variable, and the category for households without children under the age of 5 serves as the control group. The two categories (households with and without children under the age of 5) can be compared for differences in net utilization. These two groups consist of completely different households. The responses of one group have nothing to do with the responses of the other group, meaning that the two groups are independent. An investigator may be interested in comparing the proportion of net use between the two groups because differences in proportions may help explain why some households use ITNs and some do not.

Descriptive statistics can be provided to describe the sample of households with and without children under the age of 5. A table of descriptive statistics such as Table 4-7 might be helpful in describing these two types of households.

The descriptive statistics in Table 4-7 provide some interesting information for households in the study. The majority (51%) of the households are more than 50 miles from a healthcare facility and live in a rural area (53%). The average age for the head of the household is 48 (SD = 7.4). The heads of households report a median family size

RESEARCH QUESTION:
Does having a child under the age of 5 impact the utilization of insecticide-treated nets?

		Children in the Household Younger Than 5	
	Total Households (N = 1876)	No (N = 1,043)	Yes (N = 833)
Net Used the Previous Night (%)			
No	1376 (73.3%)	823 (78.9%)	553 (66.4%)
Yes	500 (26.7%)	220 (21.1%)	280 (33.6%)
Roof Type (%)			
Thatched	623 (33.2%)	334 (32.0%)	289 (34.7%)
Corrugated metal	795 (42.4%)	444 (42.6%)	351 (42.1%)
Other	458 (24.4%)	265 (25.4%)	193 (23.2%)
Distance to Healthcare Facility (%)			
<15 miles	552 (29.4%)	301 (28.9%)	251 (30.1%)
15–50 miles	371 (19.8%)	200 (19.2%)	171 (20.5%)
50 + miles	953 (50.8%)	542 (52.0%)	411 (49.3%)
Household in Rural Area (%)			
Yes	993 (52.9%)	557 (53.4%)	436 (52.3%)
No	883 (47.1%)	486 (46.6%)	397 (47.7%)
Wealth Index of Household (%)			
Lowest 25%	479 (25.5%)	264 (25.3%)	215 (25.8%)
Next Lowest	536 (28.6%)	312 (29.9%)	224 (26.9%)
Next highest	541 (28.8%)	302 (29.0%)	239 (28.7%)
Highest 25%	320 (17.1%)	165 (15.8%)	155 (18.6%)
Age (years)			
Mean (SD)	48.5 (7.42)	48.8 (7.16)	48.2 (7.72)
Median (Q1, Q3)	49 (44, 54)	49 (44, 54)	48 (43, 53)
Minimum, maximum	20, 73	20, 73	20, 72
Family Size			
Mean (SD)	5.6 (1.79)	5.5 (1.72)	5.8 (1.87)
Median (Q1, Q3)	6 (4, 7)	5 (4, 7)	6 (4, 7)
Minimum, Maximum	1, 12	1, 10	1, 12

© Cengage Learning, 2012.

of 6 with a range of 1–12. Most (73%) of the households did not use an insecticide-treated net the previous night. Although the households with and without children under 5 are similar with respect to age and family size, there are some differences between them. In particular, those with children under 5 in the household report more net use than those without children under 5 (34% versus 21%).

This example includes more than one categorical variable to investigate: having children under the age of 5 and whether ITNs were used. When the study involves more than one categorical variable (the outcome and the group), there is more than one way to construct a table of descriptive statistics. Specifically, the table depends on the variable used for the columns. For example, in addition to comparing households based on whether they have children under the age of 5, comparing households that used nets versus those that did not is also interesting (Table 4-8).

	Total Households (N = 1876)	Used Insecticide-Treated Nets in the Previous Night	
		No (N = 1376)	Yes (N = 500)
Children Under 5 (%)			
No	1043 (55.6%)	823 (59.8%)	220 (44.0%)
Yes	833 (44.4%)	553 (40.2%)	280 (56.0%)
Roof Type (%)			
Thatched	623 (33.2%)	394 (28.6%)	229 (45.8%)
Corrugated Metal	795 (42.4%)	643 (46.7%)	152 (30.4%)
Other	458 (24.4%)	339 (24.6%)	119 (23.8%)
Distance to Healthcare Facility (%)			
<15 miles	552 (29.4%)	352 (25.6%)	200 (40.0%)
15–50 miles	371 (19.8%)	262 (19.0%)	109 (21.8%)
50 + miles	953 (50.8%)	762 (55.4%)	191 (38.2%)
Household in Rural Area (%)			
No	993 (52.9%)	785 (57.0%)	208 (41.6%)
Yes	883 (47.1%)	591 (43.0%)	292 (58.4%)
Wealth Index of Household (%)			
Lowest 25%	479 (25.5%)	406 (29.5%)	73 (14.6%)
Next lowest	536 (28.6%)	403 (29.3%)	133 (26.6%)
Next highest	541 (28.8%)	367 (26.7%)	174 (34.8%)
Highest 25%	320 (17.1%)	200 (14.5%)	120 (24.0%)
Age (years)			
Mean (SD)	48.5 (7.42)	50.1 (6.84)	44.3 (7.33)
Median (Q1, Q3)	49 (44, 54)	50 (46, 55)	44 (40, 49)
Minimum, maximum	20, 73	28, 73	20, 62
Family Size			
Mean (SD)	5.6 (1.79)	5.1 (1.53)	7.1 (1.61)
Median (Q1, Q3)	6 (4, 7)	5 (4, 6)	7 (6, 8)
Minimum, maximum	1, 12	1, 9	3, 12

© Cengage Learning, 2012.

It is evident that there are differences between the households that used an insecticide-treated net in the previous night (4–8). In particular, households using insecticide-treated nets report a higher percentage of children under 5, are more likely to live in a thatched roof, have a higher percentage of households living within 15 miles of a healthcare facility, and are more likely to live in a rural area. Furthermore, the average age of the household head is younger and the families are larger in the households using insecticide-treated nets.

Tables 4-7 and 4-8 provide a description of how other variables are related to the group or exposure variable (children under the age of 5 in the household) and the outcome variable (use of ITNs), respectively. Depending on the research question, one or both of these tables may be useful.

Proportions in a Contingency Table

When dealing with relationships between categorical variables, one of the more challenging tasks is determining the denominator for the calculation of the proportion or percentage. When dealing with one sample, the determination is fairly straightforward: The denominator is typically the number of subjects. However, with more than one categorical variable, the calculation of the proportions can get more complicated because there are more choices for the denominator. Multiple-group studies entail three types of proportions (or percentages): total, row, and column proportions (or percentages). These three different types of proportions are often displayed as a **contingency table**. A contingency table is simply a table in which the categories of one variable make up the rows and the categories of another variable make up the columns (Table 4-9). The cells of the contingency table provide the number of subjects belonging to a particular category (level) of the row variable *and* a particular category (level) of the column variable.

Most statistical software packages also provide the total, row, and column percentages for each cell. In this example, having children under the age of 5 is the column variable, and utilization of insecticide-treated nets is the row variable. Because there are two categories in the children-under-the-age-of-5 variable and two categories for the use-of-ITNs variable, the contingency that results is a 2 × 2 (2 rows × 2 columns) table (Table 4-10).

TABLE 4-9 **CONTINGENCY TABLE (2 × 2 EXAMPLE)**

	Column Variable Level 1	Column Variable Level 2	Totals
Row Variable Level 1	Number of subjects with row level 1 *and* column level 1	Number of subjects with row level 1 *and* column level 2	**Total number of subjects with row level 1**
Row Variable Level 2	Number of subjects with row level 2 *and* column level 1	Number of subjects with tow level 1 *and* column level 2	**Total number of subjects with row level 2**
Totals	**Total number of subjects with column level 1**	**Total number of subjects with column level 2**	**Total number of subjects**

© Cengage Learning, 2012.

TABLE 4-10 **EXAMPLE OF A CONTINGENCY TABLE (2×2)**

Table of Net by Child			
Frequency Percentage Row Percentage Column Percentage	**Column Variable: Child**		
	0	1	Total
Row Variable: Net Use 0	823 43.87 59.81 78.91	553 29.48 40.19 66.39	1376 73.35
1	220 11.73 44.00 21.09	280 14.93 56.00 33.61	500 26.65
Total	1043 55.60	833 44.40	1876 100.00

© Cengage Learning, 2012.

In this example,

- 280 households are in column 2 (Child = 1) *and* row 2 (net = 1), or 280 households have children under the age of 5 *and* did use an insecticide-treated net.
- 1376 households did not use an insecticide-treated net, and 500 households did.
- 1043 households are without children under the age of 5, and 833 households have children under the age of 5.

The total percentage is provided as the first proportion in each of the cells. The denominator for each of these percentages is 1876. For example, the total percentage of households that have children under the age of 5 *and* that used an insecticide-treated net is 280 ÷ 1876 = 14.93%.

The row percentages are next. For each row percentage, the row total is used as the denominator. The row percentage for households with children under the age of 5 who did use nets, for example, is 280 ÷ 500 = 56.00%.

Finally, the last percentage provided is the column percentage. For each column percentage, the column total is used as the denominator. The column percentage for households with children under the age of 5 who did use nets, for example, is 280 ÷ 833 = 33.61%.

Application of Formula: CONTINGENCY TABLE PROPORTIONS

What you need to calculate the proportions:

The total proportion, $\hat{p}$:

a. *Cell Count:* The number of subjects with a particular row and column characteristic. In this example, the number of subjects who did use an insecticide-treated net *and* who do have a child under 5 years old is 280.
b. *Total sample size: n* = 1876

To calculate the total proportion: Divide (a) by (b) = 280 ÷ 1876 = 0.1493 (14.93%).

The column proportion $\hat{p}_c$:

a. *Cell count:* The number of subjects with a particular row and column characteristic. In this example, the number of subjects who did use an insecticide-treated net and who do have children under 5 years old is 280.
b. *The number of subjects in column c: n_c* = 833 subjects have children under 5 years old (column subset).

To calculate the column proportion: Divide (a) by (b) = 280 ÷ 833 = 0.3361 (33.61%).

The row proportion $\hat{p}_r$:

a. *Cell Count:* The number of subjects with a particular row and column characteristic. In this example, the number of subjects who did not use an insecticide-treated net and(italics) who do have a child under 5 years old is 280.
b. *The number of subjects in row r: n_r* = 500 subjects used insecticide-treated nets (row subset).

To calculate the row proportion: Divide (a) by (b) = 310 ÷ 477 = 0.5600 (56.00%).

Notice the difference in the denominators for these proportions (and percentages). The total proportion uses all the subjects, a column proportion uses the number of subjects in the column, and a row proportion uses the number of subjects in the row. The interpretations of these proportions are also different. The observed percentage of households using an insecticide-treated net and who have children under the age of 5 is 15% (total proportion = 0.15). Of the households with children under the age of 5, 34% used an insecticide-treated net (column proportion = 0.34). Of the households that used an insecticide-treated net, 56% have children under the age of 5 (row proportion = 0.56). The proportion to use depends on the question being asked.

The row and column proportions are also known as **conditional probabilities**, which is a proportion of subjects with a particular category (level) within a certain subset of subjects. A column proportion is a conditional probability because it is the proportion of subjects with a particular category (level) given that the subjects belong to the column: the proportion of households not using insecticide-treated nets, given that the household does not have children under age 5 (the column condition). Likewise, a row proportion is a conditional probability because it is the proportion of subjects with a particular category given the subjects belong to the row: the proportion of households with children under 5, given that the household uses insecticide-treated nets (the row condition).

When the goal is to investigate multiple groups, the research question typically involves comparing proportions between groups. Therefore, the parameters of interest are conditional probabilities because the proportions are calculated using the number of subjects in each group as the denominator.

Hypothesis Test for Two Dichotomous Variables (2×2 Contingency Table)

One of the goals of this study was to determine the factors associated with using insecticide-treated nets. One potential factor is the presence of children under the age of 5 in the household.

RESEARCH QUESTION: Does having a child under the age of 5 impact the utilization of insecticide-treated nets?

To determine whether having children under the age of 5 impacts the utilization of insecticide-treated nets, the parameters of interest are p_{U5} and p_{O5}, where p_{U5} represents the true proportion of insecticide-treated net use in households with children under 5 (U5), and p_{O5} represents the true proportion of insecticide-treated net use in households with children over 5 (O5). Estimates of p_{U5} and p_{O5}, are the proportion using insecticide-treated nets in households given that the household has children under 5 and over 5, conditional probabilities. In this example, the estimates for the proportion of net use for the two groups (households with and without children under 5) are $\hat{p}_{U5} = 0.34$ and $\hat{p}_{O5} = 0.21$, respectively. A difference between these two proportions would imply that having children under the age of 5 impacts the use of insecticide-treated nets. In other words, does the information from the sample suggest that the proportion of net use in households with children under 5 (p_{U5}) is different from the proportion of net use in households with no children under 5 (p_{O5})? Hypothesis testing can help.

RESEARCH HYPOTHESIS: The true proportion of insecticide-treated net use in households with children under 5 (p_{U5}) is *different from* the true proportion of insecticide-treated net use in households with no children under 5 (p_{O5}): $p_{U5} \neq p_{O5}$.

NULL HYPOTHESIS: The true proportion of insecticide-treated net use in households with children under 5 (p_{U5}) is *equal to* the true proportion of insecticide-treated net use in households with no children under 5 (p_{O5}) or $p_{U5} = p_{O5}$.

If the two proportions (p_{U5} and p_{O5}) are equal, then having a child under the age of 5 in the household is not associated with net use. In other words, if the two proportions are equal, then having young children in the household made no difference in whether insecticide-treated nets were used. Hence, if the two proportions are equal, then the two variables (having children under the age of 5 and the use of insecticide treated nets) are independent. On the other hand, if the two proportions are different, then having children under the age of 5 makes a difference in the use of nets, and the two variables (having children under the age of 5 and insecticide-treated net use) are considered to be dependent.

Two variables are considered to be dependent when the value of one impacts the value of the other. If the two variables have nothing to do with each other, then they are considered independent. Therefore, investigating the association of having children under the age of 5 and insecticide-treated net utilization can be restated in terms of dependence.

> **RESEARCH HYPOTHESIS:** Using insecticide-treated nets and having children under the age of 5 are dependent.
>
> **NULL HYPOTHESIS:** Using insecticide-treated nets and having children under the age of 5 are independent.

The two forms of hypotheses, stated in terms of the equality of proportions or independence, are the same.

To determine whether ITN use is dependent on having children under 5 (i.e., the true proportion of ITN use is different for households with and without children under 5), the hypothesis test assumes the null hypothesis is true: The two variables are independent or the two proportions are equal. Therefore, the goal is to use the sample data to determine whether there is sufficient evidence against the null hypothesis. This hypothesis test is generally referred to as a *chi-square test of independence*. In particular, it can be used to determine whether the distribution of subjects in the cells observed in the contingency table would be expected if the null hypothesis were true.

Application of Formula

Chi-square test of independence test statistic $= \sum_{i=1}^{c} \frac{(O_{\text{cell } i} - E_{\text{cell } i})^2}{E_{\text{cell } i}}$

c = The number of cells in the contingency table

$O_{\text{cell } i}$ = The number of subjects observed in cell i

$E_{\text{cell } i}$ = The number of subjects expected if the null hypothesis were true in cell i

		Table of Net by Child		
		Column Variable: Child		
		0	1	Totals
Row Variable: Net Use	0	823	553	1376
	1	220	280	500
Totals		1043	833	1876

© Cengage Learning, 2012.

What you need to get the test statistic:

1. *The observed cell counts for each of the cells:* There are four cells ($c = 4$). The observed counts are $O_{\text{cell } 1} = 823$, $O_{\text{cell } 2} = 553$, $O_{\text{cell } 3} = 220$, and $O_{\text{cell } 4} = 280$.

continues

continued

2. *The expected cell counts for each of the cells:* The expected cell count is found by taking the row total times the column total and dividing the product by the overall total:
   a. $E_{cell\ 1} = (1376 \times 1043) \div 1876 = 1{,}435{,}168 \div 1876 = 765.0$
   b. $E_{cell\ 2} = (1376 \times 833) \div 1876 = 1{,}146{,}208 \div 1876 = 611.0$
   c. $E_{cell\ 3} = (500 \times 1043) \div 1876 = 521{,}500 \div 1876 = 278.0$
   d. $E_{cell\ 4} = (500 \times 833) \div 1876 = 416{,}500 \div 1876 = 222.0$

3. *The difference between the observed (1) and expected (2) cell counts for each of the cells:*
   a. $O_{cell\ 1} - E_{cell\ 1} = 823 - 765.0 = 58.0$
   b. $O_{cell\ 2} - E_{cell\ 2} = 553 - 611.0 = -58.0$
   c. $O_{cell\ 3} - E_{cell\ 3} = 220 - 278.0 = -58.0$
   d. $O_{cell\ 4} - E_{cell\ 4} = 280 - 222.0 = 58.0$

4. *Square the difference between observed and expected:* $(3)^2 = 58.0^2 = 3{,}364.0$

5. *Divide the square (4) by the expected count from each cell:*
   a. $3364.0 \div 765.0 = 4.4$
   b. $3364.0 \div 611.0 = 5.5$
   c. $3364.0 \div 278.0 = 12.1$
   d. $3364.0 \div 222.0 = 15.2$

To calculate the test statistic: Sum (5a) through (5d) $= 4.4 + 5.5 + 12.1 + 15.2 = 37.2$.

In this case, the test statistic is 37.2. When the null hypothesis is true, the test statistic for investigating independence with the contingency table comes from a chi-square sampling distribution with (rows $-$ 1) $\times$ (columns $-$ 1) $= 1 \times 1 = 1$ degree of freedom. Any test statistic larger than 3.84 is considered rare (only 5% of test statistics are farther away than the test statistic found here). Statistical tables or a statistical software package can be used to find the p-value associated with a test statistic of 37.

The p-value obtained from this chi-square test of independence is <0.0001 (Table 4-11).

TABLE 4-11 **RESULTS OF A 2×2 CHI-SQUARE TEST OF INDEPENDENCE**

Table of Net by Child			
Frequency Percentage Row Percentage Column Percentage	Column Variable: Child		
	0	1	Total
0	823 43.87 59.81 78.91	553 29.48 40.19 66.39	1376 73.35
1	220 11.73 44.00 21.09	280 14.93 56.00 33.61	500 26.65
Total	1043 55.60	833 44.40	1876 100.00

Row Variable: Net Use

Statistics for Table of Net by Child			
Statistic	DF	Value	Prob
Chi-square	1	37.1375	<0.0001

© Cengage Learning, 2012.

CONCLUSION: The *p*-value is small (<0.0001). Therefore, there is sufficient evidence to reject the null hypothesis. Insecticide-treated net utilization is dependent on having children under the age of 5 in the household. In other words, there is a significant difference in the rate of net use for households with children under 5 and not.

Categorical outcomes will not always be dichotomous. Because categorical variables can be dichotomous, nominal, or ordinal, various hypotheses and chi-square tests can be used to investigate associations between different types of categorical variables. Although the same chi-square test of independence can be used when the categorical variable has more than two levels (i.e., multiple groups and/or an outcome with multiple categories), different types of chi-square tests may be more appropriate for answering research questions. This is particularly true when the research question involves nominal or ordinal data. The hypotheses (and types of chi-square tests) depend on the types of categorical variables involved: two nominal or dichotomous variables, nominal and ordinal variables, two ordinal variables.

Hypothesis Test for Two Nominal Variables (R×C Contingency Table)

RESEARCH QUESTION: Is there an association between roof type and the type of net used?

Suppose the type of insecticide-treated net used (Brand A, Brand B, and Brand C) was reported. The brands have no order and could easily be listed as Brand B, Brand C, and Brand A. Likewise, roof type has no order. These are two nominal variables, and it may be of interest to determine whether these two variables have a relationship (Table 4-12).

TABLE 4-12 **CONTINGENCY TABLE EXAMPLE (3×3 NOMINAL VARIABLES)**

Table of Roof by Type					
Frequency Percentage Row Percentage Column Percentage		Column Variable: Type			
		1	2	3	Total
Row Variable: Roof	1	87 17.40 37.99 46.28	51 10.20 22.27 33.12	91 18.20 39.74 57.59	229 45.80
	2	54 10.80 35.53 28.72	67 13.40 44.08 43.51	31 6.20 20.39 19.62	152 30.40
	3	47 9.40 39.50 25.00	36 7.20 30.25 23.38	36 7.20 30.25 22.78	119 23.80
Total		188 37.60	154 30.80	158 31.60	500 100.00

© Cengage Learning, 2012.

The relationship between two variables can be described with a 3×3 contingency table (row = 3 × column = 3). Just as in the 2×2 contingency table, the cells represent the number of subjects with the characteristics of that row and column combination; and total, row, and column percentages result from using total, row, and column denominators. To determine whether there is an association between the two nominal variables, hypothesis testing can help.

RESEARCH HYPOTHESIS: There is an association between the net brand used and the type of roof.

NULL HYPOTHESIS: There is not an association between the net brand used and the type of roof.

Because each of the variables has more than two levels, there are many more proportions to compare. A significant *p*-value just means that there is a general association; it does not test whether one percentage is different from another. In this example (Table 4-13), the *p*-value is small ($p < 0.0001$).

TABLE 4-13 **RESULTS OF A GENERAL ASSOCIATION CHI-SQUARE TEST**

Summary Statistics for Roof by Type				
Statistic	Alternative Hypothesis	DF	Value	Prob
Chi-square	General Association	4	25.2760	<0.0001

© Cengage Learning, 2012.

CONCLUSION: There is sufficient evidence ($p < 0.0001$) to reject the null hypothesis. Hence, the type of roof a household has is related to the brand of net used.

Hypothesis Test for a Nominal and Ordinal Variable (R×C Contingency Table)

RESEARCH QUESTION:

Is using a net associated with increasing wealth?

Whether an insecticide-treated net was used is a nominal (dichotomous) variable. The wealth of the household has an order (lowest 25%, next lowest, next highest, highest 25%), and so it is an ordinal variable. Investigating more than just a general association between these two variables is possible. Are more nets used as wealth increases?

The relationship between two variables can be described with a 2×4 contingency table (row = 2 × column = 4). See Table 4-14. Just as in the 2×2 contingency table example, the cells represent the number of subjects with the characteristics of that row

TABLE 4-14 **CONTINGENCY TABLE EXAMPLE (NOMINAL AND ORDINAL VARIABLES)**

Table of Net by Wealth					
Frequency Percentage Row Percentage Column Percentage	Column Variable: Wealth				
	1	2	3	4	Total
Row Variable: Net Use — 0	406 21.64 29.51 84.76	403 21.48 29.29 75.19	367 19.56 26.67 67.84	200 10.66 14.53 62.50	1376 73.35
Row Variable: Net Use — 1	73 3.89 14.60 15.24	133 7.09 26.60 24.81	174 9.28 34.80 32.16	120 6.40 24.00 37.50	500 26.65
Total	479 25.53	536 28.57	541 28.84	320 17.06	1876 100.00

© Cengage Learning, 2012.

and column combination, and total, row, and column percentages result from using total, row, and column denominators. To determine whether there is an association between the two variables, hypothesis testing can help.

Because the wealth index is ordinal, it has an ordering or a ranking. To take this characteristic into account, a score can be assigned to each level of the variable and a mean taken. The test associated with these two variables is called a *row mean scores test*.

RESEARCH HYPOTHESIS: The mean scores for at least two rows are different.

NULL HYPOTHESIS: The mean scores for all the rows are not different.

Because the contingency table is larger than a 2×2 with four cells, there are many more percentages to compare. General association can be determined, but. because the column variable is an ordinal variable where order matters, more can be said. The mean scores between the levels of the nominal variable can be compared, and a higher mean score suggests that a group has a higher level of the ordinal value. In this test, a significant p-value indicates that the mean row scores for the two rows are different. In this example (Table 4-15), the p-value is small ($p < 0.0001$).

TABLE 4-15 **RESULTS OF A ROW MEAN SCORES DIFFER CHI-SQUARE TEST**

Summary Statistics for Net by Wealth				
Statistic	Alternative Hypothesis	DF	Value	Prob
Chi-square	Row mean scores differ	1	59.4380	<0.0001
Chi-square	General association	3	60.4718	<0.0001

© Cengage Learning, 2012.

CONCLUSION: There is sufficient evidence (p < 0.0001) to reject the null hypothesis. Hence, the mean scores of wealth are different for households with net use and without.

The chi-square test of general association resulted in a p-value of <0.0001, and the chi-square test of row mean squares differ resulted in a p-value of <0.0001. Although these tests resulted in similar p-values, remember that the hypothesis being tested in each of these tests is different.

Hypothesis Test for Two Ordinal Variables (R×C Contingency Table)

RESEARCH QUESTION:
Is there a correlation between wealth and distance to healthcare?

The wealth of the household has an order (lowest 25%, next lowest, next highest, highest 25%), and so it is an ordinal variable. Family size was also collected as an ordinal variable. Investigating more than just a general association and more than a difference in rows is possible. If there is a relationship by which an increase in the levels of one variable are related to the increases or decreases in the level of the other, the two variables are said to be *correlated*. Therefore, it is possible to investigate whether the two ordinal variables are correlated.

The relationship between these two variables can be described with a 4×3 contingency table (row = 4 × column = 3). Just as in the 2×2 contingency table example, the cells represent the number of subjects with the characteristics of that row and column combination, and total, row, and column percentages result from using total, row, and column denominators. To determine whether there is a relationship between the two ordinal variables, hypothesis testing can help (Table 4-16).

TABLE 4-16 **CONTINGENCY TABLE EXAMPLE (4×3 ORDINAL VARIABLES)**

Table of Wealth by Hcdist				
Frequency Percentage Row Percentage Column Percentage	Column Variable: Hcdist			Total
	1	2	3	
Row Variable: Wealth — 1	120 6.40 25.05 21.74	111 5.92 23.17 29.92	248 13.22 51.77 26.02	479 25.53
2	163 8.69 30.41 29.53	95 5.06 17.72 25.61	278 14.82 51.87 29.17	536 28.57
3	171 9.12 31.61 30.98	98 5.22 18.11 26.42	272 14.50 50.28 28.54	541 28.84
4	98 5.22 30.63 17.75	67 3.57 20.94 18.06	155 8.26 48.44 16.26	320 17.06
Total	552 29.42	371 19.78	953 50.80	1876 100.00

© Cengage Learning, 2012.

RESEARCH HYPOTHESIS: There is a correlation between wealth and distance to a healthcare facility.

NULL HYPOTHESIS: There is not a correlation between wealth and distance to a healthcare facility.

The chi-square test of general association resulted in a p-value of 0.1325, the chi-square test of row mean squares differ resulted in a p-value of 0.4122, and the chi-square test of nonzero correlation resulted in a p-value of 0.1083 (Table 4-17). All of these tests resulted in different p-values because the hypotheses associated with them are different. Again, the research question should be used to choose the appropriate hypothesis and test.

TABLE 4-17 **RESULTS OF A NONZERO CORRELATION CHI-SQUARE TEST**

Summary Statistics for Wealth by Hcdist				
Statistic	**Alternative Hypothesis**	**DF**	**Value**	**Prob**
Chi-square	Nonzero correlation	1	2.5781	0.1083
Chi-square	Row mean scores differ	3	2.8697	0.4122
Chi-square	General association	6	9.8177	0.1325

© Cengage Learning, 2012.

CONCLUSION: The p-value in this example is not quite small enough to reject the null hypothesis. Therefore, there is not enough evidence to claim that wealth index and distance from healthcare are correlated.

Multiple-Group Proportions: Exact Tests

Sometimes the sample size is not very large, and small cell counts (expected cell count smaller than five) result. In this situation, Fisher's exact test can be used to test hypotheses. As an example, suppose a subset of the data was selected, where only older, urban households were of interest.

The hypotheses to investigate this research question are the same as the hypotheses of independence in the larger sample.

RESEARCH QUESTION:
For urban households whose head of the household is greater than 55 years old, is there an association between insecticide-treated net use and having a child under 5?

RESEARCH HYPOTHESIS: Insecticide-treated net use in urban, older households is dependent on having children under the age of 5 in the household.

NULL HYPOTHESIS: Insecticide-treated net use in urban, older households is independent of having children under the age of 5 in the household.

The hypothesis test assumes that the null hypothesis is true. The goal is to use the sample data to provide evidence against the null hypothesis. Unfortunately, the chi-square test of independence cannot be used because the sample size is small

TABLE 4-18 RESULTS FROM FISHER'S EXACT TEST WITH MULTIPLE GROUPS

Table of Net by Child			
Frequency Percentage Row Percentage Column Percentage	Column Variable: Child		
	0	1	Total
Row Variable: Net Use — 0	100 56.82 60.24 95.24	66 37.50 39.76 92.96	166 94.32
Row Variable: Net Use — 1	5 2.84 50.00 4.76	5 2.84 50.00 7.04	10 5.68
Total	105 59.66	71 40.34	176 100.00

Statistics for Table of Net by Child			
Statistic	DF	Value	Prob
Chi-square	1	0.4110	0.5215

Warning: 25% of the cells have expected counts less than 5. Chi-square may not be a valid test.

Fisher's Exact Test	
Left-sided Pr <= F	0.8349
Right-sided Pr >= F	0.3727
Table probability (P)	0.2076
Two-sided Pr <= P	0.5271

Sample Size = 176

($n = 40$) and results in too few households in the sample that did not use nets and have children under the age of 5. Specifically, the cell in the contingency table for not using ITNs and having children under the age of 5 has an expected cell count of $(10 \times 24) \div 40 = 1.8$. When the expected cell count is smaller than 5, Fisher's exact test can be used to test the hypothesis (Table 4-18). Fisher's exact test considers all possible contingency tables that could have resulted from the sample and then determines the probability that this contingency table occurred. The p-value associated with Fisher's exact test is 0.5271.

> **CONCLUSION:** This fairly large p-value suggests that there is no evidence against the null hypothesis ($p = 0.5271$). Hence, in older, urban households, ITN use is not dependent on having children under the age of 5.

Fisher's exact test is not limited to contingency tables containing two rows and columns (2×2 tables). Most statistical software packages provide Fisher's exact test for contingency tables of all sizes (R×C).

Measures of Association for a Dichotomous Outcome

> **RESEARCH QUESTION:**
> Does having a child under the age of 5 impact the utilization of insecticide-treated nets?

Although the two categorical variables of interest can be of any type (dichotomous, nominal, or ordinal), the situation when the outcome is dichotomous is special. Many public health studies involve research questions whose outcome has only two levels. Therefore, special numerical summaries are needed to describe the relationship of the dichotomous outcome with other variables. Specifically, many research questions involve trying to understand how different groups relate to one another. Differences in proportions, ratios of proportions, and odds ratios are used when the goal of the study is to investigate how groups relate to each other and the outcome of interest has only two levels.

Difference in Proportions, Risks, and Prevalence Rates

A typical research question involves determining whether two population proportions are different. The parameter of interest then becomes the difference in proportions for the two populations. This difference represents an absolute measure of the actual difference in proportions, and the proportions involved in the difference are simply two conditional probabilities. The proportion for Population 1 is the probability of the outcome given that a subject belongs to Population 1 (p_1) and the proportion for Population 2 is simply the probability of the outcome given a subject belongs to Population 2 (p_2). The difference in population proportions is $p_1 - p_2$.

- When the proportions are the same, the difference in proportions is 0.
- A difference in proportions of less than 0 indicates that the proportion of Population 2 is larger than the proportion of Population 1.
- Similarly, if the difference in proportions is greater than 0, the proportion from Population 1 is larger than that of Population 2.

The difference in proportions ($p_1 - p_2$) is estimated by the difference in sample proportions $\hat{p}_1 - \hat{p}_2$, where $\hat{p}_1$ = the proportion of those with the outcome in sample (group) 1, and $\hat{p}_2$ = the proportion of those with the outcome in sample (group) 2.

As an example, consider the difference in the proportion of net use for households with and without children under 5, $p_{U5} - p_{O5}$, where p_{U5} represents the true proportion of insecticide-treated net use in households with children under 5, and p_{O5} represents the true proportion of insecticide-treated net use in households with children over 5.

Estimates of p_{U5} and p_{O5} are the conditional probabilities for using insecticide-treated nets in households with children under 5 and over 5: $\hat{p}_{U5} = 0.34$ and $\hat{p}_{O5} = 0.21$, respectively. The estimate for the risk difference $(p_{U5} - p_{O5})$ is simply the difference between these two proportion estimates.

Application of Formula: PROPORTION DIFFERENCES

Estimate of difference in proportions $= \hat{p}_1 - \hat{p}_2$

$\hat{p}_1 =$ The proportion of those with the outcome in sample 1

$\hat{p}_2 =$ The proportion of those with the outcome in sample 2

What you need to calculate the difference in proportions:

1. *Sample proportion 1, $\hat{p}_1$*: In this example, Population 1 is the population of households with children under 5: $\hat{p}_1 = \hat{p}_{U5} = 0.34$.
2. *Sample proportion 2, $\hat{p}_2$*: In this example, Population 2 is the population of households without children under 5: $\hat{p}_2 = \hat{p}_{O5} = 0.21$.

To calculate an estimate of the risk difference: (1) minus (2): $\hat{p}_1 - \hat{p}_2 = \hat{p}_{U5} - \hat{p}_{O5} = 0.34 - 0.21 = 0.13$.

For this study, the estimated proportion difference is 0.13, which is larger than 0. The fact that the proportion difference is greater than 0 implies that the proportion of ITN use in households with children under 5 is larger than the proportion for households without children under 5. However, this proportion difference estimate describes only this sample. It is a statistic, a point estimate. To answer the research question, inferences beyond this sample need to be made, and considerations need to be made for differences that could exist if different samples were used.

Although hypothesis tests allow for testing whether the proportions are different (as was the case in the chi-square test of independence), when trying to measure the absolute differences between the proportions, the emphasis is generally on estimation. The goal is to do more than indicate whether the true proportion difference is not equal to 0; it is to actually provide an estimate for how different the two proportions are. Confidence intervals provide an interval estimate for the true parameter (proportion difference) while accounting for the variability that exists between samples. In addition, having a good estimate of the true proportion difference, the confidence interval provides a set of plausible values for the true parameter and can be used to determine whether a true proportion difference of 0 is reasonable.

Confidence intervals are based on the idea of sampling distributions and on the fact that not all samples will result in the same statistic. Although another sample of 1876 households is not likely to have the same proportions of insecticide-treated net utilization, the statistics (estimates of the proportion differences) from these different samples should all pile up fairly close to the true parameter (the true proportion difference).

In this example, the sample size is fairly large, and the rate of ITN use is not too small; so the sampling distribution of the difference in proportions (like the sampling distribution of proportions) is normally distributed. Therefore, the normal distribution can be used to find a confidence interval for the difference in proportions. However, a measure of the variability of both samples is needed. The standard error for the proportion difference is fairly straightforward to calculate with estimates of the variance for each of the samples.

Application of Formula: STANDARD ERROR FOR PROPORTION DIFFERENCES

$$\text{Standard error} = \sqrt{\frac{\hat{p}_1(1 - \hat{p}_1)}{n_1} + \frac{\hat{p}_2(1 - \hat{p}_2)}{n_2}}$$

$\hat{p}_1$ = The estimated proportion of successes in sample/Group 1

$\hat{p}_2$ = The estimated proportion of successes in sample/Group 2

n_1 = The number of subjects in sample/Group 1

n_2 = The number of subjects in sample/Group 2

What you need to calculate the variance:

1. *Variance associated with each Group:*
   a. *The sample variance for Group 1:* $\dfrac{\hat{p}_1(1 - \hat{p}_1)}{n_1} = 0.000269$

   b. *The sample variance for Group 2:* $\dfrac{\hat{p}_2(1 - \hat{p}_2)}{n_2} = 0.000159$
2. *Sum the group variances (1a) + (1b):* $0.000269 + 0.000159 = 0.000428$.

To calculate the standard error: Take the square root of the sum of *(3)* $= \sqrt{0.000428} = 0.02069$.

Application of Formula

C% confidence interval for a proportion difference: $\hat{p}_1 - \hat{p}_2 \pm z^* \times SE$.

$\hat{p}_1 - \hat{p}_2$ = The sample proportion difference

C = The confidence level for a *C%* confidence interval

z^* = The number of standard deviations from the center of the sampling distribution

SE = The standard error of the proportion difference

What you need to calculate the confidence interval:

1. *The sample proportion difference or the point estimate of the proportion difference:* $\hat{p}_1 - \hat{p}_2 = 0.13$.
2. *The standard error:* $\sqrt{0.000428} = 0.02069$.
3. *The confidence level: C%* is typically 95%, but 90% and 99% are also common.
4. *The number of standard deviations from the center of the sampling distribution:* This depends on *C%* (3) and the sampling distribution. So, when the sampling distribution is a normal distribution, the z^* for a 90% confidence interval is 1.65, the z^* for a 95% confidence interval is 1.96, and the z^* for a 99% confidence interval is 2.58. Therefore, confidence intervals can be calculated as

   90% confidence interval: $\hat{p}_1 - \hat{p}_2 \pm (1.65 \times \text{standard error})$

   95% confidence interval: $\hat{p}_1 - \hat{p}_2 \pm (1.96 \times \text{standard error})$

   99% confidence interval: $\hat{p}_1 - \hat{p}_2 \pm (2.58 \times \text{standard error})$

To calculate the 95% confidence interval for the proportion difference: The number of SEs (margin of error) is added and subtracted to and from the point estimate and is $[0.13 - 1.96 \times 0.02069, 0.13 + 1.96 \times 0.02069]$, or $[0.09, 0.17]$.

Because 95% of all confidence intervals cover the true proportion difference, this interval represents a set of plausible values for the true proportion difference. The interval estimate does not cover 0 and includes only values larger than 0, suggesting that the true proportion difference is not 0 but larger than 0. Hence, the insecticide-treated net use is associated with having a child under the age of 5 and having a child under the age of 5 increases the proportion of ITN use.

When the study design is cross-sectional and the data are collected at one point in time, as it is in this example, the proportions represent prevalence rates. Therefore, the difference in proportions is really a prevalence difference, which represents an absolute measure of the actual difference in prevalence. Similarly, if the study design is prospective, the proportion is really a measure of risk. Therefore, the difference in proportions is really a risk difference. Thus, a difference in proportions for a prospective study is really an absolute measure of the difference in risk.

Ratio of Proportions, Risks, and Prevalence Rates

Public health questions often involve investigating how one group relates to another group. Although a difference in proportions provides a measure of how different the proportions are, it does not describe how the proportions relate to each other. In public health, proportions are more generally compared with a ratio or by dividing one proportion by another instead of investigating differences. Generally, the proportion corresponding to the control group is placed in the denominator.

- If the proportions of the two groups are the same, then the ratio of proportions will be 1.
- If the ratio of proportions is larger than 1, then the numerator is larger than the denominator. that is, the proportion in the numerator is larger than the proportion in the denominator.
- Similarly, if the proportion ratio is less than 1, then the denominator is larger than the numerator; the proportion in the denominator is larger than the proportion in the numerator.

Application of Formula: PROPORTION RATIOS

Estimate of the proportion ratio $= \dfrac{\hat{p}_1}{\hat{p}_2}$

$\hat{p}_1 =$ The observed proportion of the subjects in sample 1 with a characteristic

$\hat{p}_2 =$ The observed proportion of the subjects in sample 2 with a characteristic

What you need to calculate an estimate of the proportion ratio:

1. *The sample proportion for Group 1, $\hat{p}_1$:* If Group 1 are the households with children under 5, then $\hat{p}_{U5} = 280 \div 833 = 0.34$.
2. *The sample proportion for Group 2, $\hat{p}_2$:* If Group 2 are the households without children under 5, then $\hat{p}_{O5} = 220 \div 1043 = 0.21$.

To calculate the estimate of the proportion ratio: This is the Group 1 estimate (1) divided by the Group 2 estimate (2): $0.34 \div 0.21 = 1.6$.

For this sample, the estimated proportion ratio is 1.6, which is larger than 1. A proportion ratio estimated to be larger than 1 implies that the numerator proportion is larger than the denominator proportion. The denominator represents households without children under the age of 5. Thus, the estimate of the proportion ratio implies that the proportion of households using insecticide-treated nets is larger (1.6 times larger) in the households with children under 5 versus households without children under 5. However, this proportion ratio estimate describes only this sample. It is a statistic, a point estimate. To answer the research question, inferences beyond this sample need to be made, and so considerations need to be made for differences that could exist for different samples.

With a proportion ratio, the goal is to do more than to indicate whether the true proportion ratio is equal to 1; it is actually to provide an estimate for how different the two proportions are. Therefore, the emphasis is on estimation, and confidence intervals are used to provide an interval estimate for the true parameter (proportion ratio). In addition, having a good estimate of the true proportion ratio, confidence intervals will also indicate whether or not the true proportion ratio is 1.

Confidence intervals are based on the idea of sampling distributions and that not all samples will result in the same statistic. Although it would be unlikely that another sample of 1876 households would have the same insecticide-treated net utilization, the statistics (estimates of the proportion ratios) from these different samples should all pile up fairly close to the true parameter (the proportion ratio). Unfortunately, proportion ratios (and ratios in general) do not have normal sampling distributions. In fact, they are slightly more skewed than a normal distribution. However, taking the natural log (ln) of the sample proportion ratio results in a fairly normal sampling distribution. Consequently, the confidence interval for the natural log of the proportion ratio (PR), $\ln(PR)$, can be obtained using a normal sampling distribution. To provide interval estimates for the true natural log of the proportion ratio, a measure of variability must first be found. The variance associated with the natural log of the proportion ratio is fairly straightforward to calculate. Like most variances involved with proportions, an estimate of the proportion of success, the proportion of failures, and the sample size is needed.

Application of Formula: STANDARD ERROR FOR PROPORTION RATIOS

$$\text{Standard error} = \sqrt{\frac{1 - \hat{p}_1}{\hat{p}_1 \times n_1} + \frac{1 - \hat{p}_2}{\hat{p}_2 \times n_2}}$$

$\hat{p}_1 = $ The proportion of successes observed in Group 1

$\hat{p}_2 = $ The proportion of successes observed in Group 2

$n_1 = $ The number of events observed in Group 1

$n_2 = $ The number of events observed in Group 2

What you need to calculate the variance:

1. *Group 1:*
   a. The proportion of successes in sample 1: $\hat{p}_1 = \hat{p}_{U5} = \frac{280}{833} = 0.34$.
   b. The proportion of failures in sample 1, 1 − (a): $1 - \hat{p}_{U5} = 1 - 0.34 = 0.66$.
   c. The sample size in Group 1: $n_1 = n_{U5} = 833$.
   d. Multiply the proportion of successes (a) times the sample size (c): $\hat{p}_{U5} \times n_{U5} = 0.34 \times 833 = 283.22$.
   e. Divide the estimated proportion of failures (b) by (d): $0.66 \div 283.22 = 0.002$.
2. *Group 2:*
   a. The proportion of successes in sample 2: $\hat{p}_2 = \hat{p}_{O5} = \frac{220}{1043} = 0.21$.
   b. The proportion of failures in sample 2, 1 − (a): $1 - \hat{p}_{O5} = 1 - 0.21 = 0.79$.
   c. The sample size in Group 2: $n_2 = n_{O5} = 1043$.
   d. Multiply the proportion of successes (a) times the sample size (c): $\hat{p}_{O5} \times n_{O5} = 0.21 \times 1{,}043 = 219.03$.
   e. Divide the estimated proportion of failures (b) by (d): $0.79 \div 219.03 = 0.004$.
3. *Sum (1) and (2):* $0.002 + 0.004 = 0.006$.

To calculate the standard error: Take the square root of (3): $\sqrt{0.006} = 0.08$.

Application of Formula

C% confidence interval for the natural log of the proportion ratio: $\ln\left(\dfrac{\hat{p}_1}{\hat{p}_2}\right) \pm z^* \times SE$

What you need to calculate the confidence interval:

$\ln\left(\dfrac{\hat{p}_1}{\hat{p}_2}\right)$ = The natural log of the sample proportion ratio

C = The confidence level for a C% confidence interval

z^* = The number of standard deviations from the center of the sampling distribution

SE = The standard error of the natural log of the proportion ratio

What you need to calculate the confidence interval:

1. *The sample proportion ratio or the point estimate of the proportion ratio:* $\hat{p}_1/\hat{p}_2 = 1.6$.
2. *The natural log of the proportion ratio estimate or the natural log of the sample proportion ratio (1):* $\ln(1.6) = 0.47$.
3. *The standard error:* $\sqrt{0.006} = 0.08$.
4. *The confidence level:* C% is typically 95%, but 90% and 99% are also common.
5. *The number of standard deviations from the center of the sampling distribution:* This depends on C% (4) and the sampling distribution. So, when the sampling distribution is a normal distribution, the z^* for a 90% confidence interval is 1.65, the z^* for a 95% confidence interval is 1.96, and the z^* for a 99% confidence interval is 2.58. Therefore, confidence intervals can be calculated as

    90% confidence interval: $\ln(\text{ratio estimate}) \pm (1.65 \times \text{standard error})$

    95% confidence interval: $\ln(\text{ratio estimate}) \pm (1.96 \times \text{standard error})$

    99% confidence interval: $\ln(\text{ratio estimate}) \pm (2.58 \times \text{standard error})$

To calculate the 95% confidence interval for the natural log of the proportion ratio: The number of SEs (margin of error) is added and subtracted to and from the point estimate and is $[0.47 - 1.96 \times 0.08, 0.47 + 1.96 \times 0.08]$, or $[0.31, 0.63]$.

These confidence intervals, however, do not provide interval estimates for the proportion ratio, but an interval estimate of the natural log of the proportion ratio. To obtain the interval estimate for the true proportion ratio (the parameter of interest), the upper and lower limits of the confidence interval must be exponentiated. Hence, to get the interval estimate of the proportion ratio, an additional calculation [exp(lower limit), exp(upper limit)] is required.

In this example, the 95% confidence interval for the natural log of the proportion ratio is $[0.31, 0.63]$. Therefore, the interval estimate of the proportion ratio is $[\exp(0.31), \exp(0.63)] = [1.4, 1.9]$. Because 95% of all confidence intervals cover the true proportion ratio, this interval estimate provides a set of plausible values for the true proportion ratio. This set of plausible values does not include 1 and covers possible parameters that are greater than 1, suggesting that the true proportion ratio is larger than 1. Hence, insecticide-treated net use is associated with having a child under the age of 5, and an increased proportion of use is expected for households with children under 5.

When the design is cross-sectional and the data are collected at one point in time, as in this study, the proportions represent prevalence rates. Therefore, the ratio of proportions is really a prevalence ratio and provides a relative measure of how the prevalence rates of the two groups compare. When the study design is prospective, the proportion is really a measure of risk. Therefore, the difference in proportions is really a risk ratio. The risk ratio provides a relative measure of how the risks of two groups compare. Consequently, the risk ratio is also known as the *relative risk*.

Odds Ratio

Depending on the study design, obtaining a risk or prevalence ratio may not be appropriate. For example, retrospective studies do not involve risks or prevalence rates, and the most appropriate numerical summary is the odds. To investigate the odds occurring in one group relative to another, investigators need a ratio of odds, or odds ratio. The *odds ratio* is a fraction in which the odds of one group is in the numerator and the odds of another group is in the denominator. The control group is often found in the denominator.

- If the odds of the two groups are the same, then the odds ratio is 1.
- If the odds ratio is larger than 1, then the numerator is larger than the denominator, that is, the odds in the numerator is larger than the odds in the denominator.
- Similarly, if the odds ratio is less than 1, then the denominator is larger than the numerator; the odds in the denominator is larger than the odds in the numerator.

Application of Formula

$$\text{Estimate of the odds ratio} = \frac{odds_1}{odds_2} - \frac{\hat{p}_1/1-\hat{p}_1}{\hat{p}_2/1-\hat{p}_2}$$

$\hat{p}_1$ = The observed proportion of the subjects in sample 1 with a characteristic

$\hat{p}_2$ = The observed proportion of the subjects in sample 2 with a characteristic

What you need to calculate an estimate of the odds ratio:

1. *The estimated odds for Group 1:*
   a. The estimate of the proportion of successes for Group 1, $\hat{p}_1$: If Group 1 consists of the households with children under 5, then $\hat{p}_{U5} = 280 \div 833 = 0.34$.
   b. The estimate of the proportion of failures for Group 1, $1 - \hat{p}_1$: If Group 1 consists of the households with children under 5, then $1 - \hat{p}_{U5} = 1 - 0.34 = 0.66$.
   c. The estimated odds for Group 1: This is the proportion of succcesses (a) divided by the proportion of failures (b): $0.34 \div 0.66 = 0.52$.
2. *The estimated odds for Group 2:*
   a. The estimate of the proportion of successes for Group 2, $\hat{p}_2$: If Group 2 consists of the households without children under 5, then $\hat{p}_{O5} = 220 \div 1043 = 0.21$.
   b. The estimate of the proportion of failures for Group 1, $1 - \hat{p}_2$: If Group 1 consists of the households without children under 5, then $1 - \hat{p}_{O5} = 1 - 0.21 = 0.79$.
   c. The estimated odds for Group 2: This is the proportion of succcesses (a) divided by the proportion of failures (b): $0.21 \div 0.79 = 0.27$.

To calculate the estimate of the odds ratio: This is just the Group 1 odds (1) divided by the Group 2 odds (2): $0.52 \div 0.27 = 1.9$.

For this sample, the estimated odds ratio is 1.9, which is larger than 1, implying that the numerator odds is larger than the denominator odds. The denominator represents households that do not have children under 5 in the household. Thus, the estimate of the odds ratio suggests that the odds of net use is larger (1.9 times larger) in the households with children under the age of 5 versus households without children under that age. However, this odds ratio estimate describes only this sample. It is a statistic, a point estimate. To answer the research question, inferences beyond this sample need to be made, considerations need to be made for differences that could exist for different samples.

When an odds ratio is needed, the goal is to do more than to indicate whether the true odds ratio is equal to 1; it is also to actually provide an estimate for how different the two odds are. Therefore, the emphasis is on estimating the true parameter (the odds ratio). Confidence intervals provide an interval estimate for the odds ratio and can also be used to eliminate 1 as a possible parameter.

Confidence intervals are based on the idea of sampling distributions and that not all samples will result in the same statistic. Although another sample of 1876 households would be unlikely to have the same insecticide-treated net utilization, the statistics (estimates of the odds ratios) from these different samples should all be fairly close to the true parameter (the true population odds ratio). Unfortunately, odds ratios also do not have a normal sampling distributions. In fact, they are slightly more skewed than a normal distribution. However, taking the natural log (ln) of the odds ratio estimates results in a fairly normal sampling distribution. Consequently, the confidence interval for the natural log of the odds ratio, $\ln(OR)$, can be obtained using a normal sampling distribution. However, a measure of variability is needed to calculate the interval estimate. The variance and so the standard error are actually quite simple to calculate when it comes to the natural log of the odds ratio. It is simply the sum of all the inverse cell counts.

Application of Formula

$$\text{Variance } [\ln(\widehat{OR}) = \frac{1}{\text{cell}_1} + \frac{1}{\text{cell}_2} + \frac{1}{\text{cell}_3} + \frac{1}{\text{cell}_4}$$

cell_1 = The number of subjects in cell 1 of a 2×2 contingency table

cell_2 = The number of subjects in cell 2 of a 2×2 contingency table

cell_3 = The number of subjects in cell 3 of a 2×2 contingency table

cell_4 = The number of subjects in cell 4 of a 2×2 contingency table

Table of Net by Child				
		Column Variable: Child		
		0	1	Totals
Row Variable: Net	0	823	553	1376
	1	220	280	500
Totals		1043	833	1876

© Cengage Learning, 2012.

What you need to calculate the variance:

1. *The inverse of the number of subjects in cell 1:* $1 \div 823 = 0.001$
2. *The inverse of the number of subjects in cell 2:* $1 \div 553 = 0.002$
3. *The inverse of the number of subjects in cell 3:* $1 \div 220 = 0.005$
4. *The inverse of the number of subjects in cell 4:* $1 \div 280 = 0.004$
5. *The variance: The sum of the inverse cell counts:* $0.001 + 0.002 + 0.005 + 0.004 = 0.012$

To calculate the standard error: This is the square root of the variance: $\sqrt{0.012} = 0.11$.

Application of Formula

C% confidence interval for the natural log of the odds ratio: $\ln(\widehat{OR}) \pm z^* \times SE$

$\ln(\widehat{OR})$ = The natural log of the sample odds ratio

C = The confidence level for a C% confidence interval

z^* = The number of standard deviations from the center of the sampling distribution

SE = The standard error of the natural log of the odds ratio

What you need to calculate the confidence interval:

1. *The sample odds ratio or the point estimate of the odds ratio:* $\widehat{OR} = 1.9$.
2. *The natural log of the odds ratio estimate or the natural log of the sample odds ratio (1):* $\ln(\widehat{OR}) = 0.64$.
3. *The standard error:* $\sqrt{0.012} = 0.11$.
4. *The confidence level:* C% is typically 95%, but 90% and 99% are also common.
5. *The number of standard deviations from the center of the sampling distribution:* This depends on C% (4) and the sampling distribution. So, when the sampling distribution is a normal distribution, the z^* for a 90% confidence interval is 1.65, the z^* for a 95% confidence interval is 1.96, and the z^* for a 99% confidence interval is 2.58. Therefore, confidence intervals can be calculated as

90% confidence interval: $\ln(\widehat{OR}) \pm (1.65 \times \text{standard error})$

95% confidence interval: $\ln(\widehat{OR}) \pm (1.96 \times \text{standard error})$

99% confidence interval: $\ln(\widehat{OR}) \pm (2.58 \times \text{standard error})$

To calculate the 95% confidence interval for the natural log of the odds ratio: The number of SEs (margin of error) is added and subtracted to and from the point estimate and is $[0.47 - 1.96 \times 0.08, 0.47 + 1.96 \times 0.08]$, or $[0.31, 0.63]$.

These confidence intervals, however, do not provide interval estimates for the odds ratio, but an interval estimate of the natural log of the odds ratio. To obtain the interval estimate for the true odds ratio, the upper and lower limits of the confidence interval must be exponentiated. Hence, to get the interval estimate of the odds ratio, an additional calculation [exp(lower limit), exp(upper limit)] is required.

The 95% confidence interval for the natural log of the odds ratio is [0.43, 0.85]. Consequently, the interval estimate of the odds ratio is $[\exp(0.43), \exp(0.85)] = [1.5, 2.3]$. Because 95% of all confidence intervals cover the true odds ratio, this interval represents a set of plausible values for the true odds ratio, it can be used to determine whether there is evidence that the true odds ratio is 1. This set of plausible values does not include 1 and is larger than 1, so 1 is not a plausible value for the true odds ratio. Hence, net utilization is associated with having children under the age of 5, and it appears that households with children under the age of 5 have a higher odds of net usage.

In public health, odds ratios are among the most widely used numerical summaries. Unfortunately, they are often the most misinterpreted numerical summaries. The misinterpretation is due in large part to the difficulty in interpreting what an odds actually means. In general, an odds ratio should not be misinterpreted as risk ratio or a prevalence ratio. Unlike the odds ratio, risk and prevalence ratios are ratios of proportions: $\left(\frac{p_1}{p_2}\right)$. Odds ratios are ratios of odds: $\left(\frac{p_1/1-p_1}{p_2/1-p_2}\right)$.

Suppose the odds ratio estimate obtained in this study were interpreted as a risk ratio. The estimated odds ratio was 1.9 (1.5, 2.3). If this were interpreted as a risk ratio, the conclusion would be that the risk of using an insecticide-treated net in a household with children under the age of 5 is 1.9 (1.5, 2.3) times that of households without children under the age of 5. In other words, if a household has a child under the age of 5, then they are 1.9 (1.5, 2.3) times more likely to use insecticide-treated nets compared to a household without children under the age of 5. Misinterpreting odds ratios as risk ratios or even prevalence ratios will often result in overestimating the risk or prevalence of an outcome.

It is possible to interpret an odds ratio as a relative risk when the event is rare or when there are a small number of subjects with a particular outcome. To be able to use the odds ratio as the relative risk, the outcome needs to occur less than 10% of the time. When the outcome occurs at a rate than 10%, the odds ratio and proportion ratio (risk and prevalence ratios) are relatively similar.

Interpretation of Ratios: Beyond Two Groups

When there are only two groups, ratios (risk, prevalence, or odds) are fairly easy to interpret: One group is in the numerator, and the other group is in the denominator. However, ratios are not limited to studies where the other variable results in only two groups. Ratios can be calculated for nominal variables with more than two levels, ordinal variables, and continuous variables. As an example, consider the interpretation of odds ratios (The interpretation of prevalence and risk ratios is exactly the same except that the term "odds" is replaced with "prevalence" or "risk," respectively).

For dichotomous variables with only two levels, the odds ratio is interpreted as the odds in favor of success for one group OR times that of Group 2. If the odds ratio estimate is 1.5 and the outcome is using insecticide-treated nets, then the estimated odds ratio is interpreted as the estimated odds of using an insecticide-treated net in Group 1 is 1.5 times that of Group 2. This estimated odds ratio can also be interpreted that Group 1 has a 50% higher odds of net use than Group 2. Suppose, on the other hand, that the odds ratio is less than 1: $\widehat{OR} = 0.75$. In this case, the interpretation would be that the estimated odds ratio is interpreted as the estimated odds of using an insecticide-treated net in Group 1 is 0.75 times that of Group 2. Another way to state the interpretation is that Group 1 has 25% lower odds of using an insecticide-treated net when compared to Group 2.

For categorical variables with more than two levels, the interpretation is essentially the same as when there are two levels. The difference is that one of the levels of the categorical variable has to be selected as the reference. The reference group appears in the denominator. Hence, if a categorical variable has three levels, one of the levels will be the reference, and two odds ratios will result: where each of the remaining levels are in the numerator. The odds ratios are then interpreted exactly like dichotomous variable odds ratios. If the outcome is using insecticide-treated nets and the variable of interest is a categorical variable with three groups, then two odds ratios will result. Suppose that Group 3 is chosen as the reference and that the odds ratio estimate with Group 1 in the numerator is 1.5. This estimated odds ratio could be interpreted that Group 1 has a 50% higher odds of net use than Group 3. If the estimated odds ratio associated with Group 2 is 1.25, this odds ratio estimate could be interpreted that Group 2 has a 25% higher odds of net use than Group 3.

For continuous and ordinal variables, the interpretation is different because these variables have an order. An increase of 1 unit in these variables actually has meaning. Therefore, the interpretation of odds ratios associated with these variables involve how much the odds change for every unit increase in the variable. The odds ratio is interpreted as the odds in favor of success for change by a factor of *OR* for every unit increase in the continuous or ordinal variable. Assume the outcome is using insecticide-treated nets and the estimated odds ratio is 1.5. This estimated odds ratio associated with a continuous or ordinal variable would then be interpreted that, for every one unit increase in the variable, the odds of net use increase by 1.5, or 50%. If the odds ratio estimate was less than 1—0.75, for example—then for every 1-unit increase in the variable, the odds of net use decreases by 25%.

Use caution when interpreting ordinal variables like continuous variables, however. A 1-unit increase assumes that all the jumps from one level or category to another are the same. Although the jumps between levels may be the same for a variable like age where the jumps are in 1-year increments, jumps in the level educational attainment or distance to healthcare may not be equally spaced. Is the jump from <15 to 15–50 miles the same as the jump from 15–50 miles to 50+ miles? Because assuming that the increments of an ordinal variable are equal is often difficult, the order is generally ignored and ordinal variables are treated as nominal variables. Hence, the odds ratios associated with ordinal variables are often calculated and interpreted as nominal variables.

Planning a Two-Sample Study with a Dichotomous Outcome

Just as there are many analysis options for categorical variables, so there are many possibilities for sample size estimation. In public health, a dichotomous outcome is commonly compared for the different levels of another categorical variable. Generally, the research question involves comparing the proportions (the dichotomous outcome) of an exposure and control group. Providing sample size estimates for categorical data when the goal is to compare two proportions is similar to when the outcome is continuous (see Chapter 2). Like continuous outcomes, acceptable power, acceptable probability of a type 1 error, and the effect size are needed. In addition, however, if the outcome is dichotomous, an estimate of at least one of the proportions is also needed.

Determining the effect size involves finding an estimate of the difference between the proportions, which can be stated either as a difference in proportions or as an odds ratio. When the effect size is larger, the sample size required to detect this effect is smaller. However, a large effect size is not simply a large difference in proportions. How big or small the proportion is also matters. A large proportion does not require as large a sample size as a small proportion.

Typically, the planned study is novel and no historical information is available for what difference in proportion estimates (or odds ratio estimate) to expect. In the absence of published data specific to the study, published data on a similar topic may be available, providing a reasonable starting place for estimating proportions. When the outcome is dichotomous, the measure of variability is automatically obtained by having estimates of the proportions (recall the calculation of standard error for confidence intervals and hypothesis tests). Hence, to estimate effect sizes, either two estimates of the proportion are needed, or one proportion and estimate of the odds ratio is needed.

Table 4-19 provides a summary of how the sample size estimate changes with increased effect size estimates, increased power, and changes with the group proportion. These sample size estimates are much larger than the ones needed for comparing two means. The reason is that a continuous outcome contains more information than a dichotomous outcome.

As an example (from Table 4-19), with a sample size of 300 per group ($n = 600$), assuming one group has a rate of 0.5, a Chi-square test will have at least 90% power to detect an odds ratio of 1.75, two-sided $\alpha = 0.05$. This statement could also be written with an emphasis on the difference between proportions. When the sample size is 300 per group ($n = 600$), a chi-square test will have at least 90% power to detect a difference in one group proportion of 0.5 and another group proportion of 0.64, assuming a two-sided significance level of 0.05.

TABLE 4-19 **SAMPLE SIZE ESTIMATES (TESTING FOR A DIFFERENCE IN PROPORTIONS)**

Proposed Sample Size (per group)	Proportion	Effect Size	Power
1360	0.4	1.25	
1336	0.5	1.25	0.80
1423	0.6	1.25	
1827	0.4	1.25	
1794	0.5	1.25	0.90
1910	0.6	1.25	
223	0.4	1.75	
226	0.5	1.75	0.80
249	0.6	1.75	
296	0.4	1.75	
300	0.5	1.75	0.90
331	0.6	1.75	

Sample size estimates are based on conducting a two-group chi-square test ($\alpha = 0.05$).

© Cengage Learning, 2012.

SUMMARY

This chapter began with an infectious disease and health behavior problem: understanding factors related to insecticide-treated net use. In this public health application, like many others, the outcome of interest was a categorical variable. Specifically, the outcome was dichotomous; a categorical variable with only two levels. Like the public health application presented at the start of the chapter this chapter investigated factors (such as whether young children were in the household) that might be related to insecticide-treated net use.

Dichotomous variables are common in public health because research questions typically involve whether a subject has a particular characteristic. The characteristic can range from having a disease to a lifestyle choice to a physiologic trait. In addition to dichotomous variables, categorical variables that represent groups or rankings are also common. In this example, categorical variables with more than two levels were roof type, wealth index, and distance to healthcare. These variables were analyzed as nominal variables (no order to categories) and ordinal variables (categories have order). An introduction to methods for describing, comparing, and investigating associations between categorical variables was presented.

SUMMARY OF CHAPTER CONCEPTS

GOAL	COMMON TESTS	COMMON SUMMARIES	
		Graphical	**Numerical**
How do I compare my result to a known value?			
Sample size is large and proportion is not small.	One-sample *z*-test	Pie charts Bar graphs	Proportions
Sample size is small and/or proportion is small.	Exact one-sample test		
How do I compare groups when the outcome is dichotomous?			
Two groups	Chi-square test of independence	Bar graph with two variables	Proportion (risk or prevalence) difference Proportion (risk or prevalence) ratio Odds ratio
Multiple groups			
How do I investigate the association of two categorical variables?			
Both variables are nominal	Chi-square test of general association	Bar graph with two variables	Proportions
One nominal and one ordinal variable	Chi-square test for row mean scores differ		
Both variables are nominal	Chi-square test for nonzero correlation		

KEY TERMS

prevalence   odds   conditional probabilities

risk   contingency table

PRACTICE WITH DATA

1. **DESCRIBING THE DATA**

   a. Provide the odds of net use observed in rural households.

   b. Provide proportions of net use for rural and urban households.

   c. Use a bar graph to summarize the proportions found in part (c). What does the plot show?

2. **ONE-SAMPLE STUDY**

   a. Estimate (using a 95% confidence interval) the true proportion of net use. Interpret.

   b. Suppose it is reported that 25% of households with an ITN will actually use them. Is the proportion of net possession different in this sample? Use statistical inference to justify your answer.

   c. Suppose that the normal approximation could not be used for investigating the proportion of net use. Use exact methods (confidence interval or test) to determine whether the rate of net use is different from 25%. Provide an interpretation of the results.

3. **MULTIPLE-SAMPLE STUDIES**

   a. Provide the null and research hypotheses (defining all symbols) for comparing net usage rates in rural and urban households.

   b. Perform the appropriate test to investigate the hypotheses in part (a). Interpret the results.

   c. Summarize the association between net use and rural residence using the odds ratio. Using statistical inference, provide a conclusion about the relationship.

PRACTICE WITH CONCEPTS

1. Consider the following research questions/study scenarios. For each study, discuss the most appropriate methods for describing the data (graphically and numerically). What statistical method would be the *most* appropriate for addressing the research questions? Be sure to provide a justification of the statistical method. When a statistical test is needed, provide appropriate null and research hypotheses.

   a. A study was performed to determine whether steroids were effective in slowing the development of Crohn's disease (CD). In the study, 338 patients with irritable bowel syndrome (a possible precursor to CD) were randomly assigned either to receive steroids immediately or to wait until they developed further CD symptoms.

b. A study investigating the effects of second-hand smoke in working environments asked the following question: "How often do you experience second-hand smoke in a work environment/function? Never, Occasionally, Fairly Often, Very Often, Almost Always." The question was asked of managers and employees to determine whether there was an association between position and the amount of second-hand smoke exposure.

c. Stress has been related to several poor health outcomes, particularly BMI. Women will be surveyed on stress levels and will have weight assessed at a clinic visit. Weight will be categorized into the following weight groups: underweight, normal, overweight, and obese. Stress (defined as small, moderate, large, and overwhelming) will be measured on a sample of women. Is there a relationship between stress and weight?

d. An investigation of the association between drink preferences and the color of teeth is proposed. Subjects will be surveyed as to the type of drink most often consumed (coffee/tea, juice, caramel-colored soda, water, or milk). A clinical exam will be performed after dental cleaning to determine the color of the teeth (reddish brown, reddish yellow, gray, reddish gray).

2. *Hospital re-admissions for patients with congestive heart failure (CHF) are relatively common and costly occurrences within the U.S. health infrastructure, including the Veterans Affairs (VA) healthcare system. Little is known about CHF re-admissions among rural veteran patients, including the effects of socio-demographics and follow-up outpatient visits on these re-admissions. Purpose: To examine socio-demographics of U.S. veterans with CHF who had 30 day potentially preventable re-admissions and compare the effect of 30 day VA post-discharge service use on these re-admissions for rural- and urban-dwelling veterans.* (Muus, Knudson, Klug, Gokun, Sarrazin, & Kaboli, 2010)

	30 Day Re-admission	
Location of residence	Yes	No
Urban	17,872	3,792
Rural	9,428	1,906

Source: Adapted from Table 1 (Muus et al.).

a. The authors want to investigate re-admission rates for two cohorts (urban and rural residence). Based on the information in the preceding table, create a table that provides the appropriate proportions.

b. Using the table, create a bar graph to summarize the comparison of re-admission rates for rural and urban veterans.

c. When comparing the rates of re-admission for urban versus rural veterans, the authors obtained a p-value of 0.921 from a chi-square test of independence. What does this p-value indicate?

d. The authors indicated that, "A limitation of this study is the lack of information pertaining to health care provided outside of the VA system, such as an admission to a non-VA hospital following a discharge from a VA hospital." How might this impact the comparison of re-admission rates for urban and rural veterans?

3. *This paper reports the prevalence of obesity in the US based on World Health Organization's (WHO) classification of obesity. It also reports the prevalence of individuals in the general population who use dietary modifications and/or exercise to lose weight. The main objective of this paper is to assess the relationship between obesity status, HRQL, dietary modifications, and exercise. . . . Responses*

to the HRQL questions were used as dependent variables . . . by dichotomizing the number of reported days with poor physical health . . . into ≤ 14 days and >14 days. (Hassan, Joshi, Madhavan, & Amonkar, 2003)

    a. The data for this study were obtained using a survey conducted in 2000 (the Behavioral Risk Factor Surveillance System). The authors used odds ratios to summarize the relationship of obesity status (nonoverweight, overweight, obese, and severely obese) and the dichotomized poor physical health outcome. Was the choice of odds ratios appropriate? Explain why or why not.

    b. The odds ratios that result for investigating poor physical health are

        Nonoverweight: Reference
        Overweight: 1.08 (0.99–1.17)
        Obese: 1.21 (1.09–1.33)
        Severely Obese: 1.87 (1.64–2.12)

    Provide a conclusion. Be sure to include a discussion of statistical inference.

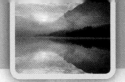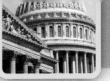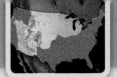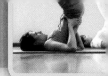

CHAPTER 5

a dichotomous outcome
confounding & regression

The statistical methods for describing and investigating two-variable associations and for making group comparisons for categorical data were described in Chapter 4. Briefly, categorical outcomes consist of three main types of variables: dichotomous, nominal, and ordinal. Categorical variables have a limited number of categories or levels, and observing values between these categories is not possible. Categorical outcomes are summarized numerically by means of descriptive statistics (counts, proportions, and percentages) and measures of association (differences in proportions, prevalence ratios, risk ratios, and odds ratios). Graphically, bar graphs and pie charts provide a picture of the distribution, and bar graphs can allow for comparing proportions (or percentages).

Generally, the effects of multiple variables (discrete and continuous) are measured on a single subject in a study. In public health, research questions investigating how multiple variables impact a dichotomous outcome are fairly common. Multiple variable relationships with a dichotomous outcome arise because multiple factors are of interest and confounding is often present.

Chapter 3, with its discussion of multiple linear regression, provided the foundations for investigating multiple variable relationships. However, the methods presented in Chapter 3 were specific to continuous outcomes. This chapter focuses on investigating multiple variable associations when the outcome is dichotomous.

LEARNING OBJECTIVES

How do I compare groups while adjusting for confounders (continuous and categorical)?

Determine whether a confounder is an effect modifier and identify appropriate statistical measures of association.

Utilize regression techniques to control for confounding.

Interpret the results (estimates and statistical tests) after controlling for confounding.

How do I investigate the association of risk factors (continuous and categorical) on the dichotomous outcome?

Utilize regression techniques to investigate risk factors.

Interpret the results (estimates and statistical tests) of the regression analysis.

How do I assess the ability of variable(s) to predict a dichotomous outcome?

Utilize the concepts of sensitivity, specificity, and ROC curves.

Identify, create, and interpret predicted probabilities.

Apply area under the curve (AUC) concepts to regression and variable selection.

What method do I use?

Identify the most appropriate method for describing the data, numerically and graphically.

Identify the most appropriate method for making comparisons.

Public Health Application

Malaria represents about 1.4% of the global burden of disease [1], and in Africa, it is the primary cause of disease burden as measured by Disability Adjusted Life Years (DALY) lost of 10.8% [2,3]. The continent bears over 90% of the global burden of about 2.7 million deaths attributable to malaria; and houses over 300 million people who suffer from this disease yearly, the worst hit being young children and pregnant women [2–4].

More than three quarters of global malaria deaths occur in under-five children living in malarious countries in sub-Saharan Africa (SSA) [5], where 25% of all childhood mortality below the age of five (about 800,000 young children [6]) is attributable to malaria [2]. Of those children who survive cerebral malaria, a severe form of the disease, more than 15% suffer neurological deficits [4,7], which include weakness, spasticity, blindness, speech problems and epilepsy. Where such children are poorly managed and do not have access to specialized educational facilities, these deficits may interfere with future learning and development [5].

About 30–40% of all fevers seen in health centers in Africa are due to malaria with huge seasonal variability between rainy and dry seasons. At the end of the dry season, it is less than 10% and more than 80% as the rainy season winds up [8].

In Nigeria, malaria is the leading cause of under-five mortality contributing 33% of all childhood deaths and 25% infant mortality. As a child will typically be sick from malaria between 3–4 times in one year, the disease is a major cause of absenteeism in school-aged children, thus impeding their educational and social development [5] and subsequently robbing the country of its future human resources.

[Korenromp E.L., Miller J., Cibulskis R.E., Kabir C.M., Alnwick D., Dye C. (2003). *Monitoring mosquito net coverage for malaria control in Africa: possession vs. use by children under 5 years. Tropical Medicine & International Health, 8(8),* *693–703. http://www.ncbi.nlm.nih.gov/pubmed/12869090*]

Data Description

In Chapter 4, the study to investigate factors related to insecticide-treated net use was described. Households ($n = 1876$) in a tropical region were selected based on whether an insecticide-treated net (ITN) was owned. Participants were asked whether the ITN had been used the previous night. The head of the household was provided a questionnaire that included the age of the head of household, a measure of household wealth, the miles to the nearest healthcare facility, whether the household was located in a rural or urban area, the family size in the household, and whether a child younger than 5 years old resided in the

household. The type of roof for the household was also recorded (thatched, corrugated metal, or other). The measure of wealth was recorded as a 4-level ordinal variable: lowest 25%, next lowest, next highest, and highest 25%. The distance to the nearest healthcare facility was categorized into three levels: within 15 miles, between 15 and 50 miles, and farther than 50 miles. All questionnaires were completed with an interviewer and conducted during the rainy season.

The primary goal of this study was to understand the factors associated with using insecticide treated nets. The primary outcome was whether an ITN was used on the previous night.

Graphical and numerical summaries that described categorical data were presented in Chapter 4. In particular, summaries for making comparisons between groups or for investigating associations between two categorical variables were described. These graphical and numerical representations are still appropriate for describing simple relationships. However, the purpose of this chapter is to provide further details on studies when the outcome is dichotomous. In addition to the numerical and graphical summaries presented in Chapter 4, numerical summaries of sensitivity and specificity describe how well a variable correctly predicts when the dichotomous outcome is one level or another. Graphically, receiver operator characteristic (ROC) curves are very useful for describing the predictive power of ordinal and continuous variables.

Numerical Summaries: Sensitivity and Specificity

When the outcome for a study is dichotomous, conditional probabilities (defined in Chapter 4) can help in understanding how well a variable performs at predicting the outcome. They are often useful when the research question involves a *screening test*. Screening tests may be used for determining whether a person has a disease or condition. Examples of screening tests are PPD (purified protein derivative) tests to screen for tuberculosis, Pap smears as screening tests for precancerous lesions, mammograms to screen for breast cancer, and x-rays at the dentist office to screen for dental caries. A good screening test does a reasonable job at identifying sick subjects as sick and healthy subjects as healthy. In statistical terms, the probability that a screening test will classify a person correctly is a conditional probability.

- The probability that a test classifies someone as sick given that the person is truly sick is known as **sensitivity**.
- The probability that a test will classify someone as healthy given that the person is truly healthy is known as **specificity**.

To further explain sensitivity and specificity, consider an unrealistic example. Suppose a screening test existed that classified all subjects as sick. Although this is not a very good screening test, it has 100% sensitivity because it would classify sick subjects as sick 100% of the time. Unfortunately, this test has 0% specificity because it would classify healthy subjects as healthy 0% of the time. Similarly, a screening test that told all patients that they were healthy has 100% specificity because it correctly identifies all healthy subjects as healthy. Unfortunately, the test also has 0% sensitivity because it incorrectly classifies all sick patients as healthy. Using the contingency tables defined in Chapter 4, conditional probabilities can be calculated to estimate the sensitivity and specificity of a test.

Suppose a new screening test is available to identify malaria cases. The test will indicate whether someone has malaria (row variable), and this can be compared to whether the subjects truly have malaria (column variable) (Table 5-1). In this example, of the subjects with malaria ($n = 804$), the test indicated that 310 had malaria. Therefore,

TABLE 5-1 **SENSITIVITY AND SPECIFICITY EXAMPLE**

Screening Test	Truth		Total
	No Malaria	Malaria	
No Malaria	905 84.42%	494 61.44%	1399
Test Malaria	167 15.58%	310 38.56%	477
Total	1072	804	1876

© Cengage Learning, 2012.

the sensitivity is $310 \div 804 = 0.39$, or 39%. On the other hand, of the subjects without malaria ($n = 1072$), the test indicated that 905 did not have the disease. Therefore, the specificity is $905 \div 1072 = 0.84$, or 84%. In this example, the test had moderate sensitivity but very good specificity. Therefore, it did a good job of determining who did not have malaria but did not perform as well determining who was actually suffering from malaria. Ideally, a screening test has both high sensitivity and high specificity.

Although sensitivity and specificity have been traditionally used in the context of screening tests, these concepts can be applied whenever the outcome is dichotomous and the goal is to determine how well variable correctly identifies whether a subject belongs to one level or another of the outcome. Later in this chapter, the concepts of sensitivity and specificity will be used to determine how well multiple variables predict a dichotomous outcome.

Graphical Summaries: Receiver Operator Characteristics (ROC) Curves

Not all screening tests or predictor variables are dichotomous. A screening test may also result in an ordinal or continuous variable. Examples of ordinal screening tests are classifications of ACL injuries from MRIs, categories of tumor volume, and level of pain measured on a Likert or visual analog scale. Continuous screening tests are also quite common: blood glucose for diabetes, hemoglobin for anemia, and PSA levels for prostate cancer. Conditional probabilities may be difficult to calculate from a contingency table when the screening test has a continuous or ordinal result. In fact, continuous screening test results require categorization before conditional probabilities (sensitivity and specificity) can be calculated. Statistical software can greatly help in these calculations because many, many categories can be created. However, whether the screening test is continuous or ordinal, summarizing sensitivity and specificity is still more complicated when the test involves more than two levels.

To evaluate the performance of an ordinal or continuous screening test, the sensitivity and specificity values for each level can be displayed graphically as a receiver operator characteristic (ROC) curve (Figure 5-1). In an ROC curve, the horizontal axis is (1 − specificity), and the vertical axis is sensitivity. A combined measure of how well the test performs is the area under the curve (AUC); the larger the area is, the better the test will be. In the example in Figure 5-1, the AUC is 0.811, which is quite good. The best possible test (Figure 5-2) would have an area under the curve of 1, and the worst possible test (Figure 5-3) would have an area of 0.5 (the same as flipping a coin).

Again, sensitivity, specificity, and ROC curves have been traditionally used in the context of screening tests, but they do not have to be limited to them. ROC curves are applicable whenever the outcome is dichotomous and the goal is to determine

Figure 5-1 Receiver operator characteristic (ROC) curve. © *Cengage Learning, 2012.*

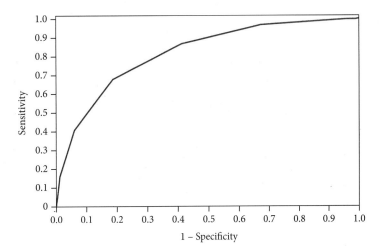

Figure 5-2 The best possible ROC curve.
© *Cengage Learning, 2012.*

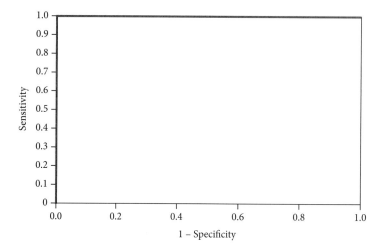

Figure 5-3 The worst possible ROC curve.
© *Cengage Learning, 2012.*

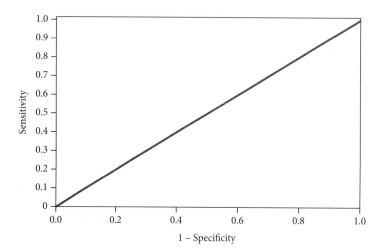

how well another variable (continuous or ordinal) correctly identifies whether or not a subject belongs to one level of the outcome. For example, ROC curves will be used later in this chapter to quantify how well multiple variables predict a dichotomous outcome.

CONFOUNDING AND EFFECT MODIFICATION

As discussed in Chapter 4, many studies in public health are conducted to compare proportions between groups. In this study, it is of interest to investigate the impact that having a child under the age of 5 has on insecticide-treated net use. If the proportions of net use between the two groups are different, then net use is dependent on whether there is a child under the age of 5 in the household. In Chapter 4, data analyses suggested that there was a dependency on ITN use and having a child under the age of 5, that the proportion of net use in households with children under 5 was not the same as households without children under the age of 5. However, this study is an observational study. The participants were not randomly assigned to have children under the age of 5 in the household or not. Therefore, factors related to ITN use might be different for households with or without children under the age of 5. Specifically, the relationship between having young children at home and insecticide-treated net use may be affected by confounding variables.

Variables that are not of primary importance but that could potentially influence the relationship between the outcome (response) variable and the exposure (explanatory) variable are called *confounding variables* (as defined in Chapter 3). For example, suppose that living in a rural area is related to both having children under the age of 5 in the household and using ITNs. This means that residing in a rural area is a potential confounding variable because it is related to both the explanatory or exposure variable (having children under the age of 5) and to the response variable (using ITNs). Potential confounding variables can be identified using the data in the study or findings from the literature. Because rural residence is expected to be a confounding variable, in determining whether having children under the age of 5 is associated with insecticide-treated net use, adjustments must be made for whether the household is in a rural area.

Stratified Contingency Tables

Rural location (the confounder) can have two possible effects:

- The relationship between having a child under the age of 5 and using insecticide-treated nets is the same for rural and urban households.
- The relationship between having a child under the age of 5 and using insecticide-treated nets is different for rural and urban households.

If the confounding variable (rural residence) alters the relationship between the two variables of interest (using ITNs and having a child under the age of 5), the confounder is called an **effect modifier.** Effect modifiers are also known as *interactions*, which exist when the relationship of two variables depends on the level or category of another variable. Effect modification occurs when there is an interaction between the explanatory and confounding variables.

To properly adjust for the impact of a confounding variable, it should be determined whether the variable is an effect modifier. This can be done by creating sets of contingency tables. In this example, three variables are potentially related: the confounder (rural residence), the response variable (use of an ITN), and the explanatory variable (children under the age of 5). Therefore, a contingency table is needed with the explanatory variable and response as the row and column variables for each level of the confounding variable (Figure 5-4). Furthermore, from each contingency table, an odds ratio estimate can be obtained; the odds ratio estimate for each level of the confounding variable is referred to as a **stratified odds ratio** estimate.

Suppose the relationship between rural residence, use of an ITN, and having children under the age of 5 results in two contingency tables: one for rural households and one for urban households (Tables 5-2 and 5-3). The estimated odds ratio for rural households is 1.0 (0.7, 1.4), and the estimated odds ratio for urban households is 2.2 (1.4, 3.4). These stratified odds ratio estimates are fairly different. In fact, the odds ratio for rural households does not appear to be significantly different from 1. On the other

Figure 5-4 Example of Stratified Contingency Tables.
© *Cengage Learning, 2012.*

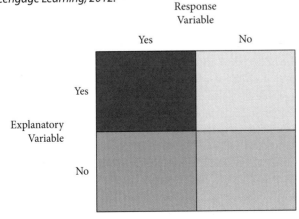

Level 1 of Confounding Variable

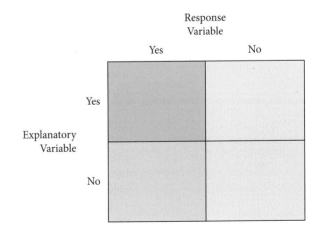

Level 2 of Confounding Variable

TABLE 5-2 STRATIFIED CONTINGENCY TABLE: URBAN HOUSEHOLDS (EFFECT MODIFICATION)

Table 1 of Child by Net, Controlling for Rural = 0			
Frequency Percentage Row Percentage Column Percentage	Column Variable: Child		
	1	0	Total
Row Variable: Net Use — 1	38 3.83 34.55 18.27	72 7.25 65.45 9.17	110 11.08
0	170 17.12 19.25 81.73	713 71.80 80.75 90.83	883 88.92
Total	208 20.95	785 79.05	993 100.00

Statistics for Table 1 of Child by Net, Controlling for Rural = 0		
	Value	95% Confidence Limits
Odds Ratio	2.2136	1.4441 3.3930

© Cengage Learning, 2012.

TABLE 5-3 STRATIFIED CONTINGENCY TABLE: RURAL HOUSEHOLDS (EFFECT MODIFICATION)

Table 2 of Child by Net, Controlling for Rural = 1			
Frequency Percentage Row Percentage Column Percentage	Column Variable: Child		
	1	0	Total
Row Variable: Net Use — 1	62 7.02 33.51 21.23	123 13.93 66.49 20.81	185 20.95
0	230 26.05 32.95 78.77	468 53.00 67.05 79.19	693 79.05
Total	292 33.07	591 66.93	883 100.00

Statistics for Table 2 of Child by Net, Controlling for Rural = 1		
	Value	95% Confidence Limits
Odds Ratio	1.0257	0.7274 1.4463

© Cengage Learning, 2012.

hand, having a child under the age of 5 more than doubles the estimated odds of using an insecticide-treated net in urban households. Therefore, the association of having a child under the age of 5 and using insecticide-treated nets is different depending on whether the household is in a rural or urban area. In this example, rural residence appears to be an effect modifier.

Now suppose that rural status had not been an effect modifier and a different set of stratified contingency tables are obtained (Tables 5-4 and 5-5), In this example, the estimated odds ratio for rural households is 1.7 (1.3, 2.2), and the estimated odds ratio for urban households is 2.2 (1.6, 3.0). These odds ratio estimates are not exactly the same, but they are similar. For both rural and urban households, there is approximately two times the increase in the estimated odds of insecticide-treated net use in households with children under 5 compared to households without children under 5. In this example, rural residence appears to be a confounder, but not an effect modifier.

In Tables 5-2 and 5-3, rural residence appears to be an effect modifier because the relationship between net use and having a child under the age of 5 is modified depending on whether the household is in a rural area or not. The odds ratio estimate for the relationship between net utilization and having children under the age of 5 for rural (R) households is $\widehat{OR}_R = 1.0$. On the other hand, the odds ratio estimate for the relationship between net utilization and having children under the age of 5 for urban (U) households is $\widehat{OR}_U = 2.2$. In contrast, Tables 5-4 and 5-5 indicate that rural residence may not modify the relationship between net use and having a child under the age of 5. The odds ratio estimate for the relationship between net utilization and having children under the age of 5 for rural (R) households is $\widehat{OR}_R = 1.7$, whereas the odds ratio estimate for the relationship between net utilization and having children under the age of 5 for urban (U) households is $\widehat{OR}_U = 2.2$.

When the outcome is dichotomous, a confounding variable is an effect modifier when the odds ratios obtained for the different levels of the confounding variable are different. In both of the preceding examples, the odds ratio estimates differ

Table 1 of Child by Net, Controlling for Rural = 0

Frequency Percentage Row Percentage Column Percentage	Column Variable: Child		
	1	0	Total
Row Variable: Net Use — 1	123 12.39 28.21 59.13	313 31.52 71.79 39.87	436 43.91
Row Variable: Net Use — 0	85 8.56 15.26 40.87	472 47.53 84.74 60.13	557 56.09
Total	208 20.95	785 79.05	993 100.00

Statistics for Table 1 of Child by Net, Controlling for Rural = 0		
	Value	95% Confidence Limits
Odds Ratio	2.1821	1.5986 2.9787

© Cengage Learning, 2012.

Table 2 of Child by Net, Controlling for Rural = 1

Frequency Percentage Row Percentage Column Percentage	Column Variable: Child		
	1	0	Total
Row Variable: Net Use — 1	157 17.78 39.55 53.77	240 27.18 60.45 40.61	397 44.96
Row Variable: Net Use — 0	135 15.29 27.78 46.23	351 39.75 72.22 59.39	486 55.04
Total	292 33.07	591 66.93	883 100.00

Statistics for Table 2 of Child by Net, Controlling for Rural = 1		
	Value	95% Confidence Limits
Odds Ratio	1.7008	1.2821 2.2563

© Cengage Learning, 2012.

depending on the level of the confounder; the odds ratio estimates just differ more in the first example. To determine whether the true odds ratios are different, hypothesis testing can be done.

Identifying Effect Modification: The Breslow-Day Test

Statistical software packages may have different names for the test to determine whether a confounder is an effect modifier, but the hypotheses are the same. Odds ratios for each level of a confounder (stratified odds ratios) are compared. If a significant difference between any of the odds ratios is found, then the confounder is an effect modifier. To determine whether rural residence is an effect modifier, two odds ratios are compared: one for rural households and one for urban households.

$$OR_R = \frac{\text{odds of net use in households with children under 5}}{\text{odds of net use in household without children under 5}}$$

$$OR_U = \frac{\text{odds of net use in households with children under 5}}{\text{odds of net use in household without children under 5}}$$

RESEARCH HYPOTHESIS: $OR_R \neq OR_U$

NULL HYPOTHESIS: $OR_R = OR_U$

In both examples (Tables 5-2, 5-3 and 5-4, 5-5), the Breslow-Day test was used to determine whether rural residence was an effect modifier (Table 5-6). In the second example (Tables 5-4 and 5-5), where the estimated odds ratios were not very different, the Breslow-Day test resulted in a p-value that was large ($p = 0.2452$). This p-value indicates that there is not enough evidence to reject the null hypothesis. Because there is not enough evidence to indicate that the odds ratios are different, rural residence is not an effect modifier. On the other hand, the example in Tables 5-2 and 5-3, where the

TABLE 5-6 BRESLOW-DAY TEST SUMMARY

	Tables 5-4 and 5-5 Odds ratio estimates are similar.	Tables 5-2 and 5-3 Odds ratio estimates are not similar.
Odds ratio estimates	$\widehat{OR}_R = 1.7$ $\widehat{OR}_U = 2.2$	$\widehat{OR}_R = 1.0$ $\widehat{OR}_U = 2.2$
p-value	0.2452	0.0056
Conclusion	No evidence of effect modification	Evidence of effect modification

© Cengage Learning, 2012.

estimated odds ratios were farther apart, the Breslow-Day test resulted in a p-value that was small ($p = 0.0056$). This small p-value indicates that there is sufficient evidence to reject the null hypothesis. Because there is sufficient evidence to indicate that the odds ratios are different, rural residence is an effect modifier.

No Evidence of Effect Modification: Mantel-Haenszel Odds Ratio

In the example of Tables 5-4 and 5-5, the odds ratios were found to be similar for rural and urban households, indicating that rural residence was not an effect modifier. However, this result does not mean that rural residence is no longer a confounder. To answer the research question, the relationship between insecticide-treated net use and having children under the age of 5 in the household needs to be investigated while accounting for the effect of rural residence.

In Chapter 3, adjusted mean differences were provided when the research question involved comparing groups while controlling for confounding variables. However, the outcome in Chapter 3 was continuous. In this example, the outcome is dichotomous (ITN use: yes/no); and means are not appropriate numerical summaries. However, odds ratios are appropriate when the outcome is dichotomous and the research question involves relationships between groups. An **adjusted odds ratio** is an odds ratio that is created while controlling for confounding variables.

One method for obtaining an estimate of the adjusted odds ratio is to provide a weighted average of the stratified odds ratio. The weighted average of the odds ratio estimates is done in a special way, and the resulting adjusted odds ratio is called a Mantel-Haenszel odds ratio (OR_{MH}). Statistical software packages can provide an estimate of the OR_{MH} (Table 5-7). The Mantel-Haenszel odds ratio estimate is calculated by considering the relationship between the explanatory (having children under the age of 5) and response (ITN use) variables for each level of the confounder (rural residence). By combining the results from each level of the confounder, the Mantel-Haenszel odds ratio (OR_{MH}) provides an odds ratio adjusted for the confounder. In this example, the estimated Mantel-Haenszel odds ratio ($\widehat{OR}_{MH}$) is 1.9. This odds ratio estimate does seem to be an average of the two stratified odds ratio estimates for rural and urban households ($\widehat{OR}_R = 1.7$ and ($\widehat{OR}_U$) =2.2). In the Mantel-Haenszel odds ratio estimate, the observed odds in the numerator is larger than the observed odds in the denominator. Households with children under 5 are in the numerator, and the denominator represents households without children under 5. In fact, for this sample the odds ratio implies that the odds of insecticide-treated net use is twice as large (1.9 times larger) in the households with children under the age of 5 compared to households without children under 5, controlling for whether the household is located in a rural location.

Although this odds ratio now accounts for a confounder, it is still only an estimate and describes only this sample. It is a statistic, a point estimate. To answer the research question about the relationship between ITN use and having children under the age of 5, inferences

TABLE 5-7 **EXAMPLE OF A MANTEL-HAENSZEL ODDS RATIO ESTIMATE**

Summary	Method	Value	95% Confidence Limits	
Odds Ratio	Mantel-Haenszel	1.9040	1.5449	2.3465

© Cengage Learning, 2012.

beyond this sample need to be made. As explained in Chapter 4, studies involving odds ratios typically emphasize estimation, and so confidence intervals are used for statistical inference. The same is true for adjusted odds ratios.

The confidence interval for a Mantel-Haenszel odds ratio can easily be obtained using statistical software (Table 5-7). In this example, the 95% confidence interval for the Mantel-Haenszel odds ratio is [1.5, 2.3]. The confidence interval provides a set of plausible values for the true adjusted odds ratios. An adjusted odds ratio of 1 is not included in this interval estimate, providing evidence that after controlling for rural residence, the true OR_{MH} is not 1 and is larger than 1.

Evidence of Effect Modification

The weighted average (Mantel-Haenszel) method used to calculate an adjusted odds ratio is a reasonable approach when the confounder is not an effect modifier. However, the OR_{MH} is not appropriate to use in the presence of effect modification. Effect modification indicates that the stratified odds ratios are different depending on the level of the confounding variable. In the example of Tables 5-2 and 5-3, $\widehat{OR}_R = 1.0$ and $\widehat{OR}_U = 2.2$. These stratified odds ratios were found to be significantly different ($p = 0.0056$). If the stratified odds ratios are different, then trying to collapse them (by averaging) into a single adjusted odds ratio does not make much sense. Therefore, when a confounder is an effect modifier, the odds ratio estimates for each level of the confounder have to be presented separately (stratified odds ratios). By doing so, the relationship between the response (ITN use) and the explanatory or exposure variable (having a child under the age of 5) can be quantified while controlling for the effect modifier (rural residence).

The estimates for rural and urban households odds ratios ($\widehat{OR}_R = 1.0$ and $\widehat{OR}_U = 2.2$) describe only this sample of urban and rural households. They are statistics, point estimates. The research goal is to investigate the relationship of ITN use and having children under the age of 5, while controlling for rural residence. So, inferences beyond this sample are required. Again, as explained in Chapter 4, studies involving odds ratios typically emphasize estimation, and so confidence intervals are used for statistical inference. The 95% confidence interval for the two odds ratios can be easily obtained using statistical software (Table 5-8). In fact, the method of calculating the confidence interval is exactly the same as when calculating the confidence interval for only one odds ratio (Chapter 4).

TABLE 5-8 **EXAMPLE OF STRATIFIED ODDS RATIO ESTIMATES**

Controlling for Rural = 0		
Summary	**Value**	**95% Confidence Limits**
Odds Ratio	2.2136	1.4441 3.3930
Controlling for Rural = 0		
Summary	**Value**	**95% Confidence Limits**
Odds Ratio	1.0257	0.7274 1.4463

© Cengage Learning, 2012.

In the example in Table 5-8, the confidence interval for the rural odds ratio is [0.7, 1.4]. Although the estimate for the rural odds ratio is slightly larger than 1, the confidence interval overlaps 1.0. Because the confidence interval represents a set of plausible values for the true rural odds ratio, the true odds ratio for rural households may be 1.0. Thus, there is not sufficient evidence to conclude that there is an association between having children under the age of 5 and insecticide-treated net use in rural households.

The confidence interval for the urban odds ratio, however, is [1.4, 3.4]. This interval does not cover 1 and provides evidence that the true odds ratio for urban households is not 1. In fact, the confidence interval suggests that the true odds ratio for urban households is greater than 1. This means that the numerator odds is larger than the denominator odds in urban households. The denominator is still the households without children under 5, and the numerator still represents households with children under 5, but the households are limited to those in urban areas Thus, the estimated urban odds ratio implies that for households in urban areas the odds of insecticide-treated net use are approximately twice as large (95% CI: 1.4, 3.4) in households with children under 5 when compared to households without children under 5.

DICHOTOMOUS DEPENDENT VARIABLE WITH MULTIPLE REGRESSORS: LOGISTIC REGRESSION

RESEARCH QUESTION:
What factors are associated with ITN use?

Chapter 4 discussed analyses for investigating a research question that asked about the factors related to insecticide-treated net use. It has been established that having children under 5 is related to ITN use; the investigation of other factors is warranted. Descriptive statistics and simple comparisons suggest that besides having children under the age of 5, family size, distance to the nearest clinic, roof type, age of household head, urban/rural location, and wealth might also help to explain why some households use ITNs and others do not (Table 5-9).

In this study, households using insecticide-treated nets tend to report a higher percentage of children under 5, have higher observed rates living under a thatched roof, within 15 miles of a healthcare facility, and in a rural area. Furthermore, the average age of the household head tends to be younger, and the families are larger in the households using insecticide-treated nets. However, these are simple two-variable or bivariate comparisons. The statistical methods presented so far cannot really investigate the relationships of multiple variables with a dichotomous response variable. Furthermore, continuous factors (family size and age of household head) may be associated with ITN use. Even simple relationships with a dichotomous response and a continuous variable cannot be explored with the methods presented so far. *Logistic regression*, however, is often used when the outcome is dichotomous. Logistic regression

- Predicts the probability of an outcome (even when the regressor is continuous)
- Simultaneously considers the relationships of multiple variables (dichotomous, nominal, ordinal and/or continuous) with a dichotomous outcome
- Investigates an explanatory (exposure) variable with a dichotomous outcome while controlling for confounding

In Chapter 3, linear regression models were used for investigating multiple explanatory variables and for comparing group means while controlling for potential confounders. Much of the discussion in Chapter 3 applies to the logistic regression model. In fact, the discussions involving inferences and interpretations of the slopes are essentially the same for linear and logistic regression. However, linear regression is no longer appropriate because the outcome now has only two levels. Logistic regression, however, can be used for dichotomous outcomes very much as linear regression was used for continuous outcomes.

TABLE 5-9 CHARACTERISTICS OF THE SAMPLE BY INSECTICIDE-TREATED NET USAGE

	Used Insecticide-Treated Nets in the Previous Night	
	No (N = 1376)	Yes (N = 500)
Children Under 5 (%)		
No	823 (59.8%)	220 (44.0%)
Yes	553 (40.2%)	280 (56.0%)
Roof Type (%)		
Thatched	394 (28.6%)	229 (45.8%)
Corrugated metal	643 (46.7%)	152 (30.4%)
Other	339 (24.6%)	119 (23.8%)
Distance to Healthcare Facility (%)		
<15 miles	352 (25.6%)	200 (40.0%)
15–50 miles	262 (19.0%)	109 (21.8%)
50 + miles	762 (55.4%)	191 (38.2%)
Household in Rural Area (%)		
No	785 (57.0%)	208 (41.6%)
Yes	591 (43.0%)	292 (58.4%)
Wealth Index of Household (%)		
Lowest 25%	406 (29.5%)	73 (14.6%)
Next lowest	403 (29.3%)	133 (26.6%)
Next highest	367 (26.7%)	174 (34.8%)
Highest 25%	200 (14.5%)	120 (24.0%)
Age (years)		
Mean (SD)	50.1 (6.84)	44.3 (7.33)
Median (Q1, Q3)	50 (46, 55)	44 (40, 49)
Minimum, Maximum	28, 73	20, 62
Family size		
Mean (SD)	5.1 (1.53)	7.1 (1.61)
Median (Q1, Q3)	5 (4, 6)	7 (6, 8)
Minimum, Maximum	1, 9	3, 12

© Cengage Learning, 2012.

The Model

The model for logistic regression is very similar to the model described in Chapter 3 for linear regression. In fact, the right-hand side is pretty much the same:

$$\alpha + \beta_1 x_1 + \beta_2 x_2 + \cdots + \beta_K x_K$$

where x represents the covariates, β_K represents the slopes (parameters of interest), and α represents the intercept. The left side of the equation, however, is not simply the response variable, as in linear regression. Whereas the right-hand side of the equation ($\alpha + \beta_1 x_1 + \beta_2 x_2 + \cdots + \beta_K x_K$) can be anything (0, negative, positive, fraction, whole number, etc.), the dichotomous response variable has only two levels. Even if the probability of the response is used (e.g., the probability of using ITNs), probabilities cannot be anything; they are restricted to be between 0 and 1. To make the left-hand side of the equation equal to the right-hand side, the left-hand side needs the flexibility to be anything (0, negative, positive, fraction, whole number, etc.). Therefore, the left-hand side of the model is the *logit(p)*. The logit(p) is the natural log of the odds or $\ln\left(\frac{p}{1-p}\right)$, where p represents the true probability of success (e.g., using an insecticide-treated net). Therefore, the logistic regression model is

$$\text{logit}(p) = \ln\left(\frac{p}{1-p}\right) = \alpha + \beta_1 x_1 + \beta_2 x_2 + \cdots + \beta_K x_K.$$

The primary assumption of the logistic regression model is that the outcome variable is a dichotomous variable such as the one in this example: the use of insecticide-treated nets (yes/no).

The logistic regression model for this study would include variables for having a child under the age of 5 (child), the wealth index (wealth1, wealth2, and wealth3), distance to healthcare (hcdist1, hcdist2), living in a rural area (rural), family size (famsize), age of household head (age), and roof type (roof1, roof3). Except for age and family size, which are continuous variables, the other variables in the model are treated as nominal categorical variables and are included in the regression as dummy variables (Chapter 3). The logistic regression model is:

$$\text{logit}(p) = \ln\left(\frac{p}{1-p}\right) = \alpha + \beta_1(\text{child}) + \beta_2(\text{wealth1}) + \beta_3(\text{wealth2}) + \beta_4(\text{wealth3})$$
$$+ \beta_5(\text{hcdist1}) + \beta_6(\text{hcdist2}) + \beta_7(\text{rural}) + \beta_8(\text{famsize})$$
$$+ \beta_9(\text{age}) + \beta_{10}(\text{roof1}) + \beta_{11}(\text{roof3})$$

where p represents the true probability of using an insecticide-treated net.

The ordinal variables (wealth and distance to healthcare) were not included in the regression model as ordinal variables. To include an ordinal variable in a regression, the jumps from one level to the next should be equal because the interpretation of the slope involves a 1-unit increase in the explanatory variable. It is not often that ordinal variables meet this criterion. Furthermore, ordinal variables are treated like nominal variables when investigators are less interested in what happens with a 1-unit increase and more interested in comparing one category to a reference. For example, there is more interest in describing how those close to healthcare compare to those farther away than there is to describe the effect of moving from one level of the distance-to-healthcare variable to the next. For this reason, wealth and distance-to-healthcare are treated as nominal variables. Similar to linear regression (Chapter 3), for a nominal variable with C categories, C − 1 dummy variables corresponding to C − 1 categories are included in the regression, with the omitted category serving as the reference.

Getting the Slopes and Intercept

Linear regression used the least squares method to estimate slopes (β's) and the intercept (α), but it is not quite as simple in logistic regression. Although the mathematical details are somewhat beyond the scope of this text, to get the estimates $\hat{\alpha}$, logistic regression uses maximum likelihood estimation. *Maximum likelihood estimation* attempts to find the values for the β's and α that maximize the likelihood function (the probability of the observed sample, where β and α are the unknown elements). The *likelihood function* is based on the fact that each subject in the sample is an independent observation. In a logistic regression, it is assumed that each subject is independent *and* that the outcomes for the subjects come from a binomial distribution. Because the subjects are independent, the probability for the whole sample is just the multiplication of the probabilities for each subject; these probabilities are written as functions of α and the β's, the likelihood function. The estimates for the α and β's are obtained by choosing $\hat{\alpha}$ and $\hat{\beta}$ to maximize the numerical value of the likelihood function for the observed sample. In most instances, these estimates (called *maximum likelihood estimates*) are obtained using an iterative process based on a numerical analysis algorithm. Sometimes this iterative process fails to converge; hence, estimates of α and β do not exist for some sets of data. When implementing a logistic regression, check to make sure the algorithm to obtain the estimates converges; this is standard output on any statistical software. In summary, this is not a calculation that can be made by hand; statistical software is needed to implement a logistic regression.

Hypothesis Tests

Three types of hypothesis tests result from any regression.

- The *overall hypothesis test* is to see whether there is a relationship between any of the variables and the outcome.
- The *hypothesis tests for the effects* are useful if the model involves nominal variables with multiple categories. Hypothesis tests for the effects are conducted to determine whether the original nominal variable, not the specific dummy variables, is related to the outcome, controlling for all other variables in the model.
- Finally, *specific hypothesis tests* involve testing that one of the variables is related to the outcome, controlling for all other variables in the model.

Overall Hypothesis Test

Whenever the model involves multiple variables, whether explanatory or confounding, an overall hypothesis test can be performed to see whether any of the variables have a relationship to the outcome. The global hypotheses associated with the overall test do not change from Chapter 3; the overall hypotheses for linear and logistic regression are exactly the same.

In this example, the logistic regression model is as follows:

$$\text{logit}(p) = \ln\left(\frac{p}{1-p}\right) = \alpha + \beta_1(\text{child}) + \beta_2(\text{wealth1}) + \beta_3(\text{wealth2}) + \beta_4(\text{wealth3})$$
$$+ \beta_5(\text{hcdist1}) + \beta_6(\text{hcdist2}) + \beta_7(\text{rural}) + \beta_8(\text{famsize})$$
$$+ \beta_9(\text{age}) + \beta_{10}(\text{roof1}) + \beta_{11}(\text{roof3})$$

where p represents the true probability of using an insecticide-treated net.

RESEARCH HYPOTHESIS: *At least one* of the true slopes is not 0 ($\beta_k \neq 0$, for at least one k, $k = 1 \ldots 11$).

NULL HYPOTHESIS: All of the true slopes are 0 ($\beta_k = 0$, for every k, $k = 1 \ldots 11$).

The overall hypotheses are not particularly interesting or exciting. If the null hypothesis can be rejected, it simply means that this model is better than nothing (Table 5-10).

TABLE 5-10 **EXAMPLE RESULTS FOR THE OVERALL (GLOBAL) TEST**

Testing Global Null Hypothesis: BETA = 0			
Test	**Chi-Square**	**DF**	**Pr > ChiSq**
Likelihood ratio	856.1337	11	<0.0001
Score	701.6489	11	<0.0001
Wald	410.0370	11	<0.0001

© Cengage Learning, 2012.

CONCLUSION: The *p*-values associated with the overall test are small ($p < 0.0001$). Hence, there is sufficient evidence to reject the null hypothesis. At least one of these regressors is related to the outcome.

A statistically significant result from the overall test means only that one or some or all of the variables are related to the outcome. It does not indicate which regressors are significantly contributing to the relationship or the direction of the association. To specifically investigate the impact of the regressors, specific inferences (hypothesis tests and confidence intervals) need to be performed. However, these more specific investigations of the contribution of each regressor should be performed only after determining that a relationship exists somewhere or that this model is better than nothing. If the overall test results in a large p-value, then the overall or global null hypothesis cannot be rejected; there is no evidence of a relationship. If there is no evidence of a relationship, then there is no reason to continue searching for the contribution of the individual regressors.

Hypothesis Test for Effects

In this example, the logistic regression model is as follows:

$$\text{logit}(p) = \ln\left(\frac{p}{1-p}\right) = \alpha + \beta_1(\text{child}) + \beta_2(\text{wealth1}) + \beta_3(\text{wealth2}) + \beta_4(\text{wealth3})$$
$$+ \beta_5(\text{miles15–50}) + \beta_6(\text{miles50}) + \beta_7(\text{rural}) + \beta_8(\text{famsize})$$
$$+ \beta_9(\text{age}) + \beta_{10}(\text{roof1}) + \beta_{11}(\text{roof3})$$

where p represents the true probability of using an insecticide-treated net.

Nominal variables are included in the regression as sets of dummy variables that correspond to certain levels of the categorical variable. The slopes associated with these dummy variables represent a comparison between one category of the nominal variable and the reference category. A nominal variable with multiple categories can result in multiple dummy variables, each with its own slope. Confusion can arise when trying to determine whether the nominal variable or the dummy variable is related to the response. For example, the research question may address the relationship between distance to healthcare and the probability of ITN use, but the regression results in parameter estimates ($\hat{\beta}$s) and p-values for each dummy variable in the model. Quite possibly, traveling more than 50 miles to healthcare might have a different effect from traveling less than 15 miles ($\beta_6 \neq 0$), but traveling between 15 and 50 miles might not be different from traveling more than 50 miles ($\beta_5 = 0$). If one p-value is significant and the other is not, how do you determine whether distance to healthcare, in general, is associated with the probability of using an insecticide-treated net? How is it possible to address the relationship between distance to healthcare and ITN use when multiple (and possibly conflicting) estimates have to be considered? Analyzing the overall effect of the nominal variable, can help (Table 5-11).

The *type 3 effects tests* presented in Table 5-11 are chi-square tests for the overall effect of each variable, controlling for all other variables in the model. These correspond to the adjusted sums of squares discussed in Chapter 3. When the p-value is small, the effect is associated with the outcome. A large p-value indicates that there is not enough evidence to assume that the effect is associated with the outcome.

TABLE 5-11 **EXAMPLE OF THE ANALYSIS OF EFFECTS**

Type 3 Analysis of Effects			
Wald			
Effect	DF	Chi-Square	Pr > ChiSq
age	1	121.2391	<0.0001
famsize	1	273.6828	<0.0001
hcdist	2	36.9434	<0.0001
child	1	25.6523	<0.0001
wealth	3	42.1425	<0.0001
roof	2	47.4428	<0.0001
rural	1	23.7546	<0.0001

© Cengage Learning, 2012.

CONCLUSION: The overall effects of distance to healthcare ($p < 0.0001$), wealth index ($p < 0.0001$), and roof type ($p < 0.0001$) are all associated with insecticide-treated net use, controlling for all other variables in the model.

Results of the type 3 effects tests are provided for continuous and dichotomous variables. However, with continuous and dichotomous variables, there is only one variable (and one β) in the model; so the p-values for the type 3 effects are exactly the same as the p-values (corresponding to specific hypothesis tests) for the individual variables. Although the results of the type 3 tests may be helpful for investigating the overall effect, they are typically not presented. Generally, the focus of a logistic regression analysis is on the statistical inference associated with specific slopes.

Specific Hypothesis Tests for the Slopes

In this example, the logistic regression model is:

$$\text{logit}(p) = \ln\left(\frac{p}{1-p}\right) = \alpha + \beta_1(\text{child}) + \beta_2(\text{wealth1}) + \beta_3(\text{wealth2}) + \beta_4(\text{wealth3})$$
$$+ \beta_5(\text{hcdist1}) + \beta_6(\text{hcdist2}) + \beta_7(\text{rural}) + \beta_8(\text{famsize})$$
$$+ \beta_9(\text{age}) + \beta_{10}(\text{roof1}) + \beta_{11}(\text{roof3})$$

where p represents the true probability of using an insecticide-treated net.

Just as in linear regression (Chapter 3), each regressor in the model has a corresponding slope (β), and the slopes (β's) are the parameters of interest. The hypotheses and confidence intervals for the slope in a logistic regression are actually exactly the same as the hypotheses and confidence intervals described in Chapter 3 for linear regression. Statistical inference for the slope means trying to determine whether there is evidence for a nonzero slope (Table 5-12). If a slope (β) is 0, then the corresponding variable does not have an association with the outcome.

Even though a research question and the corresponding hypotheses may focus on one specific variable, the other variables in the regression need to be mentioned. In a multiple variable regression analysis, the statistical tests for a specific variable are conducted assuming that all other variables are already in the model.

TABLE 5-12 **EXAMPLE OF INFERENCE FOR SLOPES**

	Parameter Estimate	Standard Error	Wald Chi-Square	Pr > ChiSq
intercept	−1.5975	0.6012	7.0592	0.0079
age	−0.1177	0.0107	121.2391	<0.0001
famsize	0.8430	0.0510	273.6828	<0.0001
hcdist 1	0.9575	0.1606	35.5529	<0.0001
hcdist 2	0.6200	0.1862	11.0928	0.0009
child 1	0.7085	0.1399	25.6523	<0.0001
wealth 1	−1.4321	0.2238	40.9622	<0.0001
wealth 2	−0.7331	0.2025	13.1121	0.0003
wealth 3	−0.5574	0.1985	7.8825	0.0050
roof 1	1.1272	0.1640	47.2677	<0.0001
roof 3	0.6594	0.1826	13.0488	0.0003
rural 1	0.6825	0.1400	23.7546	<0.0001

Analysis of Maximum Likelihood Estimates

© Cengage Learning, 2012.

RESEARCH QUESTION:
Is roof type associated with using an ITN, controlling for other variables in the regression?

As an example, consider the roof type variable. Because roof type is a nominal variable with three levels, it is included in the regression as two dummy variables. Dummy variables for corrugated metal (roof1) and for other roof material (roof3) are in the model, making thatched roof the reference. Because two slopes are associated with roof type, there are two sets of hypotheses.

NULL HYPOTHESIS: The slope (β_{10}) for having a corrugated roof is 0, after controlling for all other variables in the model.

RESEARCH HYPOTHESIS: The slope (β_{10}) for having a corrugated roof is not 0, after controlling for all other variables in the model.

NULL HYPOTHESIS: The slope (β_{11}) for having other roof material is 0, after controlling for all other variables in the model.

RESEARCH HYPOTHESIS: The slope (β_{11}) for having other roof material is not 0, after controlling for all other variables in the model.

In both sets of null and research hypotheses, the statement "after controlling for all other variables in the model" is included. The benefit of using regression analysis is that the estimates for the slopes are obtained while simultaneously adjusting for the other variables in the model. In other words, the other variables in the model are assumed to have slopes that are significantly different from 0.

CONCLUSION: Both hypothesis tests result in small p-values ($p < 0.0001$). Therefore, both null hypotheses can be rejected; both slopes are not 0. Because these are dummy variables, the parameter estimates represent the estimated change in the natural log of the odds between corrugated and thatched roofs (1.1272, $p < 0.0001$) and between other materials and thatched roofs (0.6594, $p < 0.0001$), controlling for the other variables in the model.

Although the estimates of the slopes were critical in a linear regression, slope-specific interpretations are less helpful in logistic regression because the natural log of the odds is not as meaningful an outcome. Who talks about the change in the natural log of the odds? However, the slopes in a logistic regression can be transformed into a measure that is important with dichotomous outcomes: an odds ratio. Consequently, the p-values presented with the estimates of the slopes can be transferred to the corresponding odds ratio estimates.

Adjusted Odds Ratios

Whenever multiple regressors are included in a regression, the slopes are obtained by simultaneously considering all the regressors in the model. Therefore, the slope estimates are adjusted for all the other variables. Regardless of whether the regression is conducted to predict the probability of the outcome, to understand multiple variable relationships, or simply to adjust for potential confounders, the statistical inference for the specific slopes is the same.

Just as in linear regression, the interpretation of any slope (β) is the change in the response for every unit increase in the regressor (a variable on the right-hand side of the model equation). However, the so-called response in logistic regression is not as simple to explain as in linear regression. In a logistic regression, the left side of the equation is $\text{logit}(p) = \ln\left(\frac{p}{1-p}\right)$. Explaining the change in the natural log odds for every unit increase in the regressor is difficult. Luckily, these parameters (β's) have meaningful interpretations.

In this example, the logistic regression model is as follows:

$$\text{logit}(p) = \ln\left(\frac{p}{1-p}\right) = \alpha + \beta_1(\text{child}) + \beta_2(\text{wealth1}) + \beta_3(\text{wealth2}) + \beta_4(\text{wealth3})$$
$$+ \beta_5(\text{hcdist1}) + \beta_6(\text{hcdist2}) + \beta_7(\text{rural}) + \beta_8(\text{famsize})$$
$$+ \beta_9(\text{age}) + \beta_{10}(\text{roof1}) + \beta_{11}(\text{roof3}),$$

where p represents the true probability of using an insecticide-treated net.

For the purposes of illustration, suppose all regressors were held constant (every household had the same values) except for whether a household had a child under the age of 5. Assume that having a child under the age of 5 is coded as 1 (child = 1) and not having children under the age of 5 is coded as 0 (child = 0). The outcome for households with children under the age of 5 is logit(p_{U5}), and the outcome for households without children under the age of 5 is logit(p_{O5}), where p_{U5} and p_{O5} represent the probability of using an ITN for households with and without children under 5, respectively. The logistic regression models for each type of household are as follows:

$$\text{logit}(p_{U5}) = \ln\left(\frac{p_{U5}}{1-p_{U5}}\right) = \alpha + \beta_1(1) + \beta_2(\text{wealth1}) + \beta_3(\text{wealth2}) + \beta_4(\text{wealth3})$$
$$+ \beta_5(\text{hcdist1}) + \beta_6(\text{hcdist2}) + \beta_7(\text{rural})$$
$$+ \beta_8(\text{family size}) + \beta_9(\text{age}) + \beta_{10}(\text{roof1})$$
$$+ \beta_{11}(\text{roof3})$$

and

$$\text{logit}(p_{O5}) = \ln\left(\frac{p_{O5}}{1-p_{O5}}\right) = \alpha + \beta_1(0) + \beta_2(\text{wealth1}) + \beta_3(\text{wealth2}) + \beta_4(\text{wealth3})$$
$$+ \beta_5(\text{hcdist1}) + \beta_6(\text{hcdist2}) + \beta_7(\text{rural})$$
$$+ \beta_8(\text{famsize}) + \beta_9(\text{age}) + \beta_{10}(\text{roof1})$$
$$+ \beta_{11}(\text{roof3})$$

Notice that the child variable is replaced with 1 and 0 for those with and without children under 5, respectively. The difference in outcome between these two groups is the difference in the logits: logit(p_{U5}) − logit(p_{O5}). Because all other variables are held constant, the difference in the logits for having children under the age of 5 is

$$\text{logit}(p_{U5}) - \text{logit}(p_{O5}) = \ln\left(\frac{p_{U5}}{1-p_{U5}}\right) - \ln\left(\frac{p_{O5}}{1-p_{O5}}\right) = \beta_1(1) - \beta_1(0) = \beta_1$$

The intercept "cancels out," as do all the other regressors that are held constant. The only item remaining on the right-hand side is the slope associated with whether there are children under the age of 5 in the household.

A property of natural logs is that the natural log of the differences can be written as the natural log of the quotient. In this example,

$$\ln\left(\frac{p_{U5}}{1-p_{U5}}\right) - \left(\frac{p_{O5}}{1-p_{O5}}\right) = \ln\left(\frac{\dfrac{p_{U5}}{1-p_{U5}}}{\dfrac{p_{O5}}{1-p_{O5}}}\right)$$

Therefore,

$$\beta_1 = \ln\left(\frac{\dfrac{p_{U5}}{1-p_{U5}}}{\dfrac{p_{O5}}{1-p_{O5}}}\right)$$

In Chapter 4, an odds was defined as the ratio of the probability of successes to the probability of failure, and the odds ratio was the ratio of the odds. Therefore, β_1 represents the natural log of the odds ratio for households with children under the age of 5 compared to those without. To "undo" the natural log and release the odds ratio, the slope is exponentiated. Hence $e^{\beta_1} = \dfrac{\dfrac{p_{U5}}{1-p_{U5}}}{\dfrac{p_{O5}}{1-p_{O5}}} = \dfrac{\text{odds}_{U5}}{\text{odds}_{O5}}$ and represents the true odds ratio, holding all other variables constant. Holding all other variables constant is the same as "adjusting for" or "controlling for" all other variables in the model; e^{β_1} represents the true adjusted odds ratio. Consequently, all of the β's in the regression model can be transformed and interpreted as the adjusted odds ratios. Furthermore, because the e^{β_1} represents a ratio, testing whether a regressor is associated with the outcome (i.e., testing whether the odds ratio is significantly different from 1) is the same as testing whether the slope (β) is equal to 0. The p-value for testing this hypothesis is exactly the same as the p-value for the estimate of the slope ($\hat{\beta}$).

> NULL HYPOTHESIS: The odds ratio is 1, after controlling for all other variables in the model.

> RESEARCH HYPOTHESIS: The odds ratio is not 1, after controlling for all other variables in the model.

The adjusted odds ratios for dichotomous, nominal, ordinal, and continuous regressors have the same interpretations as the odds ratios for dichotomous, nominal, ordinal, and continuous variables discussed in Chapter 4. The only difference is that an adjusted odds ratio is found by controlling for all other variables in the model.

Interpreting Adjusted Odds Ratios for Nominal Regressors

Three nominal variables are included in this logistic regression. Type of roof is a true nominal variable because the categories (thatched, corrugated metal, and other material) do not have an order. The other categorical variables of wealth index and distance to healthcare facility are actually ordinal variables. However, because the levels of these variables are not equally spaced and it is of interest to make comparisons to a reference level, these variables are treated as nominal variables. Recall from Chapter 3 that, for nominal variables, each level is made into a dummy variable, and the reference level is not included in the model. For example, roof type has 3 levels: thatched, corrugated metal, and other material. A dummy variable (with values of only 0 and 1) is created for each level.

Corrugated metal [roof1] = 1 if roof is made of corrugated metal
= 0 otherwise
Other [roof3] = 1 if roof is made of a material other than corrugated metal or thatched
= 0 otherwise

A third dummy variable for a thatched roof is not necessary because if a household has roof1 = 0 and roof3 = 0, then the household has a thatched roof. The omitted level is considered the reference.

As an example, suppose that the parameter estimates for β_{10} and β_{11} are 1.1272 ($p < 0.0001$) and 0.6594 ($p < 0.0001$). The parameter estimate for corrugated metal ($\hat{\beta}_{10}$) represents the estimated difference in the natural log odds between corrugated and thatched roofs, and the parameter estimate for other ($\hat{\beta}_{11}$) represents the estimated difference in the natural log odds between other material and thatched roofs. To get the adjusted odds ratios, these estimates need to be exponentiated: $\exp(1.1272) = 3.1$ and $\exp(0.6594) = 1.9$. Therefore, the estimated odds of ITN use is three times higher in corrugated metal compared to thatched roofs. Households with roofs of other materials have nearly double the odds of ITN use compared to households with thatched roofs, controlling for all other variables in the model.

Interpreting the Adjusted Odds Ratio for a Continuous Regressor

As an example of a continuous regressor, suppose that the parameter estimate for age is $\hat{\beta}_9 = -0.1176$, which represents the difference in the natural log odds as age increases by one year. However, the difference in the logs is not as informative as the odds ratio.

By taking exp(–0.1176), an estimate of the odds ratio can be obtained. The estimated odds ratio associated for age is $\exp(-0.1176) = 0.889$ ($p < 0.0001$). Therefore, as the age of the head of household increases by 1 year, the estimated odds of net use decrease by 11%, controlling for all other variables in the model.

Increasing the age by one year is not a very large increase, instead a larger increment may be more informative. For example, what if the investigator was interested in how the odds of ITN use changed for every 5-year increase in age? Because this is not a linear regression, the odds ratio cannot simply be multiplied by 5. However, the regression is linear with respect to the log odds; the parameter estimate ($\hat{\beta}_9$) can be multiplied by 5 to get the change in log odds for a 5-year increase in age. Exponentiating $5 \times \hat{\beta}_9$ provides the odds ratio estimate for a 5-year increase. Accompanying confidence intervals can be calculated in the same way.

Application of Formula

Estimate for odds ratio for a U-unit increase $= e^{\hat{\beta}U}$

$\hat{\beta}$ = The parameter estimate associated with the continuous variable

U = The number of units to increase

What you need to calculate the estimated odds ratio for a U-unit increase:

1. *The parameter estimate:* In this example, age is the variable of interest, and the parameter estimate associated with age is $\hat{\beta} = -0.1176$.
2. *The number of units to increase:* In this example, a 5-year increase in age is desired; so $U = 5$.
3. *Multiply the parameter estimate (1) and number of units (2):* $\hat{\beta} 5 \times U = -0.117765 \times 5 = -0.588$.

To calculate the estimated odds ratio associated with a U unit increase: Exponentiate the product found in (3), $\exp(\hat{\beta} 5 \times U) = \exp(-0.588) = 0.56$.

Application of Formula

95% confidence interval for the odds ratio for a U-unit increase $= \exp(U \times [\hat{\beta} \pm 1.96 \times SE])$

SE = The standard error of the parameter estimate associated with the continuous variable

U = The number of units to increase

What you need to calculate the confidence interval for the odds ratio with a U-unit increase:

1. *The 95% confidence interval for the parameter (β):*
   a. The lower bound for the confidence interval is $\beta \hat{\beta} - (1.96 \times SE)$. The lower bound is $-0.1176 - (1.96 \times 0.0106) = -0.1384$.
   b. The upper bound for the confidence interval is $\hat{\beta} + (1.96 \times SE)$. The lower bound is $-0.1176 + (1.96 \times 0.0106) = -0.0968$.
   c. The 95% confidence interval is $[-0.1384, -0.0968]$.
2. *Multiply the upper and lower bound found in (1) by U:*
   a. The lower bound found in (1a) is -0.1384. In this example, $U = 5$; so $-0.1384 \times 5 = -0.6920$.
   b. The upper bound found in (1b) is -0.0968. In this example, $U = 5$; so $-0.0968 \times 5 = -0.4840$.

To calculate the 95% confidence interval for an odds ratio for a U-unit increase: Exponentiate the upper and lower bounds found in (2). In this example, the 95% confidence interval is $[\exp(-0.6920), \exp(-0.4840)]$, or $[0.50, 0.62]$.

The confidence interval is not limited to a 95% confidence interval. For example, interval estimates for 90% and 99% confidence can be calculated in the same way; 1.96 is replaced by 1.645, and 2.58, respectively.

The estimated odds ratio associated with age in 5-year increments is 0.56. Therefore, the estimated odds of net use decreases by 44% for every 5-year increase in the age of the household head, controlling for all other variables ($p < 0.0001$). The 95% confidence interval [0.50, 0.62] does not cover 1, providing evidence that the true odds ratio is not 1.

Interpreting the Results of a Logistic Regression

The implementation of a logistic regression is the same regardless of whether the research question involves

- Investigating multiple variable relationships with a dichotomous outcome
- Or comparing groups while adjusting for potential confounding variables

Statistical software packages do not distinguish between these two perspectives when performing the regression. However, the research questions and the focus of the interpretation may differ.

Suppose a logistic regression is conducted using ITN use as the response variable and having a child under the age of 5, wealth, distance to health care, rural residence, family size, age of the head of household, and roof type) are included in the model as regressors.

The multiple logistic regression model is

$$\text{logit}(p) = \ln\left(\frac{p}{1-p}\right) = \alpha + \beta_1(\text{child}) + \beta_2(\text{wealth1}) + \beta_3(\text{wealth2}) + \beta_4(\text{wealth3})$$
$$+ \beta_5(\text{hcdist1}) + \beta_6(\text{hcdist2}) + \beta_7(\text{rural}) + \beta_8(\text{famsize})$$
$$+ \beta_9(\text{age}) + \beta_{10}(\text{roof1}) + \beta_{11}(\text{roof3})$$

where p represents the true probability of using an insecticide-treated net. Using statistical software, the following output results from implementing this logistic regression (Table 5-13).

The overall test (not presented in Table 5-13) resulted in a small p-value ($p < 0.0001$). Therefore, there is sufficient evidence to reject the global null hypothesis and continue on to investigate which variables are related to ITN utilization. All of the type 3 effects have small p-values, and consequently all of the slopes in the logistic regression model are significantly different from 0 ($p < 0.01$). As discussed, investigators implementing a logistic regression are typically interested not in slopes but in adjusted odds ratios. The information in Table 5-13 is helpful but would typically not be presented. The results of a logistic regression are usually presented as adjusted odds ratios with 95% confidence intervals (Table 5-14).

Regressors as Explanatory Variables

Sometimes logistic regressions are implemented in public health because the goal is to understand how factors are related to a dichotomous outcome. In this case, an investigator uses logistic regression as a way of explaining why some subjects have one level of the variable and some subjects have the other level of the variable; the regressors are considered explanatory variables.

TABLE 5-13 RESULTS OF A LOGISTIC REGRESSION WITH MULTIPLE FACTORS

Type 3 Analysis of Effects			
Effect	**DF**	**Wald Chi-Square**	**Pr > ChiSq**
age	1	121.2391	<0.0001
famsize	1	273.6828	<0.0001
hcdist	2	36.9434	<0.0001
child	1	25.6523	<0.0001
wealth	3	42.1425	<0.0001
roof	2	47.4428	<0.0001
rural	1	23.7546	<0.0001

Analysis of Maximum Likelihood Estimates				
	Parameter Estimate	**Standard Error**	**Chi-Square**	**Pr > ChiSq**
Intercept	−1.5975	0.6012	7.0592	0.0079
age	−0.1177	0.0107	121.2391	<0.0001
famsize	0.8430	0.0510	273.6828	<0.0001
hcdist 1	0.9575	0.1606	35.5529	<0.0001
hcdist 2	0.6200	0.1862	11.0928	0.0009
child 1	0.7085	0.1399	25.6523	<0.0001
wealth 1	−1.4321	0.2238	40.9622	<0.0001
wealth 2	−0.7331	0.2025	13.1121	0.0003
wealth 3	−0.5574	0.1985	7.8825	0.0050
roof 1	1.1272	0.1640	47.2677	<0.0001
roof 3	0.6594	0.1826	13.0488	0.0003
rural 1	0.6825	0.1400	23.7546	<0.0001

© Cengage Learning, 2012.

TABLE 5-14 RESULTS OF A LOGISTIC REGRESSION WITH MULTIPLE FACTORS (ODDS RATIOS)

Effect	**Point Estimate**	**95% Wald Confidence Limits**	
age	0.889	0.871	0.908
famsize	2.323	2.102	2.567
hcdist 1 vs 3	2.605	1.902	3.569
hcdist 2 vs 3	1.859	1.291	2.678
child 1 vs 0	2.031	1.544	2.672
wealth 1 vs 4	0.239	0.154	0.370
wealth 2 vs 4	0.480	0.323	0.714
wealth 3 vs 4	0.573	0.388	0.845
roof 1 vs 2	3.087	2.239	4.257
roof 3 vs 2	1.934	1.352	2.766
rural 1 vs 0	1.979	1.504	2.604

© Cengage Learning, 2012.

RESEARCH QUESTION:
How is the utilization of ITNs related to having children under 5 in the household, wealth, distance to health care, rural residence, family size, age of the head of household, and roof type?

Younger age, having a child under the age of 5 in the household, a larger family, living closer to healthcare facilities, increased wealth, not living in a house with a thatched roof, and living in an urban area are all related to an increased odds of insecticide-net utilization (Table 5-14). These variables were included in a multiple-variable logistic regression model; so the resulting odds ratio estimates for each factor has been adjusted for each of the other variables in the model. Specifically, households with children under 5 have approximately twice the odds of ITN use when compared to households without children under 5 (95% CI: 1.5, 2.7). Having a corrugated or other type of roof is associated with 3.1 (95% CI: 2.2, 4.3) and 1.9 (95% CI: 1.4, 2.8) times higher estimated odds of net use when compared to households with a thatched roof. The effect of wealth is associated with ITN use ($P < 0.0001$). In fact, the estimated odds of ITN use for those in the highest wealth group were 75%, 50%, and 40% higher than those in the lowest, next to lowest, and next to highest wealth classifications. Rural households have almost twice the estimated odds of net use compared to urban households (95% CI: 1.5, 2.6). Distance to a healthcare facility is also associated with ITN ($p < 0.0001$); a greater odds of use was observed for households living less than 15 miles and between 15–50 miles compared to those living more than 50 miles from healthcare facilities. Further, as family size increases by one person the estimated odds of net use increases by 2.3 ($p<0.0001$). Increasing age, however, is associated with decreased estimated odds in net use. In fact, as the age of the head of household increases by 1 year, the estimated odds of net use decrease by 11% (95% CI: 0.87, 0.91).

CONCLUSION: Younger age, having a child under the age of 5 in the household, a larger family, living closer to healthcare facilities, increased wealth, not living in a house with a thatched roof, and living in an rural area are all related to an increased odds in insecticide-net utilization.

Regressors as Confounders

Adjusting for confounding has been previously described using Mantel-Haenszel odds ratios when there was only one categorical confounder. However, an observational study is unlikely to result in only one confounding variable. Furthermore, the OR_{MH} cannot be provided for a continuous confounder. Logistic regression, on the other hand, can handle multiple confounders (dichotomous, nominal, ordinal, and continuous).

RESEARCH QUESTION:
Is having a child under the age of 5 associated with utilization of ITNs, controlling for wealth, distance to health care, rural residence, family size, age of the head of household, and roof type?

The results of the logistic regression (Table 5-14) indicate that having a child under the age of 5 is associated with net utilization ($p < 0.0001$). In fact, the estimated odds of using an ITN for households with children under 5 is 2.03 (95% CI: 1.5, 2.7) times that of those without children under 5 years old in the household, controlling for all other variables in the model.

CONCLUSION: Even after adjusting for potential confounding variables, wealth, distance to health care, rural residence, family size, age of the head of household, and roof type, there is an increased odds of ITN use among households with children under the age of 5 (adjusted *OR* estimate: 2.03; 95% CI: 1.5, 2.7).

The primary difference between the interpretation of the results of a logistic regression when regressors are explanatory variables and when regressors are confounders is the level of detail given to individual regressors. Unless an adjusted odds ratio for a confounding variable is particularly interesting, they are usually ignored; a confounding variable is included in the model only to better understand the relationship between explanatory and response variables. In contrast, when explanatory variables are of interest, all these variables are interesting to the investigator. Adjusted odds ratio estimates for each of these variables will be discussed and explained because the purpose of the logistic regression is to investigate how all these variables are related to the dichotomous outcome.

Interactions

Logistic regression is implemented when there are multiple variables of interest. In any multiple variable regression, the relationship between any one variable and the response is adjusted for the other variables in the model, regardless if the variables were included as confounders or explanatory variables. However, when one variable alters or modifies the relationship of a regressor and the response, the variable is an effect modifier. To account for effect modification, it is not sufficient simply to include variables in the model.

Effect modifiers are variables that alter the relationship of the dependent variable and a regressor. Effect modification was discussed earlier where a single categorical effect modifier required the use of stratified odds ratio estimates. Effect modifiers can be incorporated into a logistic regression as an *interaction*. Interactions are used whenever the relationship between a variable and the response depends on the level of another variable (effect modification). They are included in the model as if they were an additional variable. For example, suppose that an interaction between having children under the age of 5 and rural status is suspected. The model that incorporates the interaction between having children under the age of 5 (child) and rural status (rural) is

$$\text{logit}(p) = \ln\left(\frac{p}{1-p}\right) = \alpha + \beta_1(\text{child}) + \beta_2(\text{wealth1}) + \beta_3(\text{wealth2}) + \beta_4(\text{wealth3})$$
$$+ \beta_5(\text{hcdist1}) + \beta_6(\text{hcdist2}) + \beta_7(\text{rural})$$
$$+ \beta_8(\text{famsize}) + \beta_9(\text{age}) + \beta_{10}(\text{roof1})$$
$$+ \beta_{11}(\text{roof3}) + \beta_{12}(\text{rural} \times \text{child})$$

Determining whether a variable is an effect modifier is the same as determining whether the interaction of having a child under the age of 5 and rural status is significant, which is the same as determining whether the slope (β_{12}) associated with the interaction is significantly different from 0.

NULL HYPOTHESIS: The slope (β_{12}) for the interaction is 0, after controlling for all other variables in the model.

RESEARCH HYPOTHESIS: The slope (β_{12}) for the interaction is not 0, after controlling for all other variables in the model.

If the p-value associated with the slope for the interaction is large, then the interaction can be excluded. However, if the p-value associated with the slope is small ($p < 0.05$), then the interaction needs to be considered. In this example, a significant interaction means that the relationship of having children under the age of 5 and the use of nets should not be discussed without considering whether the household is located in a rural area. In other words, rural residence is an effect modifier. Therefore, if an interaction is included in the model, most statistical software packages will not provide the odds ratio estimates for any variables involved in the interaction without specifically requesting them.

To illustrate how regression estimates can be used to calculate odds ratio estimates for each level of the effect modifier, suppose rural location is an effect modifier (i.e., there is a significant interaction between rural status and having children under the age of 5). Then, for rural locations (rural = 1) and households with children under 5 (child = 1), the right-hand side of the model becomes

$$\alpha + \beta_1(1) + \beta_2(\text{wealth1}) + \beta_3(\text{wealth2}) + \beta_4(\text{wealth3}) + \beta_5(\text{hcdist1})$$
$$+ \beta_6(\text{hcdist2}) + \beta_7(1) + \beta_8(\text{famsize}) + \beta_9(\text{age}) + \beta_{10}(\text{roof1})$$
$$+ \beta_{11}(\text{roof3}) + \beta_{12}(1 \times 1)$$

Hence for rural locations (rural = 1) and households without children under 5 (child = 0), the right hand side of the model becomes

$$\alpha + \beta_1(0) + \beta_2(\text{wealth1}) + \beta_3(\text{wealth2}) + \beta_4(\text{wealth3}) + \beta_5(\text{hcdist1})$$
$$+ \beta_6(\text{hcdist2}) + \beta_7(1) + \beta_8(\text{famsize}) + \beta_9(\text{age}) + \beta_{10}(\text{roof1})$$
$$+ \beta_{11}(\text{roof3}) + \beta_{12}(1 \times 0)$$

Holding everything else constant, the difference between having children under the age of 5 and not in rural households becomes $\ln\left(\frac{p_{U5}}{1-p_{U5}}\right) - \ln\left(\frac{p_{O5}}{1-p_{O5}}\right) = \beta_1(1) + \beta_{12}(1 \times 1) - [\beta_1(0) + \beta_{12}(1 \times 0)] = \beta_1 + \beta_{12}$. Therefore, in rural households, the adjusted odds ratio for using an insecticide-treated net for households with children under 5 versus no children under 5 is $\exp(\beta_1 + \beta_{12})$.

Similarly, for urban (rural = 0) households and households with children under 5 (child = 1), the right-hand side of the model becomes

$$\alpha + \beta_1(1) + \beta_2(\text{wealth1}) + \beta_3(\text{wealth2}) + \beta_4(\text{wealth3}) + \beta_5(\text{hcdist1})$$
$$+ \beta_6(\text{hcdist2}) + \beta_7(0) + \beta_8(\text{famsize}) + \beta_9(\text{age}) + \beta_{10}(\text{roof1})$$
$$+ \beta_{11}(\text{roof3}) \times \beta_{12}(0 \times 1)$$

Hence for urban locations (rural = 0) and households without children under 5 (child = 0), the right-hand side of the model becomes

$$\alpha + \beta_1(0) + \beta_2(\text{wealth1}) + \beta_3(\text{wealth2}) + \beta_4(\text{wealth3}) + \beta_5(\text{hcdist1})$$
$$+ \beta_6(\text{hcdist2}) + \beta_7(0) + \beta_8(\text{famsize}) + \beta_9(\text{age}) + \beta_{10}(\text{roof1})$$
$$+ \beta_{11}(\text{roof3}) + \beta_{12}(0 \times 0)$$

Holding everything else constant, the difference between having children under the age of 5 and not in urban households becomes $\ln\left(\frac{p_{U5}}{1-p_{U5}}\right) - \ln\left(\frac{p_{O5}}{1-p_{O5}}\right) = \beta_1(1) + \beta_{12}(0 \times 1) - [\beta_1(0) + \beta_{12}(0 \times 0)] = \beta_1$. Therefore, in urban households, the adjusted odds ratio for using an insecticide-treated net for households with children under 5 versus no children under 5 is $\exp(\beta_1)$. Once the odds ratio estimates are found, confidence intervals can be obtained and interpreted. This example was fairly straightforward because the effect modifier (rural status) and the regressor (children under the age of 5) were both dichotomous. In the event that either variable is nominal, multiple slopes are necessary to calculate the odds ratio estimates. Similarly, if a continuous variable is involved in the interaction, odds ratio estimates are generally presented for a set of representative values of the continuous variable.

When an interaction is present, the stratified adjusted odds ratios can be provided using statistical software. As an example, suppose an interaction exists between having a child under the age of 5 and living in a rural area; rural residence is an effect modifier (Table 5-15).

TABLE 5-15 RESULTS FROM A LOGISTIC REGRESSION WITH A SIGNIFICANT INTERACTION

Type 3 Analysis of Effects			
Effect	DF	Wald Chi-Square	Pr > ChiSq
child*rural	1	7.5641	0.0060
Odds Ratios and Wald Confidence Interval			
	Estimate	95% Confidence Limits	
child 0 vs at rural = 0	2.214	1.444	3.393
child 0 vs 1 at rural = 1	1.026	0.727	1.446

© Cengage Learning, 2012.

Predicting Probabilities

The logistic regression is based on a statistical model and the estimates that result provide a prediction equation. The prediction equation for a logistic regression has the form $\ln\left(\frac{\hat{p}}{1-\hat{p}}\right) = \hat{\alpha} + \hat{\beta}_1 x_1 + \hat{\beta}_2 x_2 + \cdots + \hat{\beta}_K x_K$. The parameters are replaced with the estimates, $\hat{\alpha}$ and $\hat{\beta}$'s. Although the estimates from a linear regression (Chapter 3) were used with possible regressor values to predict the response, predicting the natural log of the odds in a logistic regression is usually not of interest. However, investigators may be interested in trying to predict the probability of a particular outcome. For example, an investigator may want to try to predict the probability of insecticide-treated net use using having children under the age of 5 and the wealth of the household as regressors (Table 5-16).

Choosing values for the regressor, the investigator can predict the probability of an outcome ($\hat{p}$), by transforming the logistic regression prediction equation $\hat{p} = \frac{e^{\hat{\alpha} + \hat{\beta}_1 x_1 \cdots + \hat{\beta}_K x_K}}{1 + e^{\hat{\alpha} + \hat{\beta}_1 x_1 + \cdots + \hat{\beta}_K x_K}}$.

TABLE 5-16 LOGISTIC REGRESSION RESULTS WITH CHILDREN UNDER 5 AND WEALTH AS REGRESSORS

Analysis of Maximum Likelihood Estimates				
	Parameter Estimate	Standard Error	Wald Chi-Square	Pr > ChiSq
Intercept	−0.8368	0.1298	41.5881	<0.0001
child 1	0.6462	0.1074	36.1864	<0.0001
wealth 1	−1.2051	0.1734	48.3184	<0.0001
wealth 2	−0.5672	0.1545	13.4797	0.0002
wealth 3	−0.2130	0.1495	2.0315	0.1541

© Cengage Learning, 2012.

Predicted probability $= \hat{p} = \dfrac{e^{\hat{\alpha} + \hat{\beta}_1 x_1 \cdots + \hat{\beta}_K x_K}}{1 + e^{\hat{\alpha} + \hat{\beta}_1 x_1 + \cdots + \hat{\beta}_K x_K}}$

$\hat{\alpha} =$ Estimate of the intercept

$\hat{\beta} =$ Estimate of the slope

$x =$ The value of the regressor

What you need to calculate the predicted probability:

1. *Estimates from the logistic regression (Table 5-16):*
   a. Estimate of the intercept: $\hat{\alpha} = -0.8368$
   b. Estimate of the slopes: $\hat{\beta}_{child} = 0.6462, \hat{\beta}_{weakth1} = -1.2051, \hat{\beta}_{wealth2} = -0.5672, \hat{\beta}_{wealth3} = -0.2130$
2. *Values for the regressors:* In this example, the predicted probability for having children under 5 (child = 1) and being in the lowest wealth group (wealth1 = 1, wealth2 = 0, and wealth3 = 0).
3. $\hat{\alpha} + \hat{\beta}_1 x_1 + \hat{\beta}_2 x_2 + \cdots + \hat{\beta}_K x_K$: In this example, the sum is $-0.8368 + 0.6462(1) - 1.2051(1) + 0.5672(0) - 0.2130(0) = -1.3957$.
4. *Exponentiate the sum obtained from (3):* $\exp(-1.3957) = 0.2477$.
5. *Add 1 to the value in (4):* $0.2477 + 1 = 1.2477$.

To calculate the predicted probability: Divide (4) by (5): $\hat{p} = \dfrac{0.2477}{1.2477} = 0.1985$.

Statistical software packages can be used to easily estimate probabilities and the confidence intervals for them. With any prediction equation, however, remember that the prediction equation is only as good as the data used to create it. To avoid unreasonable predictions, possible regressor values must be limited to those similar to the ones used to find the estimates of intercept and slope.

Why the Odds Ratio?

In linear regression, the statistical model equates the response variable to the regressors as $y = \alpha + \beta_1 x_1 + \beta_2 x_2 + \cdots + \beta_K x_K + \varepsilon$. In logistic regression, the response is dichotomous and is restricted to two levels. Even if an investigator is interested in predicting the probability of an outcome, a probability is restricted to be between 0 and 1. Since the right-hand side of the statistical model (regressors) can be anything (positive, negative, fraction, whole number), the logit$(p) = \ln\left(\dfrac{p}{1-p}\right)$ is the left-hand side of the model when the outcome is dichotomous because the logit can also take on any numerical value. So, in a logistic regression, the two sides of the statistical model are *linked* using the logit. Therefore, a logistic regression may be described as a binomial regression with a logit *link function*. The use of the logit as the link is the reason $\hat{\beta}$'s can be exponentiated into odds ratio estimates. If a different link function is used, the parameter estimates ($\hat{\beta}$'s) do not transform into odds ratio estimates.

Often, investigators are not interested in odds ratios as a measure of association, but the use of the logit results in estimates that correspond to odds ratios. Therefore, a logistic regression (and the logit link) should not be used if the odds ratio is not the desired measure of association. Many times odds ratios are incorrectly interpreted as if they were prevalence or risk ratios, but this can result in overestimating the effect (Chapter 4). Alternative regression models are available if a measure other than the odds ratio is appropriate. If a prevalence ratio is of interest, for example, then a log (not a logit) link function can be used so that the model becomes

$$\ln(p) = \ln\left(\frac{p}{1-p}\right) = \alpha + \beta_1(\text{child}) + \beta_2(\text{wealth1}) + \beta_3(\text{wealth2}) + \beta_4(\text{wealth3})$$
$$+ \beta_5(\text{hcdist1}) + \beta_6(\text{hcdist2}) + \beta_7(\text{rural}) + \beta_8(\text{famsize})$$
$$+ \beta_9(\text{age}) + \beta_{10}(\text{roof1}) + \beta_{11}(\text{roof3})$$

Holding all other variables constant, the difference between households with and without children under 5 results in $\ln(p_{U5}) - \ln(p_{O5}) = \ln(p_{U5}/p_{O5})$. Therefore, $\beta_1 = \ln(p_{U5}/p_{O5})$. Hence $e^{\beta_1} = p_{U5}/p_{O5}$ and represents the true prevalence ratio holding all other variables constant. Consequently, all of the β's in the regression model can be transformed and interpreted as adjusted prevalence ratios. This particular regression model is referred to as the *log-binomial regression model*.

Diagnostics

Regression models provide a way for investigators to understand how the data might have been produced. Therefore, a model is really helpful only if it is appropriate for the data or if the data fit well. Statistical software packages offer several options for determining whether the model fits well. A few of these methods are discussed here.

Pearson, Deviance, Hosmer-Lemeshow Hypothesis Tests

Three hypothesis tests are commonly used to determine how well the model fits in logistic regression: Pearson, deviance, and Hosmer-Lemeshow. In all three tests, the hypotheses are the same.

RESEARCH HYPOTHESIS: The model does not fit.

NULL HYPOTHESIS: The model fits.

When the sample size is not excessively large or when the number of continuous regressors is limited, the Pearson and deviance tests should be fairly similar. When a large p-value results, the model fits reasonably well. Given a larger number of continuous regressors, the assumptions of the Pearson and deviance tests may not be met. In this case, the Hosmer-Lemeshow test may be used. Similar to the other tests, a large p-value indicates model fit. Although a small p-value for any of these tests indicates a lack of model fit, keep in mind that, when the sample size is large, a small p-value is easier to obtain and using hypothesis tests to determine model fit may not be appropriate.

Using ROC Curves in Logistic Regression

Sensitivity and specificity (introduced at the beginning of this chapter) apply nicely in a logistic regression because the outcome is dichotomous. To investigate how well the regressors predict the outcome, the linear combination of regressors can be thought of as a continuous "screening test" trying to predict the outcome. Because the combination of the regressors form a continuous "screening test," ROC curves can be used to see how well the regressors predict the outcome. In this example, the regressors are having a child under the age of 5, wealth, distance to healthcare, living in a rural area, family size, age of household head, and roof type.

The ROC curve can be used to determine how well these variables predict whether an insecticide-treated net was used (Figure 5-5). The area under the curve is 0.905, which is very close to 1, indicating that these variables do a good job of predicting whether nets will be utilized. ROC curves are particularly helpful in variable selection because variables can be removed or included based on how much they impact the ROC curve and the area under the curve (AUC).

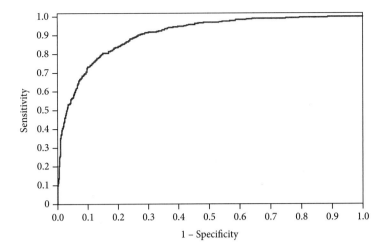

Figure 5-5 ROC curve (regression). © *Cengage Learning, 2012.*

Residuals

The residuals can also be used to determine how well the model fits the data. In particular, Pearson and deviance residuals can be used to identify extreme observations. These residuals can be used much like the residuals of a linear regression. In particular, Pearson and deviance residuals should be randomly distributed around 0, and very large or very small residuals indicate potential outliers.

Variable Selection

One of the most time-consuming tasks in completing any regression analysis is deciding which variables to include. If the purpose of the study is to investigate possible risk factors for a particular outcome, the methods for choosing risk factors or explanatory variables are slightly different from those in a study whose purpose is determining whether certain groups are different, controlling for potential confounders. When trying to investigate possible risk factors, the variables are included in the regression because they are critical to predicting the outcome. When trying to compare groups additional variables are included only because they are potential confounders, and variable selection is not necessarily based on statistical rationale. Hence, variable selection for a regression analysis depends on the goals of the analysis:

- Forecasting/prediction
- Covariate-adjustment (adjusting for confounders)

Forecasting/Prediction

When forecasting is the primary goal of the regression analysis, the research question usually involves trying to predict an outcome based on values from explanatory variables. Investigators must choose an appropriate set of explanatory variables, ones that do a good job of explaining the outcome. Therefore, model fit is particularly important. If the regression model does not fit the data, then the resulting prediction equation will not do a very good job of forecasting outcomes or predicting probabilities. In addition, outliers and influence points must be considered because they may alter the regression estimates. Furthermore, the assumptions of the regression analysis must be rigorously tested because the model is being used to predict outcomes.

Covariate-Adjustment

When adjustment for covariates or confounders is the primary goal of the regression analysis, the research question usually involves trying to compare two (or more) groups. The data are generally obtained from an observational study with groups defined by something other than random chance. To get a better estimate of the differences between groups, variables are included in the model that impact group assignment and the outcome of interest. Unlike when prediction is the primary goal, the selection of variables has much more to do with published literature and an understanding of the groups/outcome than it does with model fit. Although good model fit is important, the primary reason for including a variable is not to improve model fit measures. The rationale for selecting a variable is based more on the context of the problem and less on statistical justification.

So the first step to variable selection in covariate-adjustment is to consult the literature, and identify variables used in other analyses as potential covariates. A next step can involve data analysis, especially considering descriptive statistics, simple statistical tests, and/or simple regressions. Finding unadjusted odds ratios and conducting simple statistical tests may be helpful. Variables that are related to the outcome and group membership should be considered candidates for the regression analysis. Generally, these are variables that result in small p-values when investigating simple statistical tests. However, the p-value does not at have to be smaller than 0.05 to determine whether variables are potential candidates (e.g. p-values of 0.2–0.3 may be considered). The goal is not to determine statistical significance but to create a subset of variables. If the p-value cutoff for variable selection is too stringent (i.e., $p < 0.05$), important variables may be omitted. When trying to determine whether a variable has an impact, do not focus entirely on the p-value; consider the statistics too. Remember that good estimates are the goal and that providing them relies on using an appropriate model.

Strategies for Performing the Regression

A good strategy for performing a regression analysis is to follow the strategies for regression diagnostics.

- Plotting the data is a good first step in identifying variables that may be related to the outcome. Descriptive statistics and bar graphs are helpful. Additionally, considering one regressor at a time may also be informative.
- Once the literature has been consulted, simple tests have been performed, and plots have been created and reviewed, a set of potential variables can be identified.
- Some variables may be measuring the same thing; so potential variables can be further reduced by removing variables that demonstrate multicollinearity.
- With a potential set of regressors, the assumptions of the model can be checked and potential outlier/influence points identified. Although outlier and influence points are generally not omitted, an investigation of how removing these points affects estimates may be useful.
- In evaluating the regression output, some variables may not really contribute to the prediction of the outcome. Unnecessary variables can be removed from the model. Be careful in eliminating variables here. If a variable is removed from the model, the estimates are no longer adjusted for that variable.
- With logistic regression, ROC curves are helpful in model selection. Because these curves provide a measure of how well the variables in the model predict the outcome, variables that increase the area under the ROC curve should be included, and variables that do not impact the area under the curve may be candidates for exclusion. A logistic regression model with a high area under the ROC curve is desirable.

Using automatic model selection strategies, statistical software can provide a set of variables for the regression model. Although this strategy is reasonable if many potential variables have to be included without guidance for choosing among them, relying solely on automated model selection strategies should be avoided. Many public health problems include variables in the regression for covariate-adjustment, and the primary reason for keeping a variable may be based on the literature or on knowledge about the subject, not necessarily on statistical rationale. Hence, relying on automated model selection strategies may have little justification.

SUMMARY

This chapter began with an infectious disease and health behavior problem: understanding factors related to insecticide-treated net use. In this public health application, as in many others, the outcome of interest was a dichotomous variable. Like the public health application presented at the start of the chapter, the data for this chapter investigated different factors (such as whether young children were in the household) that might be related to insecticide-treated net use.

The most common analyses associated with dichotomous outcomes were explained in this chapter. Specifically, methods were presented for investigating associations with multiple variables. Furthermore, dealing with confounding and effect modification, with one or multiple variables, was also presented. Predicting the probability of a dichotomous outcome was also discussed in the context of screening tests and regression. The chapter concluded by considering several aspects of logistic regression models, one of the most common statistical methods in public health.

SUMMARY OF CHAPTER CONCEPTS

GOAL	METHOD
How do I compare groups while adjusting for a confounder (categorical)?	
Is there effect modification?	Stratified odds ratios Breslow-Day test
Association between two variables, controlling for a categorical confounder?	Odds ratio (MH)
How do I compare groups while adjusting for confounders (continuous or categorical)?	
Is there a difference between the groups, controlling for other variables?	Multiple logistic regression Adjusted odds ratios
How do I investigate the association of risk factors (continuous and categorical) on the outcome?	
Is there a relationship between explanatory variables and a dichotomous response?	Multiple logistic regression Adjusted odds ratios
Can variables predict an outcome?	Sensitivity Specificity Receiver operator characteristic (ROC) Curves Predicted probabilities

KEY TERMS

sensitivity	effect modifier	adjusted odds ratio
specificity	stratified odds ratio	

PRACTICE WITH DATA

1. DESCRIBING THE DATA

a. Provide the sensitivity and specificity using having a child under 5 as a screening tool for whether a household will use an ITN. Hint: Sensitivity is associated with a positive and specificity is associated with a negative.

b. Construct an ROC curve using the wealth index as a screening tool for using an ITN.

2. CONFOUNDING AND EFFECT MODIFICATION

a. Consider the relationship between ITN use and having a child under the age of 5. Suppose that roof type (thatched or corrugated metal) is a confounder. Is roof type an effect modifier? Use the data and statistical inference to support your answer.

b. Based on the response to part (a), what odds ratio estimates are most appropriate. Provide these and interpret.

3. LOGISTIC REGRESSION

a. Suppose it is of interest to determine whether wealth is related to the use of an ITN. Perform a logistic regression to investigate this relationship while controlling for potential confounders (family size, distance to healthcare, and rural residence). Based on the results, provide a conclusion.

b. Using the results from part (a), provide the predicted probability of net use for households with the highest wealth index, a family size of 4, and living in an urban area within 15 miles of a healthcare facility.

c. Describe the predictive power of the model by providing the ROC curve and the area under it. Intepret.

PRACTICE WITH CONCEPTS

1. Consider the following research questions/study scenarios. For each study, discuss the most appropriate methods for describing the data (graphically and numerically). What statistical method would be *most* appropriate for addressing the research questions? Be sure to provide a justification of the statistical method. When a statistical test is needed, provide appropriate null and research hypotheses.

a. A study was performed to determine whether steroids were effective in slowing the development of Crohn's disease (CD). In the study, 338 patients with irritable bowel syndrome (a possible precursor to CD) were randomly assigned to either receive steroids immediately or to wait until they developed further CD symptoms. Data were collected a year after randomization. In addition to evaluating whether CD developed, data on race, blood tests measurements (continuous), and the number of visits to the doctor in the last year were also collected.

b. A study investigating the effects of second-hand smoke in working environments asked the following question: "How often do you experience second-hand smoke in a work environment/function? Never, Occasionally, Fairly Often, Very Often, Almost Always." The question was asked of managers and employees to determine whether there was an association between position and the amount of second-hand smoke exposure. The responses to the questions were grouped into Little/None and Often, where Little/None was defined as responses of Never or Occasionally and Often was defined as responses of Fairly Often, Very Often, and Almost Always. Additionally, the time in which subjects were on the job (<2 years, ≥2 years) was thought to be a factor.

    c. Stress has been related to several poor health outcomes, particularly high blood pressure. Women will be surveyed on stress levels (defined as small/moderate and large/overwhelming) and will have their blood pressure assessed at a clinic. Women will be categorized as having high blood pressure or not (the outcome of interest). Weight and height will also be assessed at the clinic visit to obtain BMI. Is there a relationship between stress and high blood pressure, controlling for BMI?

2. Pap smears are a diagnostic test used to detect cervical cancer. Although the test has high specificity, it also has low sensitivity. As a result, women have to be screened often. Using the definitions of sensitivity and specificity, explain why increased frequency of screening is needed when sensitivity is low and specificity is high.

3. *"This paper reports the prevalence of obesity in the US based on World Health Organization's (WHO) classification of obesity. It also reports the prevalence of individuals in the general population who use dietary modifications and/or exercise to lose weight. The main objective of this paper is to assess the relationship between obesity status, HRQL, dietary modifications, and exercise . . . Responses to the HRQL questions were used as dependent variables . . . by dichotomizing the number of reported days with poor physical health . . . into ≤14 days and >14 days."* (Hassan et al., 2003, pp. 1227–1228)

    a. A logistic regression was used to investigate obesity and poor physical health while controlling for the following variables: age, gender, race, income, health status, education, current smoker, and diet/exercise status. Justify the use of a logistic regression.

    b. The odds ratios that result from the logistic regression defined in part (a) are

        Nonoverweight: Reference
        Overweight: 1.08 (0.99–1.17)
        Obese: 1.21 (1.09–1.33)
        Severely Obese: 1.87 (1.64–2.12)

    Provide a conclusion. Be sure to include a discussion of statistical inference.

    c. The authors state, "Our study has certain limitations. First, due to the cross-sectional nature of our study, causality cannot be inferred." Explain what this statement means and why it is an issue.

CHAPTER 6

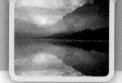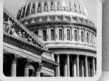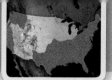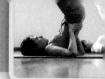

count data

Count data occur whenever the outcome is counted in whole numbers from 0 to infinity. Count data can be found in many public health applications. The number of steps taken, the number of concussions, number of dental caries, the number of cigarettes smoked, the number of swine flu cases, the number of relapses, the number of health-care utilizations (uses of urgent treatment centers, emergency room visits, and/or hospital visits), the number of lesions on body, or even the number of days in pain are just a few examples. In each of these examples, the outcome represents a count, some number of whole units. Because a count represents the number of whole units, the collected data have gaps between them; for example, a subject cannot have 0.333 relapses, 0.75 hospital visits, or 0.123 concussions. Because values between whole numbers are not observed, count data are considered discrete.

In many public health studies, investigators are interested in counting the number of events for a population at risk, but subjects can differ in their contribution to event counts. For example, in a study investigating the count of concussions among student athletes, some athletes may have played a sport longer and would have had more time to have concussions. A nutrition study counting the number of fast food restaurants in different regions may have regions of different geographic or population size. Likewise, when counting the number of swine flu cases for a county, the population size of the county would need to be considered. These examples demonstrate that investigations of count data also need to consider potential variations in the contribution of risk for an event.

This chapter provides a description of summaries, as well as methods for comparing groups and for investigating multiple variable associations when the outcome is a count, particularly count data that occur when the subjects may contribute different amounts of time, space, or subjects at risk.

LEARNING OBJECTIVES

How do I describe count data?

Identify, create, and present appropriate descriptive statistics and figures specific to count data.

How do I make comparisons?

Identify appropriate statistical tests for comparison in one and multiple samples.

Understand when it is necessary to use exact tests versus approximations.

Interpret the results of the statistical tests.

How do I compare groups while adjusting for confounders (continuous and categorical)?

Utilize regression techniques to control for confounding.

Interpret the results (estimates and statistical tests) of the regression analysis.

How do I investigate the association of risk factors (continuous and categorical) on the outcome?

Utilize regression techniques to investigate risk factors.

Interpret the results (estimates and statistical tests) of the regression analysis.

What method do I use?

Identify the most appropriate method for the data.

Public Health Application

Fractures of the vertebrae (spine), proximal femur (hip), and distal forearm (wrist) have long been regarded as the quintessential osteoporotic fractures. Osteoporosis is a systemic condition, however, and results of large prospective studies have shown that almost all types of fracture are increased in patients with low bone density, and, irrespective of type of fracture, adults who sustain a fracture are 50–100% more likely to have another one of a different type.

After allowing for the functional impairment expected in old people, fractures of the hip, spine, and distal forearm cause about 7% of women to become dependent on the basic activities of daily living and precipitate nursing home care in a further 8%. Hip fractures contribute the most to this burden. The most important long-term impairment is in the ability to walk: about 20% of patients are nonambulatory even before fracture, but of those able to walk, half cannot

do so independently afterwards. Among women who lived independently before hip fracture, about half remain in long-term care or need help with the activities of daily living a year after the event. Ultimately, up to a third of individuals who have a hip fracture can become totally dependent, and the risk of institutionalisation is great.

Osteoporosis has clinical and public health importance only because of these fractures. Osteoporotic fractures are one of the most common causes of disability and a major contributor to medical care costs in many regions of the world. Indeed, for white women, the one-in-six lifetime risk of sustaining a hip fracture is greater than the one-in-nine risk of developing breast cancer. The social burden of fractures will increase throughout the world as the population ages.
(Cummings & Melton, 2002)

Data Description

The World Health Organization has defined categories based on bone density t-scores; a woman with a t-score that is greater than -1 is considered normal, while t-scores between -1 and -2.5 and scores less than -2.5 have been classified as indicative of osteopenia and osteoporosis, respectively. A longitudinal study of postmenopausal women newly diagnosed as osteopenic or osteoporotic was conducted to investigate

- The impact of a strength training program on fracture rates
- The impact of the training program on the number of hospitalizations and emergency room visits
- Potential risk factors related to fracture rates in this population

The recruitment and enrollment period lasted for 2 years. Female patients were recruited at their primary care physician after receiving a diagnosis of either osteopenia or osteoporosis. After consent was obtained, baseline data were collected. Data elements collected at the first visit (at diagnosis) included quality of life (visual analog scale from 1–100), a pain assessment (10 point scale), a measure of physical activity (no and limited activity, somewhat active, very active), current calcium use (yes/no) history of fracture (yes/no). Age and race (white, black, other) were also collected at the first visit. A total of 6,060 women

were enrolled at the clinic visits and contributed baseline data. Approximately half (52%) had a previous history of a nontraumatic fracture.

At the initial visit, where a diagnosis of osteopenia or osteoporosis was identified, women were given a brochure describing osteopenia/osteoporosis (low bone density) and the benefits of strength training. Women were then given the opportunity to enroll in a strength training program; 3305 (54%) elected to participate in a strength training regimen.

To count the number of new fractures and the amount of healthcare utilization (emergency room, urgent treatment center, and hospital visits), women were contacted every 6 months. Contacts were made via telephone interviews with the participants, and medical records were accessed to verify information collected via telephone interviews. When a participant was unreachable, four additional attempts over the course of 6 weeks were made. A participant that had three consecutive missed contacts was considered a dropout, and no further attempts were made to collect data. Although the intent was to follow these women for 10 years after the last day of enrollment/recruitment, the average amount of follow-up time was 7.0 years (SD: 1.2). The maximum amount of follow-up time was 11.2 years, and the smallest amount of follow-up for a participant was 2.7 years.

DESCRIBING THE DATA

Depending on the type of count data collected, various descriptions are possible. If the counts are small, then describing them as a categorical variable (Chapter 4), with counts and percentages might be appropriate. However, if the count values have a considerable amount of variability for a group of subjects, the methods presented in Chapters 2 and 3 for summarizing a continuous variable may be more suitable.

Numerical and Graphical Summaries: Counts

If counting the number of hospitalizations, for example, the most a subject is hospitalized in a year might be three times; so the possible count of hospitalizations in a year would be 0, 1, 2, and 3 times. Because the count is limited, using the methods for describing categorical variables (Chapter 4) would be appropriate. On the other hand, the counts might not be limited to a few values. Consider, for example, the number of steps taken during an exercise program. The number of steps taken during an exercise program could range from 1200 to 10,978, for example, a fairly wide range of values. Because categorical data have a limited number of levels, describing the count variable as a categorical variable may not be appropriate when the counts are large and/or variable. Generally, when the counts have great variation, count data are described as continuous variables (Chapters 2 and 3) with descriptive statistics (n, mean, standard deviation, median, first and third quartile, and minimum and maximum, and correlations).

The number of fractures that this group of newly diagnosed women experience during the study period can be described with means and standard deviations or with counts and percentages. For example, the mean number of fractures experienced by this sample of 6060 women is 0.72 with a standard deviation of 1.24. The distribution of the number of fractures is graphically summarized with a histogram (Figure 6-1).

Furthermore, a categorical variable can easily be created by grouping women with similar numbers of fractures: those with no fractures, those with one to two fractures, and those with more than two fractures. In this example, 58% have no fractures, 32% have one to two fractures, and 10% have three or more fractures (Figure 6-2).

If count data could be summarized using the same statistical methods as used for continuous data (Chapters 2 and 3) or categorical data (Chapter 4), additional statistical methods would not really be necessary. However, these methods assume that each subject contributes equally to the count, e.g., that each subject is followed for the same amount of time. This assumption is not required and is not usually the case with count data. In this study of fracture counts, treating a woman who has been observed for 5 years the same as a woman who has been observed for only 1 year is unreasonable. The woman observed for 5 years has more opportunities to have fractures and may be

Figure 6-1 Histogram of the number of fractures
© *Cengage Learning, 2012.*

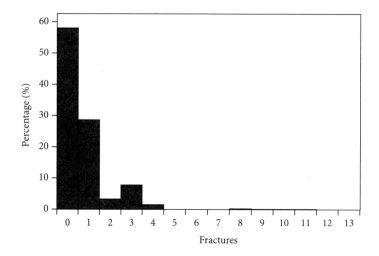

Figure 6-2 Bar graph of number of fractures
© *Cengage Learning, 2012.*

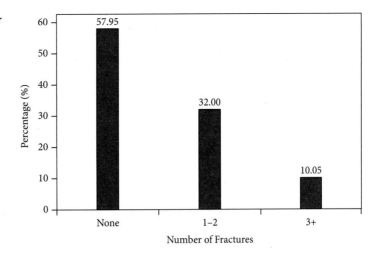

expected to have a larger fracture count than woman who had only 1 year of observation. To account for differing amounts of observation for each subject, count outcomes are often described with event rates.

Numerical Summaries for Count Outcomes

Person-Time and Event Rates

Using continuous or categorical descriptions are both reasonable ways of summarizing count data. However, these descriptions do not take into consideration the amount of risk each subject contributes to the event count (e.g., different amounts of follow-up time).

Proportions fail to provide a complete summary of count data because they are found by dividing the number of subjects with the event by the total number of subjects. The denominator represents all subjects, giving each subject an equal weight. The numerator provides the total event count and is calculated by adding the events of all the subjects, but each subject can contribute one and only one event. The components of a proportion are displayed in Figure 6-3. In the figure, each subject has the same-size square and each subject-square contains at most a single event (represented by a dot). The total rectangle, comprised of equally sized squares, represents the denominator and the sum of the dots provides the numerator of a proportion. In other words, with proportions, each subject contributes the same amount to the denominator and at most one event to the numerator; which is unlikely to be the case when the outcome is a count.

The discussion is similar for summaries when the count variable is treated like a continuous outcome. Presenting the mean count for a group of subjects describes the average count. However, doing so is misleading when different subjects can contribute multiple events to the count and may have had different opportunities for contributing to the count.

Figure 6-3 Visualization of calculating a proportion
© *Cengage Learning, 2012.*

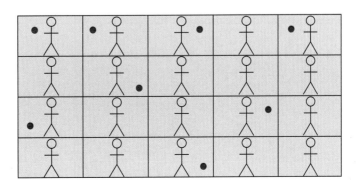

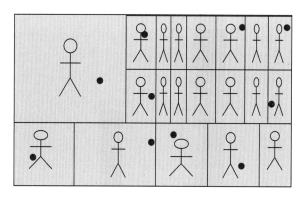

Figure 6-4 Visualization of calculating an event rate
© *Cengage Learning, 2012.*

One of the distinctions of count data is that subjects do not have to provide the same level of contribution to the count (Figure 6-4). While the entire rectangle in Figure 6-4 still represents the total number of subjects (the denominator), it is not equally divided among the subjects; some subjects contribute bigger squares. In this example, however, where women are followed over different amounts of time, the rectangle represents total **person-time**. Each woman contributes a different amount of follow-up time to the study (depicted by the different-sized squares within the rectangle) or a different amount of *person-time*. Because the women in this study contribute multiple years of observation (follow-up) times, the person-time is referred to as subject-years. For studies observed over months, person-time would be called subject-months; for a study observed over days, the person-time would be subject-days; and so on. The total amount of person-time for a study is the sum of all the individual person-times for the subjects, represented by the total rectangle in Figure 6-4, and the count is generally presented as the count per person-time.

Studies with count outcomes may have different contributions from subjects in ways other than varying follow-up times. The term "person-time" (subject-years, subject-months, subject-days, etc.) is generally reserved for studies with differing amounts of follow-up time. However, the idea holds for studies whose count outcomes need to account for differing amounts of space or units at risk. The count for these studies is presented as, for example, the count per number of square miles, the count per capita, or the count per number of teeth. This is one of the reasons why proportions (or percentages) are not ideal numerical summaries for count outcomes. Proportions (percentages) provide a description of the count of successes, assuming that each subject provides an equal contribution or the denominator represents the total number of subjects.

Another reason why proportions fall short in describing count data is that the subjects can contribute more than one event (Figure 6-5). Using a proportion to summarize the data assumes that a subject can be counted in a category once and only once, contributing at most one event (one dot) to the numerator.

Because count data may involve varying contributions from each subject, event rates (and not proportions) are best to describe count data. An *event rate* is calculated by dividing the total number of events (dots) by the total rectangle (Figure 6-5).

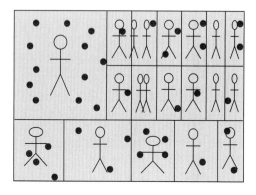

Figure 6-5 Visualization of calculating an event rate (multiple events)
© *Cengage Learning, 2012.*

The computation is similar to the calculation of a proportion, except that each subject can contribute multiple events (dots) to the numerator and the denominator (total rectangle) does not require that each subject contribute an equal share.

Application of Formula: EVENT RATES

$$\text{Estimate of the event rate} = \frac{\sum_{i=1}^{n} e_i}{\sum_{i=1}^{n} t_i}$$

e_i = The number of events for subject i

t_i = The amount of time, space, or units at risk for each subject

What you need to calculate an estimate of the event rate:

1. *The number of events for all subjects:* In this example, the total number of fractures is 4355:
$\sum_{i=1}^{6060} e_i = 4355$.
2. *The amount of time, space, or units at risk for all subjects:* In this study, where women are followed for different lengths of time, this is the total number of subject-years, which is the sum of all the follow-up times: $\sum_{i=1}^{6060} t_i = 42{,}535.6$.

To calculate the event rate: Divide the number of events (1) by (2). The fracture rate in this example is 4355 ÷ 42,535.6 = 0.10. This means that there are 0.10 fractures per 1 subject-year.

Event rates involving follow-up or observation time are typically presented as the number of events (the count) per a unit of person-time. The number of person-time units depends on the size of the event rate. Because counts are observed as whole numbers, the number of person-time units may be modified so that the event rate can be presented as a whole number per an amount of person-time. In this example, the event rate for fractures is 0.10. Because part of a fracture is not possible, it may make more sense to discuss the event rate as 10 fractures per 100 subject-years or 100 fractures per 1000 subject-years.

Although this example considers differing amounts of follow-up time, event rates can also be used to describe count data when time is not a factor. For example, if 275 fast-food restaurants are in a region with a total area of 5000 square feet, the event rate is 275 ÷ 5000 = 0.055. Therefore, there are 55 fast-food restaurants per 1000 square feet. Suppose, on the other hand, a pediatric dentistry study counted the number of white spot lesions in each child's mouth. Each child may have a different number of erupted teeth. A child with only 6 erupted teeth has fewer surfaces for white spot lesions than a child with 20 erupted teeth. If a total of 260 white spot lesions are observed on a total of 1236 teeth, the event rate is 0.21. In this example, the event rate might be presented as 2.1 white spot lesions per 10 teeth. Although 2.1 is not a whole number, presenting the data this way is more helpful to the pediatric dentist than describing the rate as 21 white spot lesions per 100 teeth.

Age-Adjusted Event Rates

Research questions in public health often involve the comparison of events and event rates between different populations. For example, much research has been done to investigate the outcomes of osteoporosis in different geographical regions. It may be of interest to compare the fracture rate for the United States to countries in the European Union or Asia. However, if the age distributions of the populations differ, then simply comparing the event rates is not accurate. In fact, if the differences in population ages are not considered, the comparison of event rates between populations or within a population across time can be misleading. To account for differences in population age, standardized, age-adjusted rates should be calculated. **Age-adjusted rates** are event rates that have been standardized using a reference population, which may vary depending on the event. However, a common reference population is the 2000 U.S. population obtained from the U.S. 2000 census. Estimates of age-adjusted rates are typically obtained by

- Dividing the sample according to age groups
- Weighting the unadjusted or crude event rates for each group according to the size of the reference population age group

Using a table of event counts and population sizes (Table 6-1) can be helpful in the calculation of age-adjusted rates. Table 6-1 provides the number of events (b) and the number of subjects in the population (c) by age group (a) for an example region. By using the U.S. 2000 population (e) as the standard population, the weighted average of the age-specific rates can be calculated to provide an age-adjusted rate for this region.

Using age-adjusted rates allows for the comparison of event rates across different geographical regions where the age of the population may be distributed differently. Note, however, that comparisons between age-adjusted rates are useful only if the *same* standard population is used to create the age-adjusted rates.

Application of Formula: AGE-ADJUSTED RATES

Age-adjusted event rate $= \sum_{i=1} w_i p_i$

w_i = The weight (proportion of the standard population in age group i) for age group i

p_i = The age-specific event rate for age group i

What you need to calculate the age-adjusted event rate (*direct method*):

1. *Age groups:* Column (a) of Table 6-1.
2. *Number of events in each age group:* Column (b) of Table 6-1.
3. *The number of people in the age group:* Column (c) of Table 6-1.
4. *The crude, age-specific rate:* Column (b) is divided by Column (c) for each age group.
5. *The number of people in the age group in the standard population:* Column (e) of Table 6-1.
6. *The weight for each age group:* This is the proportion of the standard population in each age group; column (e) is divided by the total number in the standard population.
7. *The weighted rate:* This is the crude, age-specific rate (p_i) times the weight (w_i), or column (d) times column (f).

To calculate the age-adjusted rate: Sum all the weighted rates (7) for all the age groups (column (g).) In this case, the age-adjusted event rate is 0.048. Often this age-adjusted rate is multiplied by 1000 so that it is a whole number. So the age-adjusted event rate for this region is 48 per 1000.

> **Point to Ponder**
>
> Age-adjusted rates are event rates that are standardized for a specific population. They can be used to compare rates for populations that may have different age distributions. The term "adjusted" is also used when discussing regression results. What is the difference between age-adjusted rates and estimates from a regression that have been adjusted for age?

TABLE 6-1 AGE-ADJUSTED RATE CALCULATION

Age Group (a)	Event Count (b)	Specific Population (c)	Age-Specific Rate (Crude Rate) (d)	Standard Population* (e)	Weight (f)	Weighted Rate (g)
Under 5 years	0	463,283	0	19,175,798	0.06813897	0
5–9 years	2	596,961	0.000003	20,549,505	0.07302028	0.0000002
10–14 years	4	575,005	0.000007	20,528,072	0.07294412	0.0000005
15–19 years	6	506,636	0.000012	20,219,890	0.07184903	0.0000009
20–24 years	10	518,546	0.000019	18,964,001	0.06738637	0.0000013
25–29 years	15	593,658	0.000025	19,381,336	0.06886932	0.0000017
30–34 years	54	634,586	0.000085	20,510,388	0.07288128	0.0000062
35–39 years	65	621,853	0.000105	22,706,664	0.08068549	0.0000084
40–44 years	378	585,463	0.000646	22,441,863	0.07974455	0.0000515
45–49 years	648	586,001	0.001106	20,092,404	0.07139602	0.0000789
50–54 years	1035	648,199	0.001597	17,585,548	0.0624882	0.0000998
55–59 years	1252	573,274	0.002184	13,469,237	0.04786137	0.0001045
60–64 years	1040	436,920	0.002380	10,805,447	0.0383959	0.0000914
65–69 years	777	379,735	0.002046	9,533,545	0.03387634	0.0000693
70–74 years	497	364,024	0.001365	8,857,441	0.03147389	0.0000430
75–79 years	249	343,439	0.000725	7,415,813	0.02635123	0.0000191
80–84 years	105	241,047	0.000436	4,945,367	0.01757279	0.0000077
85 years and over	12	203,476	0.000059	4,239,587	0.01506488	0.0000009
All Ages	**6149**	**8,872,106**		**281,421,906**		**0.0476**

*The standard population is based on the 2000 Census.

© Cengage Learning, 2012.

Graphical Summaries: Bar and Line Graphs

Graphical summaries of event rates are particularly useful when comparing different event rates. *Bar graphs* whose bar heights represent the event rates are helpful in describing how rates compare (Figure 6-6). In this example, the fracture rate for women in the strength training group is $1748 \div 23{,}304.6 = 0.08$, and the fracture rate for women in the control group is $2607 \div 19{,}231.0 = 0.14$. The graph of the rates suggests that the rates in the two groups may be different.

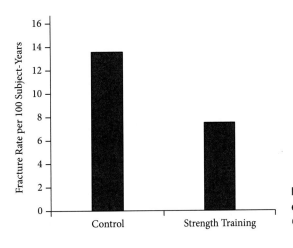

Figure 6-6 Example of bar graph for event rates
© *Cengage Learning, 2012.*

Figure 6-7. Example of rates over time (line graph) © *Cengage Learning, 2012.*

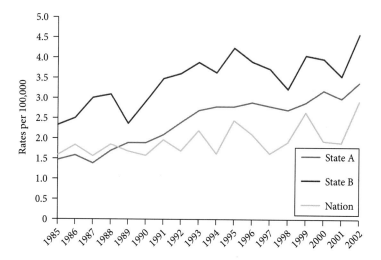

Studies investigating how rates change over time may be presented in a *line graph*, where the vertical axis represents the event rate and the horizontal axis represents time. Comparing rates over time is quite popular in population studies, and rates are often summarized graphically in line graphs. The event rates for different groups are plotted for each time point, and lines are used to connect the event rates belonging to the same group (Figure 6-7). State health departments are often interested in tracking how their state compares to a benchmark state or to the nation. A line graph is a visual representation of how rates change over time and how groups compare.

ONE-GROUP STUDIES WITH A COUNT OUTCOME

Probably more than any other type of study, a study collecting count data may not involve collecting data on a comparison group; that is, it is a one-sample or single-cohort study. When a count is the outcome, the emphasis is on the number of events; so there has to be enough time and enough subjects to observe enough events so that statistical analysis is reasonable. If the event rate, for example, is 0.1 per 100 subject-years, it will be a long wait (or require a lot of subjects) to observe even a small number of events. Examples of rare outcomes in public health are birth defects, safety concerns (adverse events), and cases of certain types of bacterial infections. When the rate of an event is low, more subjects and/or more time are required to observe enough events for analysis. So investigating fairly rare events can be very costly. For this reason, studies investigating the number of rare events may be feasible only as a one-sample study. However, investigating only one group usually means that no control groups are available for comparison. When a one-sample study is conducted because an independent comparator group is not practical, historical information or historical controls can be used to make comparisons and inferences.

Although the observed fracture rate differs from the historical control (100 versus 85 fractures per 1000 subject years), this rate estimate may be specific to this sample. *Historical controls* are estimates of the true parameter (event rate) based on data from a different study. This could include studies from a different time period, a different region, different population, or a different exposure. This study, for example, includes only women who have been diagnosed with osteopenia or osteoporosis, low bone density. The fracture rate in this sample is 100 per 1000 subject-years, but is this rate different from women who do not have such low *t*-scores? Suppose that the fracture rate in women with "normal" *t*-scores is reported to be 85 per 1000 subject-years.

Attempting to answer the research question involves determining whether there truly is a difference between the fracture rates of women recently diagnosed with low bone density and those with "normal" *t*-score outcomes. Hypothesis testing can help.

RESEARCH HYPOTHESIS: The true event rate in women recently diagnosed with low bone density is not 85 per 1000 subject-years (0.085).

NULL HYPOTHESIS: The true event rate in women recently diagnosed with low bone density is 85 per 1000 subject-years (0.085).

Statistical Inference for an Event Rate

To test this hypothesis, the true parameter (the true event rate in recently diagnosed women) is assumed to be 85 per 1000 subject-years. In other words, the historical control of 0.085 serves as the null parameter. The data from the sample ($n = 6060$) provides a statistic (an estimate of the event rate: 0.102), and it must be determined whether this statistic would be expected if the null parameter (0.085) were the true parameter. Therefore, the goal is to use the sample data to provide evidence against the null hypothesis.

Because this sample is somewhat large and fractures are not rare events, the chi-square distribution may be used to perform the hypothesis test. In particular, the test statistic used to determine whether there is enough evidence against the null comes from a chi-square distribution with 1 degree of freedom.

Application of Formula: ONE-SAMPLE TEST FOR THE EVENT RATE

$$\text{Test statistic} = \frac{(e - \mu_0)^2}{\mu_0}$$

$e = $ The total number of events

$\mu_0 = $ The null event rate times the number of subject-years observed $=$ null number of events

What you need for a one-sample test:

1. *The total number of events observed in the sample:* $e = 4355$.
2. *The expected number of events if the null hypothesis were true:* The null parameter (the event rate according to the null hypothesis) is 0.085. If this were the event rate, then after 42,535.6 subject years, $0.085 \times 42{,}535.6 = 3616$ events would be expected.
3. *The numerator is the difference between the total number of events (1) and the expected number of events (2), squared:* $(e - \mu_0)^2 = (4{,}355 - 3616)^2 = 739^2 = 546{,}121$.

To calculate the test statistic: Divide the numerator (3) by the number of events expected if the null were true that was calculated in (2): $546{,}121 \div 3616 = 151.0$.

When the null is true, the sampling distribution is a chi-square distribution with 1 degree of freedom, and any test statistic larger than 3.84 is considered rare (only 5% of test statistics are farther away than the test statistic found here); this is evidence against the null hypothesis. Furthermore, the *p*-value associated with this one-sample test is <0.0001.

CONCLUSION: There is sufficient evidence to reject the null hypothesis. The rate of fractures for women recently diagnosed with osteoporosis/osteopenia is different from the rate of fractures for a healthy population.

Confidence Interval for an Event Rate

While hypothesis tests are helpful for determining whether the true event rate is equal to some value or not, they do not provide an estimate for the true event rate. Based on the one-sample hypothesis test, it is fair to assume that the true event rate (fracture rate) is not 85 per 1,000 subject-years. However, to estimate the event rate, confidence intervals are used.

Like hypothesis tests, confidence intervals take sampling variability into account. In other words, it would be unlikely that another sample of 6060 recently diagnosed women in the United States would have 4355 fractures out of 42,535.6 subject-years. The estimate of 100 fractures per 1000 subject-years is a point estimate and describes only this sample. To have an estimate that is likely to capture the true event rate, an interval estimate is required. Like hypothesis tests, confidence intervals are based on the idea that, if many more samples of the same size are selected, the statistics (the estimates of the event rates) should all pile up fairly close to the true parameter (the true event rate). Hypothesis tests assume that a null parameter is the true parameter and use a sampling distribution based on the null parameter, but confidence intervals are based on the idea that most of the statistics will pile up fairly close to the *true* parameter. Therefore, the estimates of the event rates should be fairly close to (within a certain distance of) the true event rate. Because this sample has a fairly large number of events, the normal approximation can be used so that confidence intervals are easily calculated.

Application of Formula

C% confidence interval for the events: $e \pm z^* \times SE$

e = The number of events in the sample

C = The confidence level for a C% confidence interval

z^* = The number of standard deviations from the center of the sampling distribution

SE = The standard error

What you need to calculate the confidence interval:

1. *The number of events in the sample:* $e = 4355$.
2. *The standard error:* This is the square root of the number of events = $\sqrt{4355} = 66$.
3. *The confidence level:* C% is typically 95%, but 90% and 99% are also common.
4. *The number of standard deviations from the center of the sampling distribution:* This depends on C% (3) and the sampling distribution. So, when the sampling distribution is a normal distribution, the z^* for a 90% confidence interval is 1.65, the z^* for a 95% confidence interval is 1.96, and the z^* for a 99% confidence interval is 2.58. Therefore, confidence intervals can be calculated as

90% confidence interval: $e \pm (1.65 \times$ standard error$)$

95% confidence interval: $e \pm (1.96 \times$ standard error$)$

99% confidence interval: $e \pm (2.58 \times$ standard error$)$

To calculate the 95% confidence interval for the number of fractures: Add and subtract the margin of error (1.96 multiplication sign 66) or $[4355 - 1.96 \times 66, 4355 - 1.96 \times 66]$, or $[4226, 4485]$.

However, these confidence intervals do not provide interval estimates for the event rate, but an interval estimate of the count. To obtain the interval estimate for the true event rate, the upper and lower limits of the confidence interval must be divided by the number of subject-years (t). Hence, to get the interval estimate of the event rate, an additional calculation [lower limit/t, upper limit/t] is required. Therefore, the 95% confidence interval for the event rate is $[4226/42{,}535.6, 4484/42{,}535.6] = [0.099, 0.105]$.

Because 95% of all confidence intervals cover the true event rate, the confidence interval represents a set of plausible values for the true event rate. Therefore, because this interval does not include 0.085 and covers possible parameters that are larger than

0.085, the historical control is eliminated as a possible parameter, suggesting that the rate of fractures in newly diagnosed low-bone-density women is larger than that of healthy women.

Event Rate in One-Sample: Exact Test

The hypothesis test and confidence interval for providing inferences for the sample of women in the control group used a chi-square test statistic and normal sampling distribution, respectively, because the expected number of events was relatively large. However, when the event is rare, the expected event count may not be sufficiently large (at least 10) to use these approximations. In this example, the null event rate is 0.085; so the expected number of events when the null is true is $0.085 \times 42,535.6 = 3616$. This is definitely larger than 10, and using approximations is justified.

There may not always be a sufficient number of events (studies investigating severe birth defects and rare adverse events are good examples). Recall from Chapter 1 that the distribution of the count is the Poisson distribution. When approximations are not appropriate, statistical inference can still be performed using the properties of the Poisson distribution. A hypothesis test that cannot use the large sample approximation and must use the Poisson distribution is referred to as an *exact test*.

RESEARCH QUESTION: Is cervical cancer associated with a diagnosis of osteopenia/osteoporosis?

Suppose health outcomes including new cancer diagnoses were also collected in this study. If five cases of cervical cancer were diagnosed during the study period the observed cervical cancer rate (event rate) would be $5/42,535.6 = 0.000118$, or 11.8 per 100,000 subject-years. If the cervical cancer rate for women in the United States is 8.3 per 100,000 subject-years, is the rate of cervical cancer greater in women with low bone density?

RESEARCH HYPOTHESIS: The true event rate in women with osteopenia/osteoporosis is not 8.3 per 100,000 subject-years (0.000083).

NULL HYPOTHESIS: The true event rate in women with osteopenia/osteoporosis is 8.3 per 100,000 subject-years (0.000083).

Now the event rate is quite small, 8 per 100,000 subject-years. If the null hypothesis were true, four ($0.000083 \times 42,535.6 = 3.5$) cervical cancer diagnoses would be expected. Because this number is smaller than 10, exact tests and not approximations are needed to test the hypotheses. In the exact test, the *p*-value can be obtained directly from the Poisson distribution.

Application of Formula: EXACT TEST

What you need to get the *p*-value for an exact test:

1. *The expected number of events if the null hypothesis were true:* This is the null event rate times the number of subject-years observed μ_0. The null parameter (the event rate according to the null hypothesis) is 0.000083. If this were the event rate, then, after 42,535.6 subject-years, $0.000083 \times 42,535.6 = 3.5$ or 4 events would be expected.
2. *Whether the observed number of events in the sample is less than the number of events expected if the null hypothesis were true (1):*
   a. If the number of events in the sample is smaller than the expected null number of events, use the Poisson distribution to find the probability of getting even fewer events than what was observed. Statistical or online calculators can provide the probability that the count is less than the observed count for a Poisson distribution with a mean of the null count (1).

continues

continued

b. If the number of events in the sample is greater than or equal to the expected null number of events (1), use the Poisson distribution to find the probability of getting even more events than what was observed. Statistical or online calculators can provide the probability that the count is greater than or equal to the number of events observed.

To calculate the p-value: For a one-tailed test, the *p*-value is the probability obtained from either (a) or (b). For a two-tailed test, the *p*-value is simply 2 times the probability found either (a) or (b). The probability is multiplied by 2 because this is a two-tailed test. If multiplying by 2 results in a value greater than 1, the *p*-value is just 1.

In this example, the number of events if the null hypothesis were true is 4. The actual number of events observed was 5. Because 5 is greater than 4, the *p*-value has to be found using the method described in part (2b). The mean (or rate) of the Poisson distribution is 4. Using this distribution, the probability of observing 5 or more events is 0.2149. Therefore, the *p*-value for this hypothesis test is $2 \times 0.2149 = 0.4298$.

CONCLUSION: The *p*-value for this test is not small ($p = 0.4298$). Therefore, there is not enough evidence ($p > 0.05$) to reject the null hypothesis; that is, there is not enough evidence to conclude that the cervical cancer rate of women diagnosed with osteopenia/osteoporosis is the same as the U.S. average.

MULTIPLE GROUP STUDIES

RESEARCH QUESTION: Does strength training impact the rate of fractures?

Point to Ponder
In this example, the subjects self-selected whether to participate in a strength training program. Should the investigator randomly assign the women to enroll in strength training? What are the advantages and disadvantages to this approach? What issues would the investigator need to consider for implementing this randomized experiment?

A comparison of event rates is often necessary to address a research question. If a study involves collecting data on more than one group, comparisons can be made directly, often with one group serving as the control group. For example, this study was conducted to see how strength training affected the rate of fractures. The hypothesis is that women in the control group experience more fractures. These two groups, strength training and not, consist of completely different women; the measurements of one group have nothing to do with the measurements of the other. Therefore, these two groups represent independent samples. If the outcomes of the two independent groups differ, the differences may be attributable to the strength training. Because two independent samples are of interest, the study is often referred to as a two-sample study.

Descriptive statistics can be provided to describe the samples of low bone density women based on whether they chose the strength training protocol. A table of descriptive statistics such as Table 6-2 might be helpful in describing the women.

The two groups of women were similar at diagnosis in terms of pain rating, quality of life index, fracture history, calcium use, and race. However, the two groups differed at diagnosis in age and physical activity level. On average, the strength training cohort tended to be younger and more physically active. Whereas the participants in both groups provided follow-up measures for an average of 7 years (SD = 1.2), the average number of fractures in the strength training group is almost half that of the control group.

Rate Ratio: Two Groups

This study is an analysis of count data, and the primary outcome is the number of fractures. However, because the amount of time the subjects are observed varies, the fracture rate becomes of primary interest. The research question—whether strength training has an impact on fracture rates—can be answered by estimating

244 Biostatistics

Public Health Professional

TABLE 6-2 CHARACTERISTICS OF THE SAMPLE

	All (N = 6060)	Strength Training (N = 3305)	Control (N = 2755)
Age (years)			
Mean (SD)	58.6 (9.66)	56.9 (9.74)	60.7 (9.15)
Median (Q_1, Q_3)	58 (52, 65)	56 (50, 63)	61 (54, 67)
Minimum, maximum	31, 85	31, 85	39, 85
Pain Score (1–10)			
Mean (SD)	5.7 (2.52)	5.5 (2.71)	5.9 (2.25)
Median (Q_1, Q_3)	6 (4, 7)	6 (4, 7)	6 (5, 7)
Minimum, maximum	0, 10	0, 10	0, 10
Quality of Life (0–100)			
Mean (SD)	44.7 (15.16)	44.8 (14.93)	44.5 (15.44)
Median (Q_1, Q_3)	45 (34, 55)	45 (34, 55)	45 (34, 55)
Minimum, maximum	0, 97	0, 96	0, 97
Fracture History (%)			
Yes	3172 (52.3%)	1705 (51.6%)	1467 (53.3%)
No	2888 (47.7%)	1600 (48.4%)	1288 (46.8%)
Calcium Use (%)			
Yes	4520 (74.6%)	2456 (74.3%)	2064 (74.9%)
No	1540 (25.4%)	849 (25.7%)	691 (25.1%)
Physical Activity Level (%)			
None	2159 (35.6%)	1047 (31.7%)	1112 (40.4%)
Limited	1623 (26.8%)	945 (28.6%)	678 (24.6%)
Moderate	1698 (28.0%)	849 (25.7%)	849 (30.8%)
Rigorous	560 (9.6%)	464 (14.0%)	116 (4.2%)
Race (%)			
White	3988 (65.8%)	2184 (66.1%)	1804 (65.48%)
Black	1199 (19.8%)	657 (19.9%)	542 (19.7%)
Other	873 (14.4%)	464 (14.0%)	409 (14.9%)
Number of Fractures			
Mean (SD)	0.7 (1.24)	0.5 (1.13)	0.9 (1.33)
Median (Q_1, Q_3)	0 (0, 1)	0 (0, 1)	1 (0, 1)
Minimum, maximum	0, 13	0, 11	0, 13
Amount of Follow-up (years)			
Mean (SD)	7.0 (1.18)	7.1 (1.19)	7.0 (1.18)
Median (Q_1, Q_3)	7.0 (6.2, 7.8)	7.1 (6.3, 7.9)	7.0 (6.2, 7.75)
Minimum, maximum	2.7, 11.2	2.7, 11.1	3.0, 11.2

how the fracture rate in the strength training group compares to the rate in the control group. Just as prevalence, risk, and odds ratios quantify relationships between two variables when the outcome is dichotomous (Chapter 4), rate ratios can be used to investigate relationships between groups when the outcome is a rate. The *rate ratio* is the ratio of two rates. Generally, the rate corresponding to the control group is denominator.

- If the rates of the two groups are the same, then the rate ratio is 1.
- A rate ratio that is larger than 1 means that the numerator is larger than the denominator; that is, the event rate in the numerator is larger than the event rate in the denominator.
- If the rate ratio is less than 1, then the denominator is larger than the numerator, or the event rate in the denominator is larger than the event rate in the numerator.

Application of Formula: RATE RATIOS

$$\text{Estimate of the rate ratio} = \frac{\text{Estimate of the event rate for Group 1}}{\text{Estimate of the event rate for Group 2}}$$

What you need to calculate an estimate of the rate ratio:

1. *The event rate estimate for Group 1:* The estimated event rate for the strength training group is $1748 \div 23,304.6 = 0.075$.
2. *The event rate estimate for Group 2:* The event rate for the control group is $2607 \div 19,231.0 = 0.136$.

To calculate the estimate of the rate ratio: Divide the Group 1 event rate estimate (1) by the Group 2 event rate estimate (2): $0.075 \div 0.136 = 0.55$.

For this sample the estimated rate ratio is 0.55, which is smaller than 1. An estimated rate ratio smaller than 1 implies that the estimated numerator rate is smaller than the denominator. The denominator is the control group. Thus, the estimate of the rate ratio implies that the observed rate of fractures is smaller (approximately 50% smaller) in the group with the strength training versus those without. However, this rate ratio estimate describes only this sample. It is a statistic, a point estimate. To answer the research question, inferences beyond this sample are needed, and so sampling variability (differences between samples) has to be considered.

Although hypothesis tests allow for testing whether the rates are different, with a rate ratio, the emphasis is on estimation. The goal is not just to indicate whether the true rate ratio is equal to 1, but to provide an actual estimate of how different the two rates are. Confidence intervals allow for statistical inference by providing an interval estimate for the true parameter (rate ratio) that accounts for sampling variability. Because the confidence interval provides a set of plausible values for the true rate ratio, the confidence interval can also be used to determine whether or not it is reasonable to assume that the true rate ratio is 1.

Confidence intervals are based on the idea of sampling distributions and the fact that not all samples will result in the same statistic. Although, another sample of the same size would be unlikely to have the same number of fractures over the same number of subject-years, the statistics (estimates of the rate ratios) from these different samples should all pile up fairly close to the true parameter (the rate ratio).

Unfortunately, rate ratios (and ratios in general) do not have normal sampling distributions. In fact, they are slightly more skewed than a normal distribution. However, taking the natural log (ln) of the rate ratio estimates results in a fairly normal sampling distribution. Consequently, the confidence interval for the natural log of the rate ratio, $\ln(RR)$, can be obtained using a normal sampling distribution.

Before the confidence interval can be computed, the standard error is needed. The standard error is actually quite simple to calculate because counts are involved and counts are Poisson variables. Recall from Chapter 1, that, for Poisson variables, the mean and the variance are the same and the mean is just the number of events. Therefore, the number of events is also an estimate of the variance.

Application of Formula: STANDARD ERROR

$$S = \sqrt{\frac{1}{e_1} + \frac{1}{e_2}}$$

e_1 = The number of events observed in Group 1

e_2 = The number of events observed in Group 2

What you need to calculate the variance:

1. *The inverse of the number of events observed in Group 1:* There were 1748 fractures observed in the strength training group, so $\frac{1}{1748} = 0.00057$.
2. *The inverse the number of events observed in Group 2:* There were 2607 fractures observed for the control group, so $\frac{1}{2607} = 0.00038$.
3. *Sum of the fractions found in (1) and (2):* $\frac{1}{1748} + \frac{1}{2607} = 0.00057 + 0.00038 = 0.00095$.

To calculate the standard error: Take the square root of the (3), $\sqrt{0.00095} = 0.031$.

Application of Formula

C% confidence interval for the natural log of the rate ratio: $\ln(\widehat{RR}) \pm z^* \, SE$

$\ln(\widehat{RR})$ = The natural log of the sample rate ratio

C = The confidence level for a C% confidence interval

z^* = The number of standard deviations from the center of the sampling distribution

SE = The standard error of the natural log of the rate ratio

What you need to calculate the confidence interval:

1. *The sample rate ratio or the point estimate of the rate ratio:* $\widehat{RR} = 0.55$.
2. *The natural log of the rate ratio estimate or the natural log of (1):* $\ln(\widehat{RR}) = -0.60$.
3. *The standard error:* The standard error is $\sqrt{0.00095} = 0.031$.
4. *The confidence level:* C% is typically 95%, but 90% and 99% are also common.
5. *The number of standard deviations from the center of the sampling distribution:* This depends on C% (4) and the sampling distribution. So, when the sampling distribution is a normal distribution, the z^* for a 90% confidence interval is 1.65, the z^* for a 95% confidence interval is 1.96, and the z^* for a 99% confidence interval is 2.58. Therefore, confidence intervals can be calculated as

90% confidence interval: $\ln(\widehat{RR}) \pm (1.65 \times \text{standard error})$

95% confidence interval: $\ln(\widehat{RR}) \pm (1.96 \times \text{standard error})$

99% confidence interval: $\ln(\widehat{RR}) \pm (2.58 \times \text{standard error})$

To calculate the 95% confidence interval for the natural log of the rate ratio: Add and subtract the margin of error (1.96 multiplication sign 0.031), $[-0.60 - 1.96 \times 0.031, -0.60 + 1.96 \times 0.031]$, or $[-0.66, -0.54]$.

These confidence intervals, however, provide interval estimates not for the rate ratio, but for the natural log of the true rate ratio. To obtain the interval estimate for the true rate ratio, the upper and lower limits of the confidence interval must be exponentiated. Hence, to get the interval estimate of the rate ratio, an additional calculation [exp(lower limit), exp(upper limit)] is required.

Consequently, the interval estimate of the rate ratio is [exp(−0.66); exp(−0.54)] = [0.52, 0.58]. Because 95% of all confidence intervals cover the true rate ratio, this interval represents a set of plausible values for the true rate ratio. A rate ratio of 1 is not included in this set. In fact, the rate ratios in this set are all less than 1. Therefore, there is evidence that the true rate ratio is not 1 and is smaller than 1. Hence, the fracture rate in the strength training group is approximately half (0.52, 0.58) the fracture rate of the group without strength training.

Rate Ratios: Multiple Groups

<aside>
RESEARCH QUESTION:
Is the fracture rate associated with race?
</aside>

Comparisons between groups are not limited to two sample studies. The same methods used to determine whether two groups are different can be used to determine whether a difference exists among multiple groups. Because one of the goals of this study is to better understand factors associated with fracture rate, comparisons between racial groups (white, black, other) may help to answer the research question.

Rate ratios can be used to quantify the relationship between fracture rates and race. In Chapter 4, ratios were used to investigate relationships between nominal variables (like race) and a dichotomous outcome. Details were provided for creating dummy variables out of the levels of the nominal variable and choosing one of the levels as a reference for comparison. The same holds true for rate ratios. To investigate the rate ratios, one of the groups is chosen as the comparator or reference group (the denominator of the rate ratio). If the fracture rate of white women is the denominator, then two rate ratio estimates result: one where black women comprise the numerator and one where women of other races comprise the numerator. In this study, the estimates for the rates of fractures for white, black, and other races are $2972 \div 28008.9 = 0.110$, $797 \div 8382.2 = 0.095$, and $586 \div 6144.5 = 0.095$, respectively. Therefore, the rate ratio estimates for black race compared to white race and for other race compared to white race are both $0.095 \div 0.110 = 0.86$. Both of these rate ratio estimates are less than 1. Therefore, for this sample, the fracture rate in white women is larger than the rate for black women and for women of other races. Confidence intervals can be calculated for these rate ratios in the same way as the two-sample comparison. As an example, the 95% confidence interval for the rate ratio comparing black and white women is [0.80, 0.93], suggesting a difference in the fracture rates of black and white women.

COUNT DEPENDENT VARIABLE WITH MULTIPLE REGRESSORS: POISSON REGRESSION

<aside>
RESEARCH QUESTION:
What factors are related to fracture rates in low bone density women?
</aside>

In this example, it is of interest to consider whether strength training has an association with the rate of new fractures. Women in this study self-selected to participate in strength training; so it is possible that confounding factors could bias the comparison of fracture rates between women participating in strength-training or not. Furthermore, differences were observed between the groups with respect to race and calcium use. Because these variables may also be related to fracture rates, these could be potential confounding variables. Beyond confounding variables, investigators may also be interested in the impact of additional factors related to the event rate. In this example, activity level and pain scores may also help to explain differences in fracture rates.

The linear and logistic regressions, presented in Chapters 3 and 5, were used to investigate the research question involving the relationship between multiple variables and a response. These regressions were used when investigators wanted to

- Compare groups while controlling for potential confounding variables.
- Investigate multiple variable relationships.

Unlike linear and logistic regression, however, the response is now a count where the subjects in the study could contribute different amounts of time, space, or units at risk. Therefore, the regression model needs to be appropriate for this type of outcome. Because count data come from a Poisson distribution, the distribution of the outcome needs to be considered in the regression model. Poisson regression can be used to investigate relationships between regressors (dichotomous, nominal, ordinal, and/or continuous) and count outcomes, while accounting for differences in person-time, space, or units at risk. Many of the principles applied in linear and logistic regression are the same for Poisson regression. Also, just as linear and logistic regressions resulted in estimates that were appropriate for the outcome (adjusted slopes and mean differences in linear regression, adjusted odds ratios in logistic regression), the estimates of the Poisson regression are appropriate for count data: adjusted rate ratios. Regardless of whether the research question involves assessing multiple variable relationships or comparing groups while controlling for confounding, Poisson regression can be used when the outcome is a count.

The Model

The model for the Poisson regression is very similar to those described in Chapters 3 and 5 for linear and logistic regression. Like the other regression models, the right-hand side is $\alpha + \beta_1 x_1 + \beta_2 x_2 + \cdots + \beta_K x_K$, where x_k represents the covariates, β_k represents the slopes, and α represents the intercept. The left side of the equation, similar to logistic regression, however, cannot simply be the count. The count can be only whole, positive numbers, and the right-hand side of the equation can be anything (0, negative, fractions, etc.). Therefore, the left-hand side has to be transformed so that the right- and left-hand sides can be equal. So the left side of the model in a Poisson regression is $\ln(\mu)$, where μ represents the true mean count of events. Therefore, the Poisson regression model is

$$\ln(\mu) = \alpha + \beta_1 x_1 + \beta_2 x_2 + \cdots + \beta_K x_K$$

The primary assumption of the Poisson regression is that the outcome variable comes from a Poisson distribution, meaning that the dependent variable represents a count. It also means that the outcome should have a mean and variance that are approximately the same.

In this example, in addition to strength training (strint), possible regressors include pain score (pain), quality of life (qol), activity level (act), race (race), calcium use (cal), fracture history (frachx), and age (age). The Poisson regression model is

$$\begin{aligned} \ln(\mu) = \ &\alpha + \beta_1(\text{strint}) + \beta_2(\text{pain}) + \beta_3(\text{qol}) + \beta_4(\text{act1}) + \beta_5(\text{act2}) \\ &+ \beta_6(\text{act3}) + \beta_7(\text{race2}) + \beta_8(\text{race3}) + \beta_9(\text{cal}) \\ &+ \beta_{10}(\text{frachx}) + \beta_{11}(\text{age}) \end{aligned}$$

This model, however, does not account for the different follow-up times of the participants. This model would be appropriate if only the count or only the number of fractures was of interest, but in this study the fracture rate is of primary interest. The rate of fractures has been defined as the count of fractures divided by the number of subject-years. When the event rate is of interest, the Poisson regression model is

$$\ln(\mu/t) = \alpha + \beta_1 x_1 + \beta_2 x_2 + \cdots + \beta_K x_K,$$

where t represents the number of subject-years.

Because the natural log of a fraction is the difference of the natural logs of the numerator and denominator, $\ln(\mu/t)$ becomes $\ln(\mu) - \ln(t)$. So the model can be written as

$$\ln(\mu) - \ln(t) = \alpha + \beta_1 x_1 + \beta_2 x_2 + \cdots + \beta_K x_K$$

or

$$\ln(\mu) = \alpha + \beta_1 x_1 + \beta_2 x_2 + \cdots + \beta_K x_K + \ln(t).$$

When accounting for the amount of follow-up time each subject contributed, the model investigating the rate of fractures becomes

$$\begin{aligned} \ln(\mu) = \alpha &+ \beta_1(\text{strint}) + \beta_2(\text{pain}) + \beta_3(\text{qol}) + \beta_4(\text{act1}) + \beta_5(\text{act2}) \\ &+ \beta_6(\text{act3}) + \beta_7(\text{race2}) + \beta_8(\text{race3}) + \beta_9(\text{cal}) + \beta_{10}(\text{frachx}) \\ &+ \beta_{11}(\text{age}) + \ln(t) \end{aligned}$$

where t represents the subject-years for each participant.

Notice that nominal variables are included in the regression model as sets of dummy variables. For nominal variables, each level is made into a dummy variable, and the reference level is omitted from the model (Chapters 3 and 5). For example, race has three levels: white race (race=1), black race (race=2), and other race (race=3). A dummy variable (with values of only 0 and 1) can be created for each level.

$$\begin{aligned} \text{race2} &= 1 \text{ if race} = 2 \\ &= 0 \text{ otherwise} \\ \text{race3} &= 1 \text{ if race} = 3 \\ &= 0 \text{ otherwise} \end{aligned}$$

A third dummy variable for white race is not necessary because if race2 = 0 and race3 = 0, then the race must be white. Because the white race dummy variable is omitted, white race is considered the reference.

Getting the Intercept and Slopes

Linear regression (Chapter 3) used the least squares method to estimate β. Like logistic regression (Chapter 5), however, Poisson regression uses maximum likelihood estimation to estimate β. To get the estimates for β and α, the likelihood function is used. The likelihood function is the probability of the observed sample, where β and α are the unknown elements of this function. As in logistic regression, the likelihood function is based on the fact that each subject in the sample is an independent observation. In a Poisson regression, it is believed that each subject is independent *and* that the count for this subject comes from a Poisson distribution (a Poisson distribution with a mean of μ). Because the subjects are independent, the probability for the whole sample is just the multiplication of the probabilities for each subject. These probabilities are written as functions of α and the β's. The estimates for the α and β's are obtained by choosing $\hat{\alpha}$ and $\hat{\beta}$ to maximize the numerical value of the likelihood function for the observed sample. In most instances, these estimates (called *maximum likelihood estimates*) are obtained using an iterative process based on a numerical analysis algorithm. Sometimes the iterative process fails to converge; hence, the estimates of α and β do not exist for some sets of data. When implementing a Poisson regression, make sure the algorithm converges; this is standard output on any statistical software.

Hypothesis Tests

Three types of hypothesis tests result from any regression: the overall test, tests of effects, and specific tests about the slopes. The overall hypothesis test simply tests whether there is a relationship between any of the variables and the outcome. The hypothesis tests for the effects are useful if the model contains nominal variables entered into the model as dummy variables. Finally, specific hypothesis tests involve testing that one of the variables is related to the outcome, controlling for all other variables in the model. Generally, the results of the specific tests are the ones reported.

Overall Hypothesis Test

Whenever the model contains multiple variables, whether explanatory or confounding, an overall hypothesis test can be performed to see whether any of the variables have a relationship to the outcome. The global hypotheses associated with the overall test do not change from Chapters 3 and 5; the overall hypotheses for linear, logistic, and Poisson regression are exactly the same.

In this example, the Poisson regression model is

$$\ln(\mu) = \alpha + \beta_1(strint) + \beta_2(pain) + \beta_3(qol) + \beta_4(act1) + \beta_5(act2)$$
$$+ \beta_6(act3) + \beta_7(race2) + \beta_8(race3) + \beta_9(cal) + \beta_{10}(frachx)$$
$$+ \beta_{11}(age) + \ln(t)$$

> **RESEARCH HYPOTHESIS:** At least one of the true slopes is not 0 ($\beta_k \neq 0$, for at least one k, $k = 1 \dots 8$).

> **NULL HYPOTHESIS:** All of the true slopes are 0 ($\beta_k = 0$, for every k, $k = 1 \dots 8$).

The overall hypothesis test is not particularly interesting or exciting. If the null hypothesis can be rejected, it simply means that this model is better than nothing. A significant result from the overall test means only that one or some or all of the variables are related to the outcome. It does not indicate which regressors are significantly contributing to the relationship or the direction of the association. To specifically investigate the impact of the regressors, specific inferences (hypothesis tests and confidence intervals) need to be performed. However, these more specific investigations of the contribution of each regressor should be performed only after determining that a relationship exists or that this model is better than nothing. If the overall test results in a large p-value, then the overall or global null hypothesis cannot be rejected; there is no evidence of a relationship. In that case, there is no reason to continue searching for the contributions of the individual regressors.

Hypothesis Test for Effects

In this study, race is a nominal variable, and, although activity level has an order, the investigators prefer to treat it as a nominal variable as well. Therefore, the Poisson regression model includes dummy variables for the categories of race and activity level.

$$\alpha + \beta_1(strint) + \beta_2(pain) + \beta_3(qol) + \beta_4(act1) + \beta_5(act2) + \beta_6(act3)$$
$$+ \beta_7(race2) + \beta_8(race3) + \beta_9(cal) + \beta_{10}(frachx) + \beta_{11}(age) + \ln(t)$$

Whenever dummy variables correspond to nominal variables, investigating these variables can be confusing. The research question may address the relationship between the effect (e.g. race) and the outcome (fracture rate), but the regression analysis results in an estimate for each dummy variable. For example, black race could quite possibly be different from white race, but other race may not necessarily differ from white race. Because race has two dummy variables, it has two β's (and two $\hat{\beta}$'s). If one is significant and the other is not, how do you determine whether race, in general, is associated with fracture rate? Just like the type 3 effects discussed with logistic regression (Chapter 5), the type 3 effects tests can be obtained from statistical software (Table 6-3). They are chi-square tests for the overall effect of each variable, controlling for all other variables in the model. If the p-value is small, this indicates that the variable (the effect) is associated with the outcome. If the p-value is large, this indicates that there is not enough evidence to assume that the variable (the effect) is associated with the outcome.

TABLE 6-3 **EXAMPLE OF TYPE 3 EFFECTS**

LR Statistics for Type 3 Analysis			
Source	DF	Chi-Square	Pr > ChiSq
cal	1	147.51	<0.0001
race	2	7.60	0.0224
frachx	1	959.03	<0.0001
act	3	8.19	0.0422
strint	1	293.76	<0.0001
age	1	36.42	<0.0001
pain	1	5.49	0.0192
qol	1	4.82	0.0281

© Cengage Learning, 2012.

CONCLUSION: Race ($p < 0.0001$) and activity level ($p = 0.0422$) are associated with fracture rates, controlling for all other variables in the model.

Type 3 effects are also provided for continuous variables and categorical variables with only 2 levels, however, because there are not multiple indicators involved with these values, the p-values for the type 3 effects are exactly the same as the p-values (corresponding to specific hypothesis tests) for the individual variables.

Specific Hypothesis Tests for the Slopes

Just as in linear and logistic regression (Chapters 3 and 5), each regressor in the model has a corresponding slope (β). The slopes (β's) are the parameters. If a slope (β) is 0, then the corresponding variable does not have an association with the outcome. Although the overall research question is whether the regressors are related to the number of fractures, a specific hypothesis test relates only to a specific research question pertaining to a specific variable and specific slope. In this regression model, there are 11 slope parameters, corresponding to 11 specific variables. For the purposes of illustration, consider the specific hypothesis test for the first slope, β_1.

$$\ln(\mu) = \alpha + \beta_1(\text{strint}) + \beta_2(\text{pain}) + \beta_3(\text{qol}) + \beta_4(\text{act1}) + \beta_5(\text{act2})$$
$$+ \beta_6(\text{act3}) + \beta_7(\text{race2}) + \beta_8(\text{race3}) + \beta_9(\text{cal}) + \beta_{10}(\text{frachx})$$
$$+ \beta_{11}(\text{age}) + \ln(t)$$

> **RESEARCH QUESTION:** Is strength training associated with the rate of fractures, while controlling for other variables in the model?

Determining whether strength training is associated with fracture rates is the same as determining whether the slope (β_1) associated with strength training is significantly different from 0.

RESEARCH HYPOTHESIS: The slope (β_1) for the strength training is not 0, after controlling for all other variables in the model.

NULL HYPOTHESIS: The slope (β_1) for the strength training is 0, after controlling for all other variables in the model.

In both the null and the research hypotheses, the statement "after controlling for all other variables in the model" is included. The benefit of using regression analysis is that the estimates for the slopes are obtained while simultaneously adjusting for the other covariates in the model. In other words, it is assumed that the slopes of the other variables in the model are significantly different from 0.

TABLE 6-4 **EXAMPLE OF INFERENCE FOR SLOPES**

	Level	Parameter Estimate	Standard Error	Wald 95% Confidence Limits		Wald Chi-Square	Pr > ChiSq
				Analysis of Maximum Likelihood Parameter Estimates			
Intercept		−3.0490	0.1285	−3.3008	−2.7971	563.19	<0.0001
cal	0	0.4004	0.0322	0.3374	0.4635	155.00	<0.0001
cal	1	0.0000	0.0000	0.0000	0.0000	—	—
race	2	−0.0747	0.0399	−0.1530	0.0035	3.50	0.0613
race	3	−0.1047	0.0452	−0.1934	−0.0161	5.36	0.0206
race	1	0.0000	0.0000	0.0000	0.0000	—	—
frachx	0	−1.0153	0.0351	−1.0842	−0.9464	835.03	<0.0001
frachx	1	0.0000	0.0000	0.0000	0.0000	—	—
act	1	0.1160	0.0611	−0.0037	0.2357	3.61	0.0574
act	2	0.0493	0.0628	−0.0737	0.1723	0.62	0.4321
act	3	0.0213	0.0630	−0.1021	0.1448	0.11	0.7348
act	4	0.0000	0.0000	0.0000	0.0000	—	—
strint	1	−0.5453	0.0322	−0.6084	−0.4822	286.56	<0.0001
strint	0	0.0000	0.0000	0.0000	0.0000	—	—
age		0.0097	0.0016	0.0066	0.0128	36.62	<0.0001
pain		−0.0145	0.0062	−0.0266	−0.0024	5.51	0.0189
qol		0.0022	0.0010	0.0002	0.0041	4.82	0.0281
Scale	0	1.0000	0.0000	1.0000	1.0000		

Note: The scale parameter was held fixed.

© Cengage Learning, 2012.

CONCLUSION: The specific hypothesis test (Table 6-4) for the intervention slope results in a small p-value ($p < 0.0001$); reject the null hypothesis. The parameter estimate represents the estimated change in the natural log of the rates between the strength training and control groups (−0.5453, $p < 0.0001$), controlling for the other variables in the model. Therefore, the slope associated with strength training is significantly different from 0, controlling for all other variables in the model.

Adjusted Rate Ratios

Whenever multiple regressors are included in a regression, the slopes are obtained by simultaneously considering all the regressors in the model. Therefore, the slope estimates are adjusted for all other variables in the model. Regardless of whether the regression is conducted for predicting an outcome, understanding multiple variable relationships, or simply adjusting for potential confounders, the statistical inference for the specific slopes is the same.

Just as in linear regression, the interpretation of any slope (β) is the change in the response for every unit increase in the regressor. Although the slopes are of primary importance in a linear regression, slope-specific interpretations are less helpful in Poisson regression because interpreting the change in the $\ln(\mu)$ for every unit increase in the regressor is not meaningful. However, the slopes in a Poisson regression can be transformed into a measure that is important with count outcomes: a rate ratio. Consequently, the p-values presented with the estimates of the slopes can be transferred to the corresponding rate ratio estimates.

For example, suppose all other regressors are held constant except for whether the woman participated in strength training. Assume the strength training variable is coded as 1 for those who participated in training and 0 for those who did not. The model for those in the strength training group (ST) is

$$\ln(\mu_{ST}) = \alpha + \beta_1(1) + \beta_2(\text{pain}) + \beta_3(\text{qol}) + \beta_4(\text{act1}) + \beta_5(\text{act2})$$
$$+ \beta_6(\text{act3}) + \beta_7(\text{race2}) + \beta_8(\text{race3}) + \beta_9(\text{cal}) + \beta_{10}(\text{frachx})$$
$$+ \beta_{11}(\text{age}) + \ln(t)$$

The model for those in the control group (C) is

$$\ln(\mu_C) = \alpha + \beta_1(0) + \beta_2(\text{pain}) + \beta_3(\text{qol}) + \beta_4(\text{act1}) + \beta_5(\text{act2})$$
$$+ \beta_6(\text{act3}) + \beta_7(\text{race2}) + \beta_8(\text{race3}) + \beta_9(\text{cal}) + \beta_{10}(\text{frachx})$$
$$+ \beta_{11}(\text{age}) + \ln(t)$$

The difference between those with strength training and those in the control is $\ln(\mu_{ST}/t) - \ln(\mu_C/t) = \beta_1(1) - \beta_1(0) = \beta_1$. The intercepts "cancel out," as do all the other variables that were held constant. The only item remaining on the right-hand side is the slope associated with the intervention variable (strint).

Recall that the difference in natural logs is equivalent to the natural log of the quotient. In other words, $\ln\left(\frac{\mu_{ST}}{t}\right) - \ln\left(\frac{\mu_C}{t}\right) = \ln\left(\frac{\frac{\mu_{ST}}{t}}{\frac{\mu_C}{t}}\right)$. Therefore, $\beta_1 = \ln\left(\frac{\frac{\mu_{ST}}{t}}{\frac{\mu_C}{t}}\right)$. Hence $e^{\beta_1} = \left(\frac{\frac{\mu_{ST}}{t}}{\frac{\mu_C}{t}}\right)$ and represents the true rate ratio, holding all other variables constant. Holding all other variables constant is the same as adjusting for or controlling for all other variables in the model; so e^{β_1} represents the true adjusted rate ratio. Consequently, all of the β's in the regression model can be transformed and interpreted as the adjusted rate ratio.

Because the e^{β_1} represents a ratio, determining whether the variable of strength training is associated with the fracture rate is the same as determining whether the rate ratio is significantly different from 1.

RESEARCH HYPOTHESIS: The rate ratio is not 1, after controlling for all other variables in the model.

NULL HYPOTHESIS: The rate ratio is 1, after controlling for all other variables in the model.

Adjusted rate ratios for dichotomous, nominal, ordinal, and continuous regressors have similar interpretations as the adjusted odds ratios for dichotomous, nominal, ordinal, and continuous variables (Chapter 5). The only difference is that interpretations involve rates, not odds.

Interpreting Adjusted Rate Ratios for Nominal Regressors

Two nominal variables are included in the Poisson regression. Race is a true nominal variable because the categories (white, black, and other) do not have an order. The other categorical variable of activity level is actually an ordinal variable. However, because the levels of this variables are not equally spaced and it is of interest to make comparisons to a reference level, activity level is treated as a nominal variable. Recall from Chapter 3 that, for nominal variables, each level is made into a dummy variable, and the reference level is not included in the model. For example, race has 3 levels: white, black, and other. A dummy variable (with values of only 0 and 1) is included in the model for black (race2) and other (race3) races, leaving white race as the reference.

The parameter estimate for black race $(\hat{\beta}_7)$ represents the estimated difference in the natural log fracture rate between black and white races and the parameter estimate for other $(\hat{\beta}_8)$ represents the estimated difference in the natural log fracture rate between other and white races. Based on the results presented in Table 6-4, the parameter estimates for β_7 and β_8 are -0.0747 ($p = 0.0613$) and -0.1047 ($p = 0.0206$). To get the adjusted rate ratios, these estimates need to be exponentiated: $\exp(-0.0747) = 0.93$ and $\exp(-0.1047) = 0.90$. Therefore, controlling for all other variables in the model, the estimated fracture rate for black and other races is approximately 10% lower than that of white women.

Interpreting the Adjusted Rate Ratio for a Continuous Regressor

As an example of a continuous factor, the results provided in Table 6-4 indicate that the parameter estimate for age is $\hat{\beta}_{11} = 0.0097$, which represents the difference in the natural log of fracture rates as the age increases by one year. However, the difference in the logs is not as informative as the rate ratio. By taking $\exp(0.0097)$, an estimate of the rate ratio can be obtained. The estimated rate ratio associated for age is $\exp(0.0097) = 1.01$ ($p < 0.0001$). Therefore, as the age at diagnosis increases by 1 year, the estimated fracture rate increases by 1%, controlling for all other variables in the model.

It is not expected that increasing age by 1-year would have a large impact on the fracture rate because a 1-year increase is not very large. Instead, a larger increment may be more informative. For example, what if the investigator was interested in how the fracture rate changed for every 10-year increase in age? Because this is not a linear regression, the rate ratio cannot simply be multiplied by 10. However, the regression is linear with respect to the log rate; the parameter estimate $\hat{\beta}_{11}$ can by multiplied by 10 to get the change in log rate for a 10-year increase in age. Exponentiating $10 \times \hat{\beta}_{11}$ provides the rate ratio estimate for a 10-year increase. Accompanying confidence intervals can be calculated in the same way.

Application of Formula

Estimate for rate ratio for a U-unit increase $= e^{\hat{\beta}U}$

$\hat{\beta}$ = The parameter estimate associated with the continuous variable

U = The number of units to increase

What you need to calculate the estimated rate ratio for a U-unit increase:

1. *The parameter estimate:* In this example, age is the variable of interest, and the parameter estimate associated with age is $\hat{\beta}_{11} = 0.0097$.
2. *The number of units to increase:* In this example, a 10-year increase in age is desired; so $U = 10$.
3. *Multiply the parameter estimate(1) and number of units (2):* $\hat{\beta}_{11} 10 \times U = 0.0097 \times 10 = 0.0970$.

To calculate the estimated rate ratio associated with a U unit increase: Exponentiate the product found in (3), $\exp(\hat{\beta}_{11} 10 \times U) = \exp(0.0970) = 1.10$.

In a similar way, the confidence interval for the rate ratio associated with age in 10-year increments can be found. Multiplying the upper and lower bounds of the confidence interval for the slope (β_{11}) by 10, provides the lower and upper bounds for the slope associated with a 10-year increase. The confidence interval for the rate ratio is then obtained by exponentiating these new lower and upper bounds. For example, the 95% confidence interval for β_{11} is (0.0066, 0.0128). Therefore, the 95% confidence interval for $10*\beta_{11}$ is (0.0660, 0.1280), and the corresponding 95% confidence interval for the rate ratio is ($\exp(0.0660)$, $\exp(0.1280)$) = (1.07, 1.14). The estimated rate ratio associated with age in 10-year increments is 1.1. Therefore, the estimated fracture rate increases by 10% for every 10-year increase in age, controlling for all other variables ($p < 0.0001$). The 95% confidence interval [1.07, 1.14] does not cover 1, providing evidence that the true rate ratio associated with 10-year increases in age is not 1 and is greater than 1.

Interpreting the Results of a Poisson Regression

A Poisson regression was performed to investigate the association of fracture rates with strength training, pain, quality of life, activity levels, race, calcium use, fracture history, and age using the following model.

$$\ln(\mu) = \alpha + \beta_1(\text{strint}) + \beta_2(\text{pain}) + \beta_3(\text{qol}) + \beta_4(\text{act1}) + \beta_5(\text{act2})$$
$$+ \beta_6(\text{act3}) + \beta_7(\text{race2}) + \beta_8(\text{race3}) + \beta_9(\text{cal}) + \beta_{10}(\text{frachx})$$
$$+ \beta_{11}(\text{age}) + \ln(t)$$

where t represents the number of subject-years.

Using statistical software, the following output results from implementing this Poisson regression (Table 6-5).

TABLE 6-5 RESULTS OF THE POISSON REGRESSION

	Slope β		Rate Ratio		
	Estimate	95% Confidence Interval	Estimate	95% Confidence Interval	p-value
ST versus control	−0.545	(−0.608, −0.482)	0.58	(0.54, 0.62)	<0.0001
Pain score	−0.015	(−0.027, −0.002)	0.99	(0.97, 1.00)	0.0189
QoL	0.002	(0.000, 0.004)	1.00	(1.00, 1.00)	0.0281
Activity Level					
None versus Very	0.116	(−0.004, 0.236)	1.12	(1.00, 1.27)	0.0574
Limited versus Very	0.051	(−0.074, 0.172)	1.05	(0.93, 1.19)	0.4321
Moderate versus Very	0.021	(−0.102, 0.145)	1.02	(0.90, 1.16)	0.7348
Race					
Black versus white	−0.075	(−0.153, 0.004)	0.93	(0.86, 1.00)	0.0613
Other versus white	−0.105	(−0.193, −0.016)	0.90	(0.82, 0.98)	0.0206
Calcium use versus not	−0.400	(−0.46, −0.34)	0.67	(0.63, 0.71)	<0.0001
Fracture hx versus not	1.015	(0.946, 1.084)	2.76	(2.58, 2.96)	<0.0001
Age	0.010	(0.007, 0.013)	1.01	(1.01, 1.01)	<0.0001

© Cengage Learning, 2012.

Regressors as Explanatory Variables

RESEARCH QUESTION:
What factors are related to fracture rates in low bone density women?

One of the goals of this study was to investigate risk factors for fractures. Many times Poisson regression is used in public health as a way of explaining why subjects have different event counts; the regressors are considered explanatory variables.

Participating in the strength training regimen as well as engaging in rigorous physical exercise, and taking calcium are all associated with lower fracture rates. In contrast, older women and women with previous fracture history have higher fracture rates (Table 6-5). These variables were included in a multiple-variable Poisson regression model; so the resulting rate ratio estimates for each factor has been adjusted for each of the other variables in the model. The results of the Poisson regression indicate that strength training is associated with the fracture rate, even after controlling for other variables. In fact, the parameter estimate is −0.55, representing the difference in the log rates between those who did and did not participate in the strength training regimen. However, the difference in the logs is not as informative as the rate ratio. By taking $\exp(-0.55)$, an estimate of the rate ratio can be obtained. In this example, the rate ratio estimate associated with strength training is 0.58, indicating that the estimated fracture rate for those with strength training is 0.6 times (40% smaller) than that of those in the control group, controlling for all other variables in the model.

The confidence limits for the rate ratio can be found by exponentiating the confidence limits associated with the slope (-0.61, -0.48). Therefore, the confidence limits for the strength training rate ratio is (0.54, 0.62). Because this 95% confidence interval does not cover 1.0, 1.0 is not a plausible value for the true rate ratio. In fact the true rate ratio is smaller than 1.0, indicating that the fracture rate in the strength training groups is smaller. Furthermore, the p-value ($p < 0.0001$) is quite small. Therefore, there is sufficient evidence to reject the null hypothesis that the rate ratio is not 1, controlling for all other variables in the model.

In addition to strength training, calcium intake, previous fracture, race, and age are associated with the fracture rate. As previously reported, older age and previous fracture are associated with increased fracture rate. Also consistent with the literature, women reporting white race experienced a higher rate of fractures. When compared to white race, the black-race and other-race variables are associated with 0.93 (95% CI: 0.86, 1.00) and 0.90 (95% CI: 0.82, 0.98) times lower estimated adjusted rates of fractures. Furthermore, women taking calcium at the time of diagnosis had 0.67 (0.63, 0.71) times the fracture rate of women not taking calcium. These results are statistically significant at the 0.05 level.

> **CONCLUSION:** Strength training, calcium use, younger age at diagnosis, nonwhite race, and no previous fracture experience are all related to a decreased rate of fractures, controlling for all variables in the model.

Regressors as Confounders

> **RESEARCH QUESTION:** Is strength training associated with the number of fractures, controlling for age, fracture history, race, physical activity, pain, quality of life, and calcium intake?

If an investigator wants to make comparisons between groups not randomly assigned, the groups could differ on the outcome simply because the groups are comprised of subjects that are systematically different. In other words, confounding makes group comparisons more complicated. In this example, one of the goals is to investigate the association between strength training and fractures. Regression models provide estimates adjusted for all variables in the model; so a Poisson regression is an option for investigating differences in counts and event rates while controlling for confounding.

The results of the Poisson regression (Table 6-5) indicate that strength training is associated with fracture rate ($p < 0.0001$). In fact, the estimated fracture rate for strength training participants is 0.58 (95% CI: 0.54, 0.62) times that of those without strength training, controlling for all other variables in the model.

> **CONCLUSION:** Even after adjusting for potential confounding variables, age, fracture history, race, physical activity, pain, quality of life, and calcium intake, there is a decreased rate of fractures among women participating in strength training (aRR: 0.58; 95% CI: 0.54, 0.62).

The primary difference between the interpretation of the results of a regression when regressors are explanatory variables and when regressors are confounders is the level of detail given to individual regressors.

Diagnostics

Regression models provide a way for investigators to understand how the data might have been produced. Therefore, a model is really helpful only if it is appropriate for the data or if the model fits the data well. Hypothesis tests and examination of the residuals can help to determine how well the model fits the data.

A hypothesis test can be performed to determine whether the model fits.

> **NULL HYPOTHESIS:** The model fits.

> **RESEARCH HYPOTHESIS:** The model does not fit.

Hypothesis Tests for Model Fit

The fit of the model can be assessed by using chi-square statistics provided by the statistical software. A statistic called the *deviance chi-square* provides a mechanism for testing the model fit (Table 6-6).

TABLE 6-6 **DEVIANCE CHI-SQUARE FOR POISSON REGRESSION**

Criteria for Assessing Goodness of Fit			
Criterion	DF	Value	Value/DF
Deviance	6045	8158.9323	1.3497

© Cengage Learning, 2012.

When testing for model fit, having a large *p*-value is desirable. Ideally, this test does not provide evidence against the null. In this case, the deviance statistic is 8158.93 with 6045 degrees of freedom. Using the statistical software program or an online chi-square probability calculator, the *p*-value associated with a chi-square value of 8158.9 with 6045 degrees of freedom is very small, which suggests that there might be issues with the fit of this model.

Overdispersion

Assessing whether the model fits the data is particularly important with Poisson regression models. Because a Poisson regression is being used, the assumption is that the data arose from a Poisson distribution; so the data should exhibit the properties of the Poisson distribution. In particular, the mean and the variance must be the same (or approximately the same). If there is evidence that the variance is not similar to the mean, the Poisson distribution may not be appropriate, and the model has a problem. The variance is used in the calculation of standard errors, and the standard errors are used in the calculation of *p*-values and confidence intervals. If there is a problem with the assumption that the mean and variance are equal, the model may not be appropriate, and the inferences associated with the model could be wrong. When the variance is larger than what would be expected, the model suffers from the problem of **overdispersion**. The deviance statistic used to test for model fit (Table 6-6) can also help in determining whether overdispersion is a problem. The ratio of the deviance statistic with the degrees of freedom provides a numerical check for overdispersion. If that ratio is close to 1, then overdispersion is not a problem. If, however, the ratio is large, then overdispersion could be a problem, and a different regression model may be more appropriate. The ratio of deviance/df can also be used to determine whether **underdispersion** is a problem. Underdispersion occurs when the variance is smaller than expected and results in a ratio much smaller than 1.

As an example, the deviance statistics corresponding to the Poisson regression output in Table 6-7 indicate that overdispersion might be a problem. The ratio of the deviance statistic to the degrees of freedom is 8.9.

TABLE 6-7 **OVERDISPERSION IN POISSON REGRESSION**

Criteria for Assessing Goodness of Fit			
Criterion	DF	Value	Value/DF
Deviance	6045	53519.8715	8.8536

© Cengage Learning, 2012.

Point to Ponder

One of the reasons, besides an ill fitting model, that overdispersion is a problem is that it can influence statistical inferences? How? If overdispersion is corrected, how might the correction change the *p*-value? Explain.

Residuals

The residuals can also be used to help in assessing whether the Poisson regression is appropriate. The Pearson residuals can be used much like the residuals of a linear regression. In particular, Pearson residuals should be randomly distributed around 0. Very large or very small residuals indicate potential outliers. However, very large or very small residuals for many data points—not just a few outliers—indicate that using the Poisson regression might not be appropriate for the data.

What if Poisson Regression Is not Appropriate?

Because the Poisson distribution is somewhat restrictive (e.g., requiring the mean and variance to be the same), the Poisson model may not be ideal for every count outcome. In such a case, other distributions (and other regression models) are available. In particular, a *negative binomial regression* is often used as an alternative to the Poisson regression. The model and interpretation of the regression analysis are similar to the Poisson regression, but the distribution associated with it is the negative binomial instead of the Poisson. For example, whenever data are overdispersed, a regression based on the negative binomial is more appropriate because it has a separate dispersion parameter (variance) that can vary (up or down) separately from the mean.

The statement of the negative binomial regression model does not differ from the Poisson regression model:

$$\ln(\mu) = \alpha + \beta_1(\text{intervention}) + \beta_2(\text{pain}) + \beta_3(\text{qol}) + \beta_4(\text{act1})$$
$$+ \beta_5(\text{act2}) + \beta_6(\text{act3}) + \beta_7(\text{race2}) + \beta_8(\text{race3}) + \beta_9(\text{calcium})$$
$$+ \beta_{10}(\text{fracture history}) + \beta_{11}(\text{age}) + \ln(t)$$

where μ represents the mean number of fractures, and t represents the amount of follow-up time contributed by each participant.

The main difference between the Poisson and negative binomial models is the distribution used. As a result, the dispersion parameter is now estimated (Table 6-8). If the dispersion parameter were 0, the regression model would simply be a Poisson regression.

RESEARCH QUESTION:
Is strength training associated with the rate of fractures, while controlling for other variables in the model?

TABLE 6-8 **NEGATIVE BINOMIAL REGRESSION RESULTS**

	Slope β		Rate Ratio		
	Estimate	95% Confidence Interval	Estimate	95% Confidence Interval	p-value
ST versus control	−0.54	(−0.62, −0.46)	0.58	(0.54, 0.63)	<0.0001
Pain score	−0.01	(−0.03, 0.00)	0.99	(0.97, 1.00)	0.0767
QoL	0.002	(−0.00, 0.00)	1.00	(1.00, 1.00)	0.1501
Activity Level					
None versus very active	0.13	(−0.02, 0.28)	1.13	(0.98, 1.32)	0.0959
Limited versus very active	0.04	(−0.12, 0.19)	1.04	(0.89, 1.21)	0.6263
Somewhat versus very active	0.01	(−0.14, 0.16)	1.01	(0.87, 1.18)	0.8916
Race					
Black versus white	−0.09	(−0.19, 0.01)	0.92	(0.83, 1.01)	0.0847
Other versus white	−0.12	(−0.23, −0.01)	0.89	(0.79, 0.99)	0.0348
Calcium use versus not	−0.42	(−0.5, −0.34)	0.66	(0.60, 0.71)	<0.0001
Fracture hx versus not	1.01	(0.93, 1.09)	2.74	(2.53, 2.98)	<0.0001
Age	0.01	(0.01, 0.01)	1.01	(1.01, 1.01)	<0.0001
Dispersion	0.72	(0.63, 0.81)			

(continues)

TABLE 6-8 (*continued*)

LR Statistics for Type 3 Analysis			
Source	DF	Chi-Square	Pr > ChiSq
cal	1	96.05	<0.0001
race	2	6.28	0.0433
frachx	1	574.31	<0.0001
act	3	7.20	0.0658
strint	1	172.85	<0.0001
age	1	23.51	<0.0001
pain	1	3.13	0.0768
qol	1	2.07	0.1502
Scaled Pearson chi-square	6045	10961.0409	1.8132
Criteria for Assessing Goodness of Fit			
Criterion	DF	Value	Value/DF
Deviance	6045	5411.9001	0.8953

Note: The negative binomial dispersion parameter was estimated by maximum likelihood.

© Cengage Learning, 2012.

The results of the negative binomial regression (Table 6-8) indicate that strength training is associated with fracture rate ($p < 0.0001$). In fact, the estimated fracture rate for strength training participants is 0.58 (95% CI: 0.54, 0.63) times that of those without strength training, controlling for all other variables in the model. Note that this is essentially the same result that was found in Poisson regression.

> **CONCLUSION:** Even after adjusting for potential confounding variables, there is a decreased rate of fractures among women participating in strength training (adjusted *RR* estimate: 0.58; 95% CI: 0.54, 0.63).

Variable Selection

In a Poisson (and negative binomial) regression, model fit is generally more concerned with the choice of distribution. However, the variables that need to go into the regression also impact model fit. One of the most time-consuming tasks in completing any regression analysis is deciding which variables to include, and the strategy differs depending on whether the regressors are explanatory variables or confounders. If the purpose of the study is to investigate possible risk factors (explanatory variables) for the event, the methods for choosing explanatory variables are slightly different from those of a study for the purpose of trying to determine whether certain groups are different, controlling for potential confounders. When trying to investigate possible explanatory variables, the variables are included in the regression because they are critical to predicting the outcome. When trying to make comparisons between groups and additional variables are only included because they are confounders, deciding variable selection may not necessarily based on statistical rationale.

Hence, variable selection a regression analysis depends on the goals of the analysis:

- Forecasting/prediction
- Covariate-adjustment (adjusting for confounders)

The strategies employed in variable selection differ depending on the purpose.

Forecasting/Prediction

When forecasting is the primary goal of the regression analysis, the research question usually involves trying to predict an outcome based on values from explanatory variables. Choosing an appropriate set of explanatory variables is very important. These variables need to do a good job of explaining changes in the outcome; so model fit is particularly important. If the regression model does not fit the data, then the resulting prediction equation will not do a very good job of forecasting outcomes. In addition, outliers and influence points must be considered because they may alter the regression estimates. Furthermore, the assumptions of the regression analysis must be rigorously tested because the model is being used to predict outcomes. In fact, other regression models may quite possibly be more appropriate than the Poisson regression and should be considered. This is particularly true when over- or underdispersion is suspected.

Covariate-Adjustment

When adjustment for covariates or confounders is the primary goal of the regression analysis, the research question usually involves trying to compare two (or more) groups. The data are generally obtained from an observational study whose groups are defined by something other than random chance. To get a better estimate of the differences between groups, variables are included in the model that impact group assignment and the outcome of interest. Unlike regression analyses where the primary goal is prediction, the selection of variables has much more to do with published literature and an understanding of the groups/outcome than model fit. Although good model fit is important, the rationale for selecting a variable is based more on the context of the problem and less on statistical justification. Accordingly, the first step to variable selection in covariate adjustment is to consult the literature and identify variables used in other analyses as potential confounders. A next step can involve data analysis, especially considering descriptive statistics, simple statistical tests, and/or simple regressions. Finding unadjusted rate ratios and conducting simple statistical tests may be helpful. Variables that are related to the outcome and group membership should be considered candidates for the regression analysis. Generally, these are variables that result in small p-values when investigating simple statistical tests. However, the p-value does not at have to be smaller than 0.05 to determine whether variables are potential candidates (e.g., p-values of 0.2–0.3 may be considered). The goal is not to determine statistical significance but to create a subset of variables. If the p-value cutoff for variable selection is too stringent (i.e., $p < 0.05$), important variables may be omitted. When trying to determine whether a variable has an impact, do not focus entirely on the p-value; consider the statistics too.

The issue of under- or overdispersion should still be evaluated to determine whether a different model is necessary. Remember that good estimates are the goal and that providing them relies on using an appropriate model.

Strategies for Performing the Regression

A good strategy for performing a regression analysis is to follow the strategies for regression diagnostics.

- Plotting the data is a good first step in identifying variables that may be related to the outcome. Descriptive statistics and bar graphs are helpful. Additionally, considering one regressor at a time may also be informative.
- Once the literature has been consulted, simple tests have been performed, and plots have been created and reviewed, a set of potential variables can be identified.
- Some variables may be measuring the same thing; so potential variables can be further reduced by removing variables that demonstrate multicollinearity.

- With a potential set of regressors, the assumptions of the model can be checked and potential outlier/influence points identified. Although outlier and influence points are generally not omitted, an investigation of how removing these points affect estimates may be useful.
- Particularly in the case of Poisson regression, distributional assumptions need to be assessed. Evidence of under- or overdispersion may suggest a different regression model.
- In evaluating the regression output, some variables may not really contribute to the prediction of the outcome. Unnecessary variables can be removed from the model. Be careful in eliminating variables here. If a variable is removed from the model, the estimates are no longer adjusted for that variable.

Using automatic model selection strategies, statistical software can provide a set of variables for the regression model. Although this strategy is reasonable if many potential variables have to be included without guidance for choosing among them, relying solely on automated model selection strategies should be avoided. Many public health problems include variables in the regression for covariate-adjustment and the primary reason for keeping a variable may be based on the literature or on knowledge about the subject, not necessarily on statistical rationale. Hence, relying on automated model selection strategies may have little justification.

SUMMARY

This chapter began with a public health problem that is likely to grow as the population becomes older: understanding factors related to fractures in women with osteoporosis or osteopenia. In this public health application, the outcome of interest is a count: the number of fractures. Like the public health application presented at the start of the chapter, the data for this chapter involved different variables that might be related to the number of fractures an individual experiences.

Although the methods for summarizing continuous and categorical data can be applied to count outcomes, count data are best summarized using event rates. Event rates summarize counts and account for different contributions of person-time (or space or units at risk). When the outcome is a count, event rates can be compared to historical controls or between concurrently collected comparison groups. Because count data naturally arises from the Poisson distribution, Poisson regression provides a way of investigating multiple variable relationships with counts and event rates. Furthermore, Poisson regression can be used to produce estimates of adjusted rate ratios. The Poisson distribution, however, can be problematic because a key assumption is that the mean and the variance are the same. If the data can be more or less dispersed than would be expected under the Poisson distribution, alternative regression models (negative binomial regression) can be utilized.

SUMMARY OF CHAPTER CONCEPTS

GOAL	COMMON TESTS	COMMON SUMMARIES	
		Graphical	Numerical
How do I compare my result to a known value?			
Sample size is large and rate is not small.	One-sample chi-square test	Histograms Bar graphs Line graphs	Event rates
Sample size is small and/or rate is small.	Exact one-sample test		
How do I compare different populations or regions?			
At a single point in time		Bar graph	Age-adjusted rates
Over time		Line graph	
How do I investigate the association explanatory variables with a count (rate) outcome?			
Mean and the variance of outcome are the same	Poisson regression		Adjusted rate ratios
Overdispersion	Negative binomial regression		
Both variables are nominal	Chi-square test for nonzero correlation		
How do I compare a count (rate) while controlling for confounding?			
Mean and the variance of outcome are the same	Poisson regression		Adjusted rate ratios
Overdispersion	Negative binomial regression		

KEY TERMS

person-time   overdispersion   underdispersion

age-adjusted rates

PRACTICE WITH DATA

1. DESCRIBING THE DATA

   a. Provide appropriate graphical and numerical summaries for the number of healthcare utilizations (urgent treatment center, emergency room, specialist, and hospital visits) in this study.

   b. Provide the overall healthcare utilizations (HCU) rate and the HCU rate for the strength training and control groups.

2. ONE-GROUP STUDIES

   a. Suppose that the HCU rate in a healthy population has been reported as 206 per 100 subject-years. Using the data, determine whether the rate of HCU is similar in the sample of women with osteoporosis/osteopenia.

   b. Complete the following table and provide the age-adjusted rate of fractures for a sample of women in a county in State A.

AGE GROUP	NUMBER OF EVENTS OBSERVED	POPULATION	AGE-SPECIFIC RATE	U.S. POPULATION (STANDARD)	WEIGHT	WEIGHTED RATE
Under 1 year	2	18,303	0.000109272	3,795	0.013818	0.000002
1–4 years	7	38,423	0.000182183	15,192		0.000010
5–14 years	245	37,282		39,977	0.145564	0.000957
15–24 years	1400	33,399	0.041917423	38,077	0.138646	
25–34 years	542	36,379	0.014898705	37,233	0.135573	0.002020
35–44 years	94	27,805	0.003380687	44,659		0.000550
45–54 years	212	23,080		37,030	0.134834	0.001239
55–64 years	567	21,043	0.026944827	23,962	0.087250	
65–74 years	759	12,646	0.060018978	18,136	0.066037	0.003963
75–84 years	889	4,108		12,315	0.044841	0.009704
85 years and over	978	18,303	0.053433863	4,259	0.015508	0.000829
Totals				274,635		

© Cengage Learning, 2012.

3. MULTIPLE-GROUP STUDIES

a. Summarize the association between strength training and the rate of HCU using the rate ratio. Using statistical inference, provide a conclusion about the relationship.

b. Summarize the association between race and the rate of HCU using the rate ratio. Using statistical inference, provide a conclusion about the relationship.

c. Using the adjusted rate ratio, summarize the association between strength training and the rate of HCU, controlling for age and physical activity level. Using statistical inference, provide a conclusion about the relationship.

PRACTICE WITH CONCEPTS

1. Consider the following research questions/study scenarios. For each study, discuss the most appropriate methods for describing the data (graphically and numerically). What statistical method would be *most* appropriate for addressing the research questions? Be sure to provide a justification of the statistical method. When a statistical test is needed, provide appropriate null and research hypotheses.

   a. A study was performed to describe invasive cervical cancer rates between two states.

   b. A comparison of smoking habits for menthol and nonmenthol smokers is conducted. The outcome of interest is the number of cigarettes smoked, and race was considered to be a potential confounder.

   c. To investigate factors related to violence, a recent questionnaire asked participants, "Within the past 12 months, how many people have you known personally that were victims of homicide?" A total of 1308 subjects responded to the question and were identified as being white or nonwhite, residing in an urban or rural area, ever been arrested, male or female, employment status, and age.

2. *Estimated numbers of new diagnoses of HIV/AIDS for 2005 indicate that young people under the age of 25 account for 14% of new cases, with those aged 25–29 accounting for an additional 13% of new cases (Centers for Disease Control and Prevention, 2007). Given a lag between infection and diagnosis, the case estimates suggest that nearly a quarter of those with HIV are infected as adolescents and young adults. Homeless youth have been recognized as one group of young people at particularly high risk for contracting HIV and other sexually transmitted diseases (STDs; Noell et al., 2001; Pfeifer & Oliver, 1997; Stricoff et al., 1991). . . . The goal of the current study was to identify potential individual and environmental protective factors for sex risk behavior among homeless youth. We explored gender differences in the prediction of unprotected sex and number of sex partners. (Tevendale, Lightfoot, & Solcum, 2009)*

   a. A Poisson regression was used to investigate how religious service attendance, expectations for the future, and decision-making skills were related to the number of sexual partners, controlling for age, gender, and ethnicity. Justify the use of a Poisson regression.

   b. The authors presented the following $\hat{\beta}$'s (95% CI). Use these to create adjusted rate ratios. What can you conclude?

   Have decision-making skills: -0.44 ($-.86$, -0.03)
   Have expectations for the future: -0.03 (-0.06, 0.00)
   Attend religious services: 0.27 (0.11, 0.44)

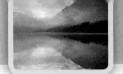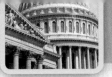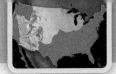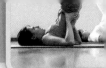

CHAPTER 7

time-to-event analysis

Research questions can involve waiting for an event to happen.

- Mortality studies, for example, often involve investigating whether one group has a longer time until death, called *survival times*, than another.
- A researcher may be interested in determining whether those on an alternative therapy regimen have a longer time until relapse than those on the standard therapy.
- A fertilization study may be interested in determining which factors influence the time until conception.
- Athletic trainers may be interested in determining how long it takes for an athlete to return to play after an injury.

These outcomes are classified as *time–to-event data* because the outcome consists of two pieces: the time until the event and whether the event happens. The two-component outcome of time-to-event data requires different types of statistical methods than the methods discussed in previous chapters. Approaches to investigating time-to-event data are often referred to as *survival analysis*. Although the term "survival" suggests that it is desirable to "survive" the events (death, relapse, loss of employment, heart attack, and so on), survival analysis can relate to "good" events as well (returning to play, obtaining medical treatment, becoming debt free, obtaining training). Because both good and bad events are appropriate for the methods described in this chapter, the phrase "time-to-event" will be used rather than "survival analysis."

LEARNING OBJECTIVES

How do I describe time-to-event data?

Identify, create, and present appropriate descriptive statistics and figures specific for time-to-event data.

How do I compare groups?

Identify appropriate statistical tests for comparing groups.

Interpret the results of the statistical tests.

How do I compare groups while adjusting for confounders (continuous and categorical)?

Utilize regression techniques to control for confounding.

Interpret the results (estimates and statistical tests) of the regression analysis.

How do I investigate the association of risk factors (continuous and categorical) on the outcome?

Utilize regression techniques to investigate risk factors.

Interpret the results (estimates and statistical tests) of the regression analysis.

How do I plan for a study when the research question involves a time-to-event outcome?

Understand the roles that power, effect size, and sample size play in designing a study.

What method do I use?

Identify the most appropriate time-to-event method for the data.

Public Health Application

To combat the epidemic of obesity among youth in the United States (U.S.), adolescents must be encouraged to get up off the couch and participate in physically active sports, recreation, and leisure activities. Participation in high school sports, one of the most popular physical activities among adolescents, has grown rapidly from an estimated 4.0 million participants in 1971–72 to an estimated 7.0 million in 2004–2005. While the health benefits of a physically active lifestyle including participating in sports are undeniable, high school athletes are at risk of sports-related injury because a certain endemic level of injury can be expected among participants of any physical activity. The challenge to injury epidemiologists is to reduce injury rates among high school athletes to the lowest possible level without discouraging adolescents from engaging in this important form of physical activity. This goal can best be accomplished by investigating the etiology of preventable injuries; by developing, implementing, and evaluating protective interventions using such science-based evidence; and by responsibly reporting epidemiologic findings while promoting a physically active lifestyle among adolescents.

(http://injuryresearch.net/resources/1/rio/2005-06HighSchoolRIOSummaryReport.pdf)

Data Description

To investigate the factors related to returning to play after injury for high school athletes, local high schools have agreed to participate in an injury surveillance program. At each of these high schools, a certified athletic trainer is employed to provide daily medical coverage at all scheduled practices and/or games. The athletic trainer is responsible for data collection for the injury surveillance system. Data elements include pain score, previous history of injury, and the cause of the injury. Age and gender for each student athlete are also collected. In addition, the date the injury occurred and the date the student athlete returns to play are recorded. All reportable injuries are entered into the injury surveillance database. All injuries, regardless of time lost from sports participation, are considered reportable. Any reportable injury is documented on a standardized injury electronic evaluation form. These evaluations are uploaded into an Internet-based, secured-access electronic database. Within a season, 137 student athletes experienced an injury that prevented them from participation. Only nine of these injured athletes were not able to return to play before the study (season) ended.

DESCRIBING THE DATA

Time-to-event data are comprised of two pieces: a time piece and a discrete piece (i.e., the occurrence of the event). The *time piece* is generally summarized as a continuous variable. The methods for describing continuous outcomes were presented in Chapter 2. Briefly, histograms and descriptive statistics (*n*, mean, standard deviation, median, first and third quartiles, and minimum and maximum) are appropriate. However, waiting times are generally not symmetric but skewed to the right due to longer wait times. For this reason, the mean and standard deviation may not be appropriate for describing the time until an event. Instead, the median and the range (first and third quartile or minimum and maximum) may be more appropriate. The *discrete piece* of a time-to-event variable (the occurrence of the event) is a dichotomous variable (the event happened: yes/no). The methods for summarizing dichotomous outcomes were discussed in Chapter 4, where numerical summaries counts and percentages were described.

However, describing the pieces of time-to-event data separately is only part of the story; the descriptions must incorporate both the time and the occurrence of the event. In public health, this description is commonly provided numerically as survival probabilities and hazard ratios and graphically through survival curves.

Numerical and Graphical Summaries: Hazard Functions

When the outcome is time-to-event, the event rate is likely to be different depending on time. (Event rates were defined in Chapter 6.) Therefore, in these types of studies, event rates are provided at different time points. A **hazard** function is a description of the event rates at different time points. Therefore, the hazard function is the collection of event (hazard) rates over time. Assuming that the hazard function does not change for 1 unit of time, it represents the number of events that would be expected in a 1-unit-long time interval. A unit of time can be seconds, hours, days, months, years, whatever is appropriate for the study.

Unlike the event rates discussed in Chapter 6, hazard rates are not constant across time and can be thought of as an event rate that changes over time. For a specific time unit, however, the hazard rate is assumed to be constant, and interpretations of the hazard rate use the fact that, for a particular time interval, the event rate is constant.

For example, suppose 1000 student athletes are observed for one season. The person-time (Chapter 6) for this study is 1000 person-seasons because season is the unit of time. Suppose that during this time period, 30 athletes sustained an injury that prevented them from participation. The study involves 1000 person-seasons, and the event rate for injury in this time period is $30 \div 1000 = 0.03$. Therefore, the hazard of a student athlete being injured at a particular point in time is 0.03, with time measured in seasons. If the hazard is constant over one season, then a student athlete can be expected to have an injury 0.03 times in a season. The interpretation of a hazard is just the same as the interpretation of an event rate (Chapter 6). The difference, however, is that, because the hazard rate can change over time, the unit of time must be considered in the interpretation. Like event rates, hazard rates are not probabilities and can be greater than 1. Also, like event rates, hazard rates can be compared.

If a student athlete who has been injured in the past has a hazard rate of 0.030 at time *t* and a second student athlete who has never suffered an injury has a hazard rate of 0.015 at time *t* then the first student athlete's risk of injury would be two times greater at time *t*. Because hazard functions are simply the collection of event rates at particular points in time, plots of these functions are very useful, providing a graphical description of how the functions change over time.

In this example, as depicted in Figure 7-1, the estimated hazard function for returning to play starts off fairly high and then progressively gets smaller as time goes on. This pattern is somewhat expected because less serious injuries require shorter times before the athlete can return to play, whereas more serious injuries entail longer times to return to play.

Figure 7-1 Example of hazard function.
© *Cengage Learning, 2012.*

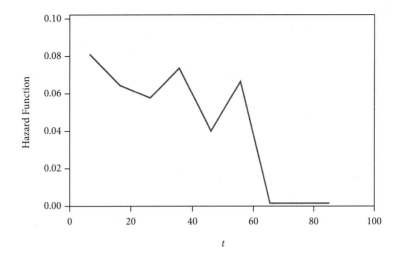

For hazard functions, "at a particular time" is an important statement. Because the hazard rate is expected to change over the time period, the specific point in time must be explicitly indicated. Consequently, hazard functions are denoted as $h(t)$, where (t) indicates that the event rate depends on the time point. The hazard functions are just the chronological collection of $h(t)$'s (event rates at time t). The hazard at time t, $h(t)$, is actually a parameter, and the hazard rates at time t obtained from a sample are statistics, $\widehat{h(t)}$. Unlike the parameters and statistics discussed in earlier chapters, there is an estimate for each time point. However, the principle remains the same: Parameters numerically describe the population, and statistics numerically describe the sample.

The term "hazard" is common in time-to-event analysis, where subjects are "at risk" for an event. However, do not be misled by the wording. "Hazard" refers to the occurrence of the event. In this example, it is preferred for students to return to play, to have the event.

Numerical and Graphical Summaries: Survival Functions

In a way, the **survival** function represents the opposite of the hazard function; it provides a description of the nonevent rate at different time points. The survival rate at any particular time is just the probability that the event will occur at a later time. Therefore, the survival function is just a series of proportions of subjects that may experience the event some time beyond the time point t.

The survival function or survival curve for return to play indicates that, at the very beginning of an injury (time = 0 days), no student athletes have returned to play (Figure 7-2). Most student athletes recover and return to play within 20 days, and there is a very low chance of having a very long time to return to play.

Figure 7-2 Example of survival curve. © *Cengage Learning, 2012.*

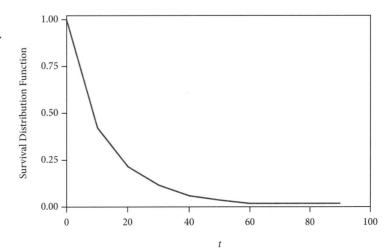

As with hazard functions, the phrase "at a particular time" is important in the interpretation of survival probabilities. The basis of time-to-event analysis is that the probability of survival is expected to change over the time period. Therefore, survival probabilities are indexed by time. For this reason, survival functions are denoted as $S(t)$, where (t) represents a specific time point. The survival function is the chronological collection of the $S(t)$'s, providing a graphical description of probability of *not* returning to play at different times. The survival probability at time t, $S(t)$, is actually a parameter, and the survival probabilities at time t obtained from a sample are statistics, $\widehat{S(t)}$. Unlike the parameters and statistics discussed in earlier chapters, there is an estimate for each time point, but the principle is the same: Parameters numerically describe the population, and statistics numerically describe the sample.

Again, do not confuse the statistical terminology with events being "bad" or "good." In this example, having short times to the event and small survival probabilities is preferred. The event is returning to play; so "survival" means that the student athlete is still waiting to return to play.

CENSORING

One of the challenges in time-to-event data analysis is that the purpose of the study is to wait for an event to occur. What if the event does not occur? What if contact is lost with the participant before the event occurs? For example, a soccer season lasts for approximately 10 weeks. If a student athlete injures her knee and requires surgery, she will not be able to return to play within the season. She will eventually be able to return to play, but the event will not occur during the season (the study period). Also possible is having a less serious injury, like an ankle sprain, a day before the season ends. Because of when the injury occurs, the athlete may not have enough time to return to play before the season ends.

Censoring Defined

When the event does not occur while the subject is being observed in the study, the subject is a censored observation. **Censoring** occurs when the event occurs outside the observation window. Events can be right-censored (the most common), left-censored, or interval-censored.

- *Right-censored events* occur when the event time is greater than the last time the subject was observed.
- *Left-censored events* occur when the event time is less than the first time the subject was observed.
- *Interval-censored events* occur when the event time is between two observation times.

Although the idea of censoring seems simple, it can be confusing. Consider the following examples (see Figure 7-3).

Example 1: The event is returning-to-play after an injury. Athletes are observed for one season. An athlete injures her knee on September 5, 2010 and is out for the season. The season ends on October 30, 2010. This is an example of right-censoring because the event happens *after* the observation period (season) ends. The time until the event (return to play) is *greater* than the time until the end of the season.

Example 2: The event is receiving medication. Rheumatoid arthritis (RA) patients are observed after diagnosis. An RA patient transfers to another physician before receiving medication. This is an example of right-censoring because the event is expected to happen *after* the patient is being observed by the original physician. The time until the event (return to play) is *greater* than the time observed. This example of right-censoring is slightly different from Example 1. In this example, the patient is not observed until the end of the study. The observation for this patient ends early because he transfers to another physician. Because the event does not occur during his observation period, he is right-censored.

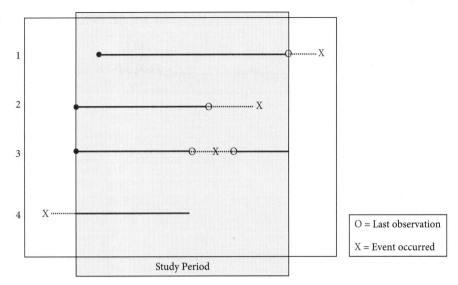

Figure 7-3 Examples of censoring.
© *Cengage Learning, 2012.*

O = Last observation

X = Event occurred

Study Period

Example 3: The event is smoking cessation. A women's health registry collects health information on participants yearly. In a 2009 survey, a participant reported smoking; for the 2010 survey, the participant reported that she had stopped smoking. This is an example of interval-censoring because the exact time of smoking cessation is not known. It is only known that it happened between 2009 and 2010.

Example 4: The event is having asthma. After well-child visits, questionnaires are given to determine whether children had a diagnosis of asthma. The child had a diagnosis of asthma prior to the first contact, when the questionnaire was administered. This is an example of left-censoring because the event occurred prior to the observation period.

Recall that the time-to-event outcome includes two pieces: (1) the time until the event and (2) whether the event occurs. It is probably more appropriate to describe piece (1) as the time until the event is observed *or* until the observation is censored. For a right-censored subject, the variable for whether the event occurs is a 0 (indicating no event). The value for the time variable is the time from the start of the study to the last observation (the point of censoring).

- If the subject does not have the event and the study period expires (as in Example 1), the time variable consists of the amount of time for the whole study and the event variable is 0.
- If, however, the subject does not have the event and does not have the full study period for observation (as in Example 2), the time until the last observation (when the subject was censored) is used as the time variable and the event variable is 0.

The most common form of censoring is right-censoring. Although there are statistical methods for handling, left- and interval-censoring, discussions of censoring in the rest of the chapter will be limited to right censoring.

Data Structure with Censored Observations

Time-to-event datasets are organized as one observation per person; there is a variable for the time and a variable for whether the event occurs (Table 7-1). The variable for whether the event occurs may be referred to as the *censoring variable.* In this example, the variable TIME represents the time until the student athlete returns to play or is censored. The variable RETURN TO PLAY represents whether the student returns to play or not, that is, has the event. Subject 25593-B, for example, has an injury that

TABLE 7-1 **AN EXAMPLE OF A TIME-TO-EVENT DATASET**

Subject ID	Cause of Injury	Pain Score	Age	History of Injury	Gender	Time	Return to Play
15664-A	Ground	6	14	0	1	0.2	1
15556-A	Repetition	8	14	1	0	1.0	1
14423-B	Ground	6	14	1	1	1.8	1
15336-C	Person	7	14	1	1	1.9	1
17885-C	Ground	7	14	1	1	2.0	1
18893-A	Ground	4	14	0	1	2.4	1
25593-B	Ground	7	14	0	1	2.5	0
25554-A	Ground	2	14	0	1	3.1	1
36645-A	Repetition	7	14	0	1	3.3	1
36788-C	Person	4	14	1	1	4.3	1
56684-A	Ground	6	14	0	1	4.5	1
89996-B	Ground	7	14	1	1	35.1	1

keeps him out of play for 2.5 days. Even though this time is less than some of the other times, he never returns to play before the season ends. Therefore, Subject 25593-B is a right-censored observation.

The Kaplan-Meier Method

Methods exist for calculating estimates of survival probabilities in the presence of censoring. One of the most common methods in public health is the Kaplan-Meier method. Subjects are observed at particular time points (which do not have to be equally spaced apart). For each time point, either a subject is still waiting for the event, the subject is censored, or the event has occurred. Therefore, for each time point, the proportion of subjects who have not had an event until that time can be calculated. These proportions are multiplied together to get an estimate of the survival probability. This method of obtaining estimates even when observations may be censored is referred to as the *Kaplan-Meier method*. Because it multiplies smaller and smaller survival probabilities, it is also known as the *product-limit method*.

Application of Formula: KAPLAN-MEIER SURVIVAL PROBABILITIES

$$\widehat{S(t_k)} = \left(1 - \frac{d_1}{s_0}\right) \times \left(1 - \frac{d_2}{s_1}\right) \times \cdots \times \left(1 - \frac{d_k}{s_{k-1}}\right)$$

t_k = Time point k

d_k = The number of subjects with events at time point k

s_{k-1} = The number of subjects without events at the previous time point (time point $k - 1$); the number of subjects still waiting for an event at time point k

continues

continued

What you need for the Kaplan-Meier estimate (using Table 7-2):

1. *An estimate of the probability of having the event at each time point,* $\frac{d_k}{s_{k-1}}$: This is the number of subjects that had the event at a certain time, divided by the number of subjects that are still waiting to have the event at that time.

   At time point 1 (t_1), 65 student athletes have returned to play out of 137: $65 \div 137 = 0.47$.
   At time point 2 (t_2), 27 student athletes have returned to play out of 72 athletes that are still waiting to return to play: $27 \div 72 = 0.38$.
   At time point 3 (t_3), 10 student athletes have returned to play out of 45 athletes that are still waiting to return to play: $10 \div 45 = 0.22$.
   At time point 4 (t_4), 8 student athletes have returned to play out of 34 athletes that are still waiting to return to play: $8 \div 34 = 0.23$. *Notice that there are not 35 athletes still waiting because 1 of the athletes was censored; so that athlete does not appear in the numerator for t_3 or the denominator for t_4.*

Proportions for the other time points are calculated in the same way.

2. An e*stimate of the probability of not having the event (survival) at each time point,* $1 - \frac{d_k}{s_{k-1}}$: 1 – the proportion calculated in (1).
   At time point 1 (t_1): $1 - 0.47 = 0.53$.
   At time point 2 (t_2): $1 - 0.38 = 0.62$.

Proportions for the other time points are calculated in the same way.

To calculate estimates for the survival probability at a particular time point: Multiply all of the probabilities for not having an event until that time [is the product of the proportions calculated in (2)]. For example, the survival estimate at time point 3, [$\widehat{S(3)}$], the proportion of those not having an event at time point 0, 1, and 2 multiplied together: $\widehat{S(3)} = 0.53 \times 0.62 \times 0.78 = 0.26$.

TABLE 7-2 KAPLAN-MEIER ESTIMATES

| Time | Event Occurred | | Waiting for Event | | | | | |
	Returned to Play	Censored	Not Returned to Play	Total	Percentage with Event	Percentage with No Event	$\widehat{S(t)}$
t_1	65	0	72	137	0.47	0.53	0.53
t_2	27	0	45	72	0.38	0.62	0.33
t_3	10	1	34	45	0.22	0.78	0.26
t_4	8	0	26	34	0.24	0.76	0.20
t_5	6	1	19	26	0.23	0.77	0.15
t_6	12	7	0	19	0.63	0.37	0.06

© Cengage Learning, 2012.

The Kaplan-Meier method for calculating survival probability estimates accounts for censoring by not counting the censored observation as a failure at time t but by removing it from the number of subjects who are still waiting for the event at time $t + 1$. However, the Kaplan-Meier estimates are just point estimates, or $\widehat{S(t)}$.

Unlike the point estimates discussed in previous chapters, however, there is no singular survival estimate. The estimates of survival probabilities are for particular time points, resulting in many estimates. This characteristic does not mean that statistical inference should be ignored. In fact, confidence intervals can be calculated for these many estimates. Like the point estimates of survival probabilities, the confidence intervals apply only to a specific time. They do not provide a confidence "interval" for the entire function or curve. The confidence interval for the survival probability at a particular time point cannot be obtained using the standard formula based on a normal sampling distribution. However, taking the natural log of the estimate of the survival probability at a particular time point permits using the standard formula, although, a measure of variability is needed first.

Application of Formula: STANDARD ERROR FOR SURVIVAL PROBABILITIES

Standard error $= \sqrt{\text{Variance}\left(\{\ln[\widehat{S(t)}]\}\right)}$

Variance $\{\ln[\widehat{S(t)}]\} = \sum\limits_{k=1}^{K} \dfrac{d_k}{s_{k-1}(s_{k-1} - d_k)}$

$d_k =$ The number of subjects with events at time point k

$s_{k-1} =$ The number of subjects without events at the previous time point (time point $k-1$); the number of subjects still waiting for an event at time point k

What you need to calculate the standard error:

1. *The number of subjects that have had the event for each time point:* d_k.
   At time point 1 (t_1), 65 student athletes have returned to play.
   At time point 2 (t_2), 27 student athletes have returned to play.
   At time point 3 (t_3), 10 student athletes have returned to play.
   At time point 4 (t_4), 8 student athletes have returned to play.
   This continues for each time point.
2. *The number of subjects without events at the previous time point (time point $k-1$):* These are the number of subjects still waiting for an event at time point $k = s_{k-1}$.
   At time point 1 (t_1), 137 student athletes started the study.
   At time point 2 (t_2), 72 student athletes have not been censored or returned to play at t_1.
   At time point 3 (t_3), 45 student athletes have not been censored or returned to play at t_2.
   At time point 4 (t_4), 34 student athletes have not been censored or returned to play at t_3.
   This continues for each time point.
3. *The difference of (2) − (1) multiplied by (2) for each time point:* $s_{k-1}(s_{k-1} - d_k)$.
   At time point 1 (t_1), $137 \times (137 - 65) = 9864$.
   At time point 2 (t_2), $72 \times (72 - 27) = 3240$.
   At time point 3 (t_3), $45 \times (45 - 10) = 1575$.
   This continues for each time point.
   The number of events found in (1) is divided by the product found in (3) for each time point: $\dfrac{d_k}{s_{k-1}(s_{k-1} - d_k)}$.
   At time point 1 (t_1), $137 \div 9864 = 0.0139$.
   At time point 2 (t_2), $72 \div 3240 = 0.0222$.
   At time point 3 (t_3), $45 \div 1575 = 0.0286$.
   This continues for each time point.
4. *The variance of* $\ln[\widehat{S(t)}]$: This is the sum of the values in *(4)*. For example, the variance of $\ln[\widehat{S(3)}] =$
   $0.0139 + 0.0222 + 0.0286 = 0.0647$.

To calculate the standard error: Take the square root of *(4)*, $\sqrt{(0.0647)} = 0.2544$

Application of Formula

C% confidence interval for the natural log of the survival probability at time t: $\ln[\widehat{S(t)}] \pm z^* \times SE$

t = The time point of interest

$\ln[\widehat{S(t)}]$ = The natural log of the sample survival probability at time t

C = The confidence level for a C% confidence interval

z^* = The number of standard deviations from the center of the sampling distribution

SE = The standard error

What you need to calculate the confidence interval (using $t = 3$ as an example):

1. *The point estimate of survival probability at time t:* $\widehat{S(3)} = 0.26$.
2. *The natural log of the estimate of survival probability at time t or the natural log of (1):* $\ln[\widehat{S(3)}] = -1.35$.
3. *The standard error:* The standard error is $\sqrt{0.0647} = 0.2544$.
4. *The confidence level:* C% is typically 95%, but 90% and 99% are also common.
5. *The number of standard deviations from the center of the sampling distribution:* This depends on C% (4) and the sampling distribution. In this case, where the sampling distribution is a normal distribution:

   The z^* for a 90% confidence interval is 1.65.
   The z^* for a 95% confidence interval is 1.97.
   The z^* for a 99% confidence interval is 2.58.

To calculate the confidence intervals:

90% confidence interval: $\ln[\widehat{S(t)}] \pm (1.65 \times$ standard error$)$
95% confidence interval: $\ln[\widehat{S(t)}] \pm (1.96 \times$ standard error$)$
99% confidence interval: $\ln[\widehat{S(t)}] \pm (2.58 \times$ standard error$)$.

The 95% confidence interval for $\ln[S(3)]$ is $-1.35 \pm (1.96 \times 0.2544)$ or $[-1.85, -0.85]$.

These confidence intervals provide interval estimates not for the true survival probability at a particular time, but for the true $\ln[S(t)]$. To obtain the interval estimate for the true $S(t)$, the upper and lower limits of the confidence interval must be exponentiated. Hence, to get the interval estimate of the $S(t)$, an additional calculation $[\exp(\text{lower limit}), \exp(\text{upper limit})]$ is required. For example, when $t = 3$, the 95% confidence interval is $[\exp(-1.85), \exp(-0.85)]$, or $[0.16, 0.43]$. These confidence intervals can also be easily obtained from statistical software packages.

Given a limited number of time points, as in the examples so far, it is easy to see how Kaplan-Meier survival estimates are calculated. However, this process can be tiresome if time is collected as a continuous variable, as it is in this study. Luckily, estimates of the survival probabilities (and confidence intervals) can be obtained for each time point easily with statistical software (Table 7-3). These estimates can then be plotted to provide a graphical description of the survival function where censored observations have been included as open circles (Figure 7-4). When the survival probabilities are estimated using the Kaplan-Meier method, the resulting curves are referred to as *Kaplan-Meier survival curves*.

Life-Table Method

Although the graphical description of the survival function is very helpful, Table 7-3 is a little too detailed to provide a good numerical summary of the survival probabilities. Therefore, the life-table method is often used to present survival probability estimates. Grouping time points into intervals, as long or as short as needed, is an

TABLE 7-3 **EXAMPLE OF KAPLAN-MEIER ESTIMATES**

t	Survival	Failure	Standard Error	Number Failed	Number Left
0.0000	1.0000	0	0	0	137
0.1000	—	—	—	1	136
0.1000	0.9854	0.0146	0.0102	2	135
0.2000	0.9781	0.0219	0.0125	3	134
0.3000	0.9708	0.0292	0.0144	4	133
0.4000	0.9635	0.0365	0.0160	5	132
0.7000	—	—	—	6	131
0.7000	—	—	—	7	130
0.7000	0.9416	0.0584	0.0200	8	129
0.8000	—	—	—	9	128
0.8000	—	—	—	10	127
0.8000	—	—	—	11	126
0.8000	0.9124	0.0876	0.0242	12	125
1.0000	—	—	—	13	124
1.0000	0.8978	0.1022	0.0259	14	123
1.1000	0.8905	0.1095	0.0267	15	122
1.2000	—	—	—	16	121
1.2000	0.8759	0.1241	0.0282	17	120
37.8000	0.0810	0.9190	0.0253	119	9
38.4000	0.0720	0.9280	0.0240	120	8
38.9000	0.0630	0.9370	0.0227	121	7
39.2000	0.0540	0.9460	0.0211	122	6
41.1000	0.0450	0.9550	0.0194	123	5
46.7000	0.0360	0.9640	0.0175	124	4
55.3000	0.0270	0.9730	0.0153	125	3
58.7000	0.0180	0.9820	0.0126	126	2
99.1000	0.00900	0.9910	0.00894	127	1
99.9000	0	1.0000	—	128	0

Note: This provides a partial table of the output obtained when using the Kaplan-Meier method.

© Cengage Learning, 2012.

Figure 7-4 Example of survival curve (censoring).
© *Cengage Learning, 2012.*

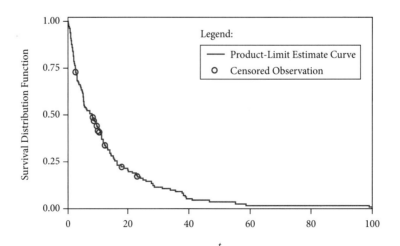

easier approach for reviewing estimates of survival probabilities. The method used to provide estimates of survival probabilities in time intervals is referred to as the *life-table method* (see Table 7-4)

Besides offering a better table of survival probability estimates, the life-table method is also able to produce estimates and plots of the hazard function, which may not be possible with some software packages using the Kaplan-Meier method. However, the life-table method loses some information because the time points are grouped into intervals, and there may not be a clear choice for defining the interval lengths.

TABLE 7-4 **EXAMPLE OF LIFE-TABLE ESTIMATES**

Interval (Lower, Upper)		Number Failed	Number Censored	Sample Size	Survival	Failure	Survival Standard Error	Hazard[1]	Hazard Standard Error[1]
0	10	78	4	135.0	1.0000	0	0	0.08125	0.008406
10	20	26	4	53.0	0.4222	0.5778	0.0425	0.065	0.012056
20	30	11	1	24.5	0.2151	0.7849	0.0362	0.057895	0.016709
30	40	7	0	13.0	0.1185	0.8815	0.0294	0.073684	0.025891
40	50	2	0	6.0	0.0547	0.9453	0.0213	0.04	0.027713
50	60	2	0	4.0	0.0365	0.9635	0.0177	0.066667	0.044444
60	70	0	0	2.0	0.0182	0.9818	0.0127	0	—
70	80	0	0	2.0	0.0182	0.9818	0.0127	0	—
80	90	0	0	2.0	0.0182	0.9818	0.0127	0	—
90	100	2	0	2.0	0.0182	0.9818	0.0127	—	—
100	—	0	0	0.0	0	1	0	—	—

[1] Evaluated at the midpoint of the interval

Note: This provides a partial table of the output obtained when using the life-table method.

© Cengage Learning, 2012.

GROUP COMPARISONS

A comparison of the hazard rates or survival functions is often necessary to address a research question. Many times one group serves as the control group. For example, student athletes who have experienced injuries in the past are expected to have longer time to return to play than athletes who have not had a previous injury. Therefore, the student athletes who have not had a previous injury serve as the control group. The two groups could be compared for differences in the time to return to play. These two groups consist of completely different student athletes, and the measurements of one group have nothing to do with the measurements of the other. Therefore, these two groups are considered to be independent. If the outcomes between the two independent groups differ, then the differences may be attributed to having a previous injury or not.

Descriptive statistics can be provided to describe the group of student athletes with a previous injury and student athletes without a history of injury. A table of descriptive statistics such as Table 7-5 might be helpful in describing the injured student athletes.

> **RESEARCH QUESTION:**
> Does previous injury impact time to return to play?

TABLE 7-5 CHARACTERISTICS OF THE SAMPLE

	All (N = 137)	History of Injury (N = 56)	First-time Injury (N = 81)
Age (years)			
Mean (SD)	16.2 (1.46)	16.2 (1.55)	16.2 (1.41)
Median (Q_1, Q_3)	16 (15, 18)	16.5 (15, 18)	16 (15, 17)
Minimum, maximum	14, 18	14, 18	14, 18
Pain Score (1–10)			
Mean (SD)	4.5 (2.15)	4.3 (2.29)	4.6 (2.05)
Median (Q_1, Q_3)	4 (3, 6)	4 (2, 6)	4 (3, 6)
Minimum, maximum	(1, 10)	1, 9	1, 10
Gender			
Males	68 (49.6%)	26 (46.4%)	42 (51.9%)
Females	69 (50.36%)	30 (53.6%)	39 (48.2%)
Cause of Injury (%)			
Repetitive	75 (54.7%)	24 (42.9%)	11 (13.6%)
Contact with ground	27 (19.7%)	18 (32.1%)	57 (70.4%)
Contact with person	35 (25.6%)	14 (25.0%)	13 (16.1%)
Returned to Play (%)			
No	9 (6.6%)	8 (14.3%)	1 (1.2%)
Yes	128 (93.4%)	48 (85.7%)	80 (98.8%)
Time to Return to Play (days)*			
Mean (SD)	12.2 (16.26)	19.5 (21.14)	7.8 (10.34)
Median (Q_1, Q_3)	6.2 (2.3, 14.8)	14.0 (5.5, 25.5)	4.7 (2.0, 9.7)
Minimum, Maximum	0.1, 99.9	0.8, 99.9	0.1, 55.3

*Time to return-to-play summary statistics are provided for only the 128 student athletes who returned to play.

© Cengage Learning, 2012.

The descriptive statistics in Table 7-5 provide interesting information on the injured student athletes. For example, approximately half of the injured athletes are male (49.6%), the average age is 16 (SD = 1.5), the athletes report median pain of 4 on a pain instrument that ranges from a low of 1 to a high of 10, the majority (54.7%) of the injuries are due to repetition, most (93.4%) injured athletes return to play by the end of the season, the time to return to play appears to be right-skewed because the mean (12.2) is considerably larger than the median, and the median time to return to play is 6.2 with a range of 0.1 to 99.9 days.

Although the student athletes with a previous injury are similar with respect to gender and age, there are some differences between student athletes who have experienced a previous injury and first-time injury athletes. In particular, those with a previous injury have a higher observed rate of injuries due to repetition (42.9% versus 13.6%). Consequently, first-time injury athletes have much higher percentages of injuries due to contact with ground than those with a previous injury (70.4% versus 32.1%). The time to return-to-play also appears to be longer for those with a previous injury. Student athletes with a previous injury have a median wait time of 14 days to return to play, while the student athletes with a first-time injury have a median wait time of only 5 days. The range of wait times is also larger for those with a previous injury compared to those without a history of injury (99.1 versus 55.2 days).

Comparing Groups with Kaplan-Meier Curves

Because this is a time-to-event analysis, the primary outcome is whether an injured student athlete returns to play *and* how long it takes the athlete to return to play. Estimates of the survival probabilities can be calculated for athletes with previous injury and for first-time injury athletes. These survival probability estimates can be calculated using the Kaplan-Meier method. Table 7-5 shows that not all injured athletes were able to return to play: 9 (6.6%) were censored. The Kaplan-Meier method can take these censored observations into account when calculating the estimated survival probabilities for each group. The same process used to calculate the survival estimates for the entire sample can be used for each group separately. The survival probability estimates for each time point t can be provided, but the output can become quite long, especially if time is measured as a continuous variable.

An easier way to examine the estimated survival probabilities for the two groups is by means of the Kaplan-Meier survival curves (Figure 7-5). The estimated survival curve for students with a history of injuries is higher than (above) the estimated survival curve for the first-time injury athletes. This pattern indicates that those with a previous injury tend to "survive" longer than the first-time athletes. In other words, those with a previous injury tend to have longer observed waiting times until the event, that is, longer observed times to return to play.

Figure 7-5 Comparison of survival curve (two groups). © *Cengage Learning, 2012.*

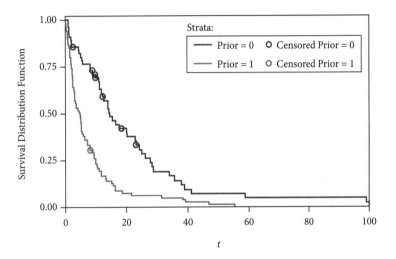

Hazard Ratios

If the estimated survival functions of the two groups are different, then the estimated hazard rates should be different too. Hazard rates can be used to investigate whether history of injury has an impact on the time to return-to-play. The comparison of hazard rates is done via the hazard ratios. The *hazard ratio* is the ratio of two hazard rates at a particular point in time. Like the ratios discussed in previous chapters (prevalence, risk, odds, and rate—Chapters 4 and 6),

- If a hazard ratio is 1, then the hazard rates are equal.
- If the hazard ratio is less than 1, then the hazard rate in the denominator is greater than the hazard rate in the numerator.
- On the other hand, if the hazard ratio is greater than 1, then the hazard rate in the numerator is greater than the hazard rate in the denominator.

The interpretation is the same as for other ratios, except instead of discussing odds, for example, hazard is described. In this example, $h_1(t)$ could represent the hazard rate at time t for student athletes with a history of injury, and $h_2(t)$ could represent the hazard rate a time t for the first-injury student athletes. The hazard ratio is $\frac{h_1(t)}{h_2(t)}$. In this study, the estimate of the hazard ratio is 0.40; the estimated hazard of returning to play is greater in the denominator (athletes that did not have a previous injury). In fact, for this sample, those without a previous injury were observed to have a 60% decrease in the risk of returning to play when compared to athletes with previous injuries.

Although the survival curves in Figure 7-5 appear to be fairly separated, with previously injured student athletes having higher estimated survival probabilities than first-injury student athletes, is the difference in the curves great enough to claim that having a previous injury is related to the time to return to play? Not only is the curve for previously injured athletes higher, the estimated hazard ratio is 0.40. Is this hazard ratio different enough from 1 to claim that having a previous injury is related to the time to return to play? Although this estimate is not equal to 1, what can be inferred about the true hazard ratio? These results are specific to this sample. Different samples result in different estimates; so hypothesis tests can help determine whether what was observed in this sample can be generalized.

The Log-Rank Test: Comparing Two Groups

Making comparisons with time-to-event data means either comparing survival curves or determining whether the hazard ratio is 1. In this example, the association between time to return to play and having a previous injury has been described with survival probability estimates (presented as a Kaplan-Meier curve in Figure 7-5) and a hazard ratio estimate. However, the question of whether these results are real or due to chance remains. A hypothesis test is needed to determine whether the true survival functions (the combination of the survival probabilities at each time point t) are equal.

> **RESEARCH HYPOTHESIS:** The survival function for first-injury student athletes is different from that for student athletes with a history of injury *at some point* in time.
>
> **NULL HYPOTHESIS:** The survival function for first-injury student athletes is the same as that for student athletes with a history of injury *for all points* in time.

Hypotheses for the survival curves are analogous to hypotheses for hazard ratios. In fact, comparing survival curves is equivalent to determining whether the hazard rate of first-injury athletes is different from the hazard rate of previous injury athletes at some point in time. To compare the hazard rates, the hazard ratio is used. If the hazard rates for the two groups are the same, then the hazard ratio will be 1. On the other hand, if the hazard rates are different, then the hazard ratio will not be 1.

> **RESEARCH HYPOTHESIS:** $\dfrac{h_1(t)}{h_2(t)} \neq 1.$
>
> **NULL HYPOTHESIS:** $\dfrac{h_1(t)}{h_2(t)} = 1.$

Regardless if the hypothesis involves survival curves or hazard ratios, hypothesis testing assumes the null hypothesis is true and uses the data from the sample to test that claim. Using the sample data, a test statistic is obtained. When the null hypothesis is true, this test statistic comes from a chi-square distribution. If the observed test statistic is one that would be expected from this sampling distribution, there is no reason to reject the null hypothesis. On the other hand, when the observed test statistic does not appear to come from this distribution, it is a rare observation, and provides evidence against the null hypothesis.

The *log-rank test* statistic is often used when comparing survival curves (or investigating hazard ratios). This test statistic was actually already discussed in Chapter 4 when Mantel-Haenszel odds ratios were presented. The same idea applies here. Mantel-Haenszel odds ratios were adjusted for a confounding variable by taking contingency tables for each level of the confounding variable and then averaging the odds ratios that resulted. The contingency table consisted of rows for the risk factor and two columns, one for each level of the outcome. For a time-to-event outcome, the rows are still the risk factor and the columns are whether or not the outcome (event) occurred. The "confounding variable," however, is time. Time is categorized into intervals small enough that the hazard rates (and survival probabilities) are constant during this period. Thus, the log-rank test involves a set of contingency tables for different points in time. The resulting test statistic (log-rank test statistic) can be used to test hypotheses about survival curves and hazard ratios. The hypothesis test is referred to as the *log-rank test*.

Application of Formula: LOG-RANK TEST

$$X^2_{LR} = \frac{(|O-E| - 0.5)^2}{\text{Variance}}$$

What you need for a log-rank test:

1. *Small time intervals:* The intervals are small enough that the event rate is constant.
2. *A contingency table for each time interval:* The rows are the levels of the categorical variable (history of injury: yes/no), and the columns are whether the event (return to play) occurred.
3. A Mantel-Haenszel test over all of these contingency tables is calculated.
   a. *The observed count for each contingency table:* The observed count is the sum of all the subjects exposed to the risk factor who have the event. So for a contingency table, it is the number of all the student athletes with a history of an injury who returned to play.
   b. *The expected count for each contingency table:* The expected count is the number of those exposed to the risk factor times the number with the event, divided by the number of subjects in the contingency table. For a contingency table, the expected count is the number of student athletes with a history of injury multiplied by the number of student athletes who returned to play, divided by number of injured student.
   c. *The observed count:* O = *the sum of all the observed counts in the contingency tables (a).*
   d. *The expected count:* E = *the sum of all the expected counts in the contingency tables (b).*
   e. *The difference between observed and expected:* O − E = *(c) − (d).* If this difference is negative, then add 0.5. If this difference is positive, then subtract 0.5.
   f. *The variance for each contingency table:* For each contingency table, multiply the number of subjects exposed and unexposed to the risk factor and the number of subjects with and without the event. In this example, this consists of those with a history of injury multiplied by those who are first-time injuries multiplied by those who return to play multiplied by those who did not return to play. This product is divided by the total number of subjects in the contingency table multiplied by the number of subjects minus 1.
   g. *The variance is the sum of the variances (f) for each contingency table.*

To calculate the test statistic: This is the difference between observed and expected (e) divided by the variance (g).

In this case, the test statistic is 24.0 (Table 7-6). It is assumed that the test statistic for a log-rank test with a categorical variable with two levels comes from a chi-square distribution with one degree of freedom. Using the chi-square distribution with one degree of freedom, is the value of 24.0 rare or common? Any test statistic greater than 3.84 is considered to be rare. The test statistic of 24.0 is pretty far from 3.84; so the test statistic is considered rare. When the test statistic is considered rare, the proportion of test statistics that are even farther away is quite small. Recall that the proportion of test statistics that are even farther away is the *p*-value; the *p*-value that results from the log-rank test is <0.0001.

TABLE 7-6 **RESULTS OF THE LOG-RANK TEST**

Test of Equality Over Strata			
Test	Chi-Square	DF	Pr > Chi-Square
Log-rank	24.0095	1	<0.0001

© Cengage Learning, 2012.

CONCLUSION: The *p*-value is small (*p* < 0.0001). This is sufficient evidence to reject the null hypothesis. Hence, the true hazard ratio is not 1, the survival curves are different at some time *t*, and so a history of injury is associated with time to return to play.

The Log-Rank Test: Comparing Multiple Groups

Comparisons between groups are not limited to two-sample studies. The same methods used to determine whether two survival curves are different can be used to determine whether a difference exists between multiple survival curves. Likewise, multiple hazard rates can also be compared via hazard ratios when more than two groups are of interest.

Because one of the goals of this study is to better understand factors associated with the time to return to play, comparisons among student athletes injured due to repetition, contact with the ground, or contact with a person may help to answer the research question. Of the three groups, student athletes injured by contact with the ground tend to have lower survival probabilities than the other causes of injuries, indicating that athletes injured by contact with the ground returned to play faster than those injured by contact with a person or repetition (Figure 7-6). However, it is of interest to determine whether the survival functions of injuries caused by repetition, contact with the ground, or contact with a person are truly different.

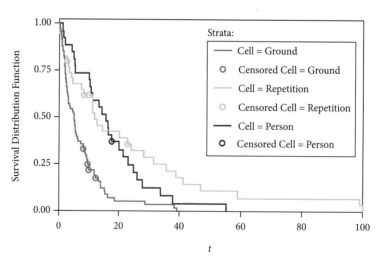

Figure 7-6 Comparison of survival curves (multiple groups). © *Cengage Learning, 2012.*

RESEARCH QUESTION: Is the cause of the injury associated with the time to return to play?

RESEARCH HYPOTHESIS: The survival functions for injuries caused by repetition, contact with the ground, and contact with a person are different *at some point* in time.

NULL HYPOTHESIS: The survival function for injuries caused by repetition, contact with the ground, and contact with a person are the same *for all points* in time.

Likewise, the hypothesis tests regarding the hazard ratio can also be used to make comparisons. The analogous null hypothesis is that all of the hazard ratios are the same and are equal to 1.

Since a ratio can only compare the hazard rates for two levels at a time (one in the numerator and one in the denominator), one level is selected as the reference category and a hazard ratio is created for each of the remaining levels. For example, injury cause has three levels: repetition, contact with the ground, or contact with a person. In this example: $h_1(t)$ represents the hazard rate at time t for student athletes with injury caused by contact with a person, $h_2(t)$ represents the hazard rate a time t for student athletes with injury caused by contact with the ground, and $h_3(t)$ represents the hazard rate a time t for student athletes with injury caused by repetition.

The hazard ratios are $\frac{h_1(t)}{h_3(t)}, \frac{h_2(t)}{h_3(t)}, \frac{h_1(t)}{h_2(t)}$. In this example, the estimates of these hazard ratios are 1.3. 2.8, and 2.3, respectively. Therefore, the observed the hazard (or risk) of returning to play is greater for those who were injured due to contact compared to those injured due to repetition. In fact, there is an observed 30% increase in the hazard of returning to play for athletes injured due to a person compared to injury by repetition and almost the triple the hazard for those who were injured by contact with the ground. Furthermore, the hazard of return to play for those who are injured from contact with the ground is more than twice that of those who are injured from contact with a person. This indicates that those injured by contact with the ground return to play faster than those injured by contact with a person or by repetition, respectively. However, are these estimates different enough from 1 to claim that cause of injury is related to returning to play?

RESEARCH HYPOTHESIS: $\frac{h_1(t)}{h_3(t)} \neq 1$ or $\frac{h_2(t)}{h_3(t)} \neq 1$ or $\frac{h_1(t)}{h_2(t)} \neq 1$.

NULL HYPOTHESIS: $\frac{h_1(t)}{h_3(t)} = 1$ and $\frac{h_2(t)}{h_3(t)} = 1$ and $\frac{h_1(t)}{h_2(t)} = 1$.

Regardless of whether the hypothesis is based on comparing survival curves or hazard ratios, the log-rank test can be used (Table 7-7).

TABLE 7-7 **RESULTS OF THE LOG-RANK TEST WHEN COMPARING MULTIPLE GROUPS**

Test of Equality over Strata			
Test	Chi-Square	DF	Pr > Chi-Square
Log-rank	25.0080	2	<0.0001

© Cengage Learning, 2012.

CONCLUSION: Because the p-value is small ($p < 0.0001$), there is sufficient evidence to reject the null hypothesis; the survival curves are different at some time point. Furthermore, at least one of the hazard ratios associated with the cause of injury is not equal to 1. These results suggest that cause of injury is related to the time to return to play.

Although comparisons between multiple groups are possible using the log-rank test, the number of groups that can be compared is limited. Moreover, the Kaplan-Meier curves are very difficult to examine if there are too many levels of a categorical variable or if more than one categorical variable is of interest. Furthermore, unless a continuous variable is categorized, log-rank tests and Kaplan-Meier curves cannot be used to investigate the relationship.

Planning a Two-Sample Study

Providing sample size estimates for time-to-event studies where the goal is to compare two hazard rates is very similar to comparing two proportions (Chapter 4). The similarity is due in part to fact that determining the sample size with time-to-event data requires having an estimate of the proportion of subjects who have the event at a particular time point. However, determining the sample size also requires estimating the number of events. Like continuous and categorical outcomes, acceptable power and significance levels (probability of a type 1 error) are also needed. Suppose an investigator wants to plan a study that has 80% power with a two-sided significance level of 0.05, the sample size will be determined by the effect size and the proportion with the event at time t.

Determining the effect size involves finding an estimate of the hazard ratio. When the effect size (hazard ratio) is larger, the sample size required to detect this effect is smaller. However, a large effect size is not simply a large hazard ratio; the size of the proportion with the event at time t also matters. If the event is rare and very few are expected to have the event at time t, then a larger sample size is required.

Table 7-8 provides a summary of how the sample size estimate changes with changing effect size (hazard ratio) estimates, power, and proportions with the event. As an example, with a sample size of 293 per group ($n = 586$), a log-rank test will have at least 80% power to detect a hazard ratio of 1.5, when one of the groups has a proportion of events of 0.6 at time t, assuming a two-sided significance level of 0.05.

TABLE 7-8 **SAMPLE SIZE ESTIMATES (TESTING FOR EQUALITY OF SURVIVAL CURVES)**

Proposed Sample Size (per Group)	Proportion with Event at Time t	Number of Events	Effect Size (Hazard Ratio)	Power
191	0.4			
232	0.5	196	1.5	0.80
293	0.6			
258	0.4			
314	0.5	265	1.5	0.90
396	0.6			
108	0.4			
131	0.5	103	1.75	0.80
166	0.6			
146	0.4			
178	0.5	139	1.75	0.90
225	0.6			

Sample size estimates are based on conducting a log-rank test ($\alpha = 0.05$),

© Cengage Learning, 2012.

PROPORTIONAL HAZARDS REGRESSION

RESEARCH QUESTION:
Are previous injury, pain, and cause of the injury associated with the time to return to play, controlling for potential confounders?

So far, previous injury and cause of injury have been investigated separately to see whether these factors have an association with the time to return to play. However, additional risk factors may also be related to an injured student athlete's time to return to play. Furthermore, considering these factors one at a time may not be adequate; multiple-variable relationships may need to be investigated.

Because this is an observational study and the student athletes with a previous injury may be different from those injured for the first time, relationships should be investigated while controlling for potential confounding variables (variables associated with both the explanatory and dependent variables). In this example, potential confounders include the age and gender of the student athlete.

To adjust for the effect of the confounding variables and to investigate multiple risk factors simultaneously, a regression is necessary. As discussed in Chapters 3, 5, and 6, regression models are useful when there are multiple regressors (dichotomous, nominal, ordinal, and/or continuous). Time-to-event data can actually be analyzed with several different types of regression models.

Model

For time-to-event outcomes in public health, the most commonly used regression model is the proportional-hazards regression model (also known as the Cox regression model). One of the advantages of the proportional-hazards regression is that the model assumptions are fairly simple: The hazards are proportional. Therefore, proportional-hazards regressions have wide applicability and use. Hence, this chapter will focus on concepts related to proportional-hazards regression.

Proportional-hazards regression is so named because the primary assumption of the regression model is that the hazards are proportional: that is, for any two different subjects, the logs of the hazard functions are parallel. The assumption refers to the relationship of the hazards over the study period:

- Proportional-hazards implies that the ratio of the hazards will be the same over time (Figure 7-7).
- Nonproportional-hazards implies that the ratio of the hazards will vary over time (Figure 7-8).

Proportional-hazards does not imply that the hazards are the same but rather that the hazards are proportional. For example, if student athletes with a first-time injury have twice the risk of returning to play compared to those with a history of injury at the start of the season, they also have twice the risk of returning to play at the end of or at any other point in the season.

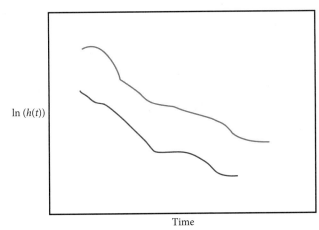

Figure 7-7 Example of proportional hazards.
© *Cengage Learning, 2012.*

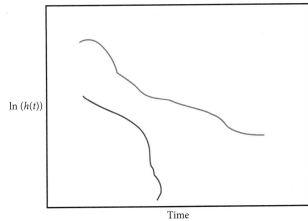

Figure 7-8 Example of nonproportional hazards.
© *Cengage Learning, 2012.*

The model for the proportional-hazards regression is very similar to the models described in Chapters 3, 5, and 6 for linear, logistic, and Poisson regression. The proportional-hazards regression model is

$$\ln[h(t)] = \alpha + \beta_1 x_1 + \beta_2 x_2 + \cdots + \beta_K x_K$$

Or

$$\ln[h(t)] = \ln[h_0(t)] + \beta_1 x_1 + \beta_2 x_2 + \cdots + \beta_K x_K,$$

where $h(t)$ represents the true hazard at time t, and $h_0(t)$ represents the unspecified (but positive) baseline hazard.

As in the other regression models, the right-hand side is simply $\alpha + \beta_1 x_1 + \beta_2 x_2 + \cdots + \beta_K x_K$, where x_k represents the covariates, β_k represents the slopes, and α represents the intercept. The intercept, however, is not a typical intercept. In the proportional-hazards model, it is actually $\ln[h_0(t)]$, where $h_0(t)$ represents an unspecified baseline hazard. In fact, the intercept is often noted as $\alpha(t)$. It represents a subject's baseline hazard and is similar to an intercept because it represents a subject's baseline hazard when all the regressors are 0. It is the same for every person. Unlike the other regression models, however, $\ln[h_0(t)]$ does not get estimated because it actually gets "canceled out."

Mathematically, if the hazards of two subjects (A and B) are proportional, then the hazard ratio $\frac{h_A(t)}{h_B(t)}$ is constant for all time points t, meaning the time point no longer matters since the ratio of the hazard functions for the two subjects does not depend on time. The fact that the ratio does not depend on time is related to baseline hazard getting canceled out.

In this example, possible regressors include previous injury (prior), cause of injury (repetition, ground, person), gender, age, and pain score (pain). The proportional-hazards regression model is

$$\ln[h(t)] = \ln[h_0(t)] + \beta_1(\text{prior}) + \beta_2(\text{ground}) + \beta_3(\text{person})$$
$$+ \beta_4(\text{gender}) + \beta_5(\text{pain}) + \beta_6(\text{age})$$

where $h(t)$ represents the true hazard at time t, and $h_0(t)$ represents the unspecified (but positive) baseline hazard. Notice that both the right and left sides of the equation involve time t. For subjects A and B, the $\ln\left[\frac{h_A(t)}{h_B(t)}\right]$ is really $\ln[h_A(t)] - \ln[h_B(t)]$. Because the intercept $\ln[h_0(t)]$ is the same for Subject A and Subject B, it cancels out. The fact that it cancels out implies that nothing depending on t is left, and the ratio of the hazards is the same at all time points—proportional hazards.

Getting the Slopes

In linear regression (Chapter 3), the least squares method was used to estimate β. In logistic and Poisson regression (Chapters 5 and 6), maximum likelihood estimation was used to estimate β. Proportional-hazards regression, however, cannot use either of these approaches. Instead it uses *partial likelihood*. This method of estimation uses the product of the likelihoods, just as in logistic and Poisson regression, but not a likelihood from every subject is included. Only the likelihoods for the subjects with events that occurred are used. So, if 128 out of 137 athletes returned to play, 128 out of 137 athletes had events; the partial likelihood is the product of these 128 likelihoods.

With partial likelihoods, what matters is not the value of the time, but rather the order in which the events occurred. The order matters because, if a subject has already had an event, then the subject is no longer at risk to have the event. In the injury example, if an athlete has returned to play, then he or she is no longer waiting to return-to-play.

The likelihood for each subject that experienced an event is the probability that the event happened to that subject rather than to the other subjects still waiting for the event. For example, the likelihood for the first student athlete to return to play is the hazard of the first student athlete divided by the sum of all the hazards for all the student athletes in the study.

Likewise, the likelihood for the second student athlete to return to play is the hazard of the second student still waiting to return to play divided by the sum of all the hazards for all the student athletes except for the first injured athlete. Because the first student athlete has already returned to play, his hazard is not included in the denominator. This continues for every subject who had an event.

According to the proportional-hazards model,

$$\ln[h(t)] = \ln[h_0(t)] + \beta_1(\text{prior}) + \beta_2(\text{ground}) + \beta_3(\text{person}) + \beta_4(\text{gender}) + \beta_5(\text{pain}) + \beta_6(\text{age})$$

This means that the hazard for a subject can be written as follows:

$$h(t) = h_0(t)\, e^{\beta_1(\text{history of injury}) + \beta_2(\text{contact with ground}) + \beta_3(\text{contact with person}) + \beta_4(\text{gender}) + \beta_5(\text{pain}) + \beta_6(\text{age})}$$

So, for every likelihood, the $h_0(t)$ ends up in the numerator and the denominator. Because it is the same for every subject, it cancels out of the fraction; so it does not matter that it is unspecified.

With partial likelihoods, the order in which events happen (or are censored) is very important. The method works only as long as every subject has different event times. However, in real data, two or more subjects can quite possibly have the same event times (i.e., *ties*). In the event of ties, special formulas are required to handle them. Four methods are Breslow, Efron, discrete, and exact. Given a small number of ties, there is not much difference between the methods and, in the absence of ties, all four methods are the same.

The *exact method* assumes that the ties occurred because continuous, untied data were grouped. The discrete method assumes that the ties are really ties and that the events happened at the same time.

Both the exact and discrete methods provide true partial likelihood methods, but they require computing time. If the dataset is very large, these methods may be too time-consuming. When the discrete and exact methods are not practical, the Efron method may be a better choice because it approximates the exact method without using as much computation time. The Breslow method, which is the default in some software packages, does the poorest job at approximation and really performs well only when there are few ties.

Hypothesis Tests

A regression with multiple regressors entails three types of hypothesis tests: the overall test, the test for effects, and the specific hypothesis tests for the slopes.

- The *overall hypothesis test* is conducted to see whether there is a relationship between any of the variables and the outcome.
- The *hypothesis tests* for the effects are useful if the model contains nominal variables with multiple categories because they test whether the nominal variable overall, not the specific dummy variables, is related to the outcome, controlling for all other variables in the model.
- Finally, *specific hypothesis tests* involve testing that one of the variables is related to the outcome, controlling for all other variables in the model.

Overall Hypothesis Test

Just as in any regression, the overall hypothesis test tests whether any of the slopes (β's) are not 0. Therefore, the rationale for the overall hypothesis is to determine whether there are any relationships between the regressors and the outcome before moving forward to investigate specific associations. In this example, the proportional-hazards regression model is

$$\ln[h(t)] = \ln[h_0(t)] + \beta_1(\text{prior}) + \beta_2(\text{ground}) + \beta_3(\text{person}) + \beta_4(\text{gender}) + \beta_5(\text{pain}) + \beta_6(\text{age})$$

where $h(t)$ represents the true hazard at time t and $h_0(t)$ represents the unspecified (but positive) baseline hazard.

RESEARCH HYPOTHESIS: At least one of the slopes (β's) is not 0.

NULL HYPOTHESIS: All of the slopes (β's) are 0.

The overall hypotheses are not particularly interesting or exciting. If the null hypothesis can be rejected, it simply means that this model is better than nothing (Table 7-9).

TABLE 7-9 **EXAMPLE RESULTS FOR THE OVERALL (GLOBAL) TEST**

Testing Global Null Hypothesis: BETA=0			
Test	**Chi-Square**	**DF**	**Pr > ChiSq**
Likelihood ratio	46.0667	6	<0.0001
Score	47.5653	6	<0.0001
Wald	44.9800	6	<0.0001

© Cengage Learning, 2012.

CONCLUSION: The p-values associated with the overall test are small ($p < 0.0001$). Hence, there is sufficient evidence to reject the null hypothesis. At least one of these regressors is related to the outcome.

Hence, a statistically significant p-value indicates that a relationship exists somewhere. It could be with one or two or all of the regressors, but the result does not indicate which regressors are significantly contributing to the relationship or the direction of the associations. To investigate the impact of individual regressors, specific inferences for slopes need to be performed. However, these more specific investigations of the contribution of each regressor can be performed only *after* it has been determined that a relationship exists between at least one of the regressors and the outcome. If the overall hypothesis test results in a large p-value, then the null hypothesis cannot be rejected; there is no evidence of a relationship between the regressors and the outcome. If there is no evidence of a relationship, then there is no reason to continue searching for the contribution of the individual regressors.

Hypothesis Test for Effects

In this example, the proportional-hazards regression model is

$$\ln[h(t)] = \ln[h_0(t)] + \beta_1(\text{prior}) + \beta_2(\text{ground}) + \beta_3(\text{person}) + \beta_4(\text{gender}) + \beta_5(\text{pain}) + \beta_6(\text{age})$$

where $h(t)$ represents the true hazard at time t and $h_0(t)$ represents the unspecified (but positive) baseline hazard.

Whenever a regression contains nominal variables, they are included in the regression as a set of dummy variables that correspond to the levels of the nominal variable (Chapter 3). However, investigating these variables can be confusing. The research question may address the relationship between injury cause (the effect) and time to return to play, for example, but the actual regression results in estimates for each indicator variable. If the dummy variable associated with contact with person results in a nonsignificant p-value but the dummy variable associated with contact with ground has a small p-value, how do you determine whether the cause of injury, in general, is associated with time to return to play? The type 3 effects tests are helpful chi-square tests for the overall effect of each variable, controlling for all other variables in the model (Table 7-10). These are similar to the adjusted sums of squares discussed in Chapter 3.

Type 3 effects are also provided for continuous variables and categorical variables with only two levels. However, because no multiple dummy variables are involved with these values, the p-values for the type 3 effects will be exactly the same as the p-values (corresponding to specific hypothesis tests) for the individual variables.

TABLE 7-10 **EXAMPLE OF TYPE 3 EFFECTS**

Effect	DF	Wald Chi-Square	Pr > ChiSq
prior	1	10.9994	0.0009
gender	1	1.7769	0.1825
age	1	0.4324	0.5108
cause	2	7.6291	0.0220
pain	1	10.5974	0.0011

© Cengage Learning, 2012.

CONCLUSION: Cause-of-injury is the only nominal variable in this model. Cause-of-injury is associated with time to return to play, controlling for all other variables in the model ($p < 0.05$).

Specific Hypothesis Tests

Although the overall and type 3 effects hypothesis tests help in determining whether a relationship exists between the response variable and the regressors, it does not provide answers for investigating specific relationships.

In this example, the proportional-hazards regression model is

$$\ln[h(t)] = \ln[h_0(t)] + \beta_1(\text{prior}) + \beta_2(\text{ground}) + \beta_3(\text{person}) + \beta_4(\text{gender}) + \beta_5(\text{pain}) + \beta_6(\text{age})$$

where $h(t)$ represents the true hazard at time t, and $h_0(t)$ represents the unspecified (but positive) baseline hazard.

Each regressor in the model has a corresponding slope β. If β is 0, then the corresponding variable does not have an association with the outcome. As an example, consider the slope associated with previous injury.

RESEARCH HYPOTHESIS: The slope (β_1) for the history of injury is not 0, after controlling for all other variables in the model.

NULL HYPOTHESIS: The slope (β_1) for the history of injury is 0, after controlling for all other variables in the model.

Both the null and research hypotheses include the statement "after controlling for all other variables in the model." The benefit of using regression analysis is that the estimates for the slopes are obtained while simultaneously adjusting for the other covariates in the model (Table 7-11). In other words, it is assumed that the other variables in the model have slopes that are significantly different from 0.

TABLE 7-11 EXAMPLE OF INFERENCE FOR SLOPES

| | | Analysis of Maximum Likelihood Estimates | | | |
	Level	Parameter Estimate	Standard Error	Chi-Square	Pr > ChiSq
prior	1	−0.71055	0.21424	10.9994	0.0009
gender	0	−0.25677	0.19263	1.7769	0.1825
age		−0.04313	0.06559	0.4324	0.5108
cause	ground	0.67013	0.27154	6.0906	0.0136
cause	person	0.15460	0.28877	0.2866	0.5924
pain		0.14216	0.04367	10.5974	0.0011

© Cengage Learning, 2012.

CONCLUSION: The hypothesis test for the previous injury slope results in a small p-value ($p = 0.0009$). Therefore, it is possible to reject the null hypothesis.

Just as in linear regression (Chapter 3), the interpretation of these parameters is the change in the "response" for every unit increase in the regressor. However, the response in a proportional-hazards regression is not as simple to explain as in linear regression. In a proportional-hazards regression, the response is the left-side of the equation, or $\ln[h(t)]$. Explaining the change in the $\ln[h(t)]$ for every unit increase in the regressor is cumbersome. Therefore, the slopes are not of particular interest for investigators. Luckily, just as in logistic (Chapter 5) or Poisson (Chapter 6) regression, these parameters (β's) can have meaningful interpretations. The slopes in a proportional-hazards regression can be transformed into a measure that is meaningful with time-to-event outcomes—an adjusted hazard ratio. Consequently, the p-values presented with the estimates of the slopes can be transferred to the corresponding hazard ratio estimates.

Adjusted Hazard Ratios

Suppose all other covariates are held constant except for the injury type (first-time injury versus history of injury). Assume first-time injury is coded as prior = 0, and those with previous history of injury are coded as prior = 1. The model for first-time (FT) injury athletes is

$$\ln[h_{FT}(t)] = \ln[h_0(t)] + \beta_1(0) + \beta_2(\text{ground}) + \beta_3(\text{person}) \\ + \beta_4(\text{gender}) + \beta_5(\text{pain}) + \beta_6(\text{age})$$

The model for those with a previous (P) injury is

$$\ln[h_P(t)] = \ln[h_0(t)] + \beta_1(1) + \beta_2(\text{ground}) + \beta_3(\text{person}) \\ + \beta_4(\text{gender}) + \beta_5(\text{pain}) + \beta_6(\text{age})$$

The difference between those with previous of injury and the first-time injured is

$$\ln[h_P(t)] - \ln[h_{FT}(t)] = \beta_1(1) - \beta_1(0) = \beta_1$$

The intercept (the baseline hazard) cancels out, as do all the other covariates that were held constant. The only item remaining on the right-hand side is the slope associated with history of injury.

Recall that the difference in natural logs is equivalent to the natural log of the quotient. In other words,

$$\ln[h_P(t)] - \ln[h_{FT}(t)] = \ln\left[\frac{h_P(t)}{h_{FT}(t)}\right]$$

Therefore,

$$\beta_1 = \ln\left[\frac{h_{\mathrm{p}}(t)}{h_{\mathrm{FT}}(t)}\right]$$

Hence $e^{\beta_1} = \frac{h_{\mathrm{p}}(t)}{h_{\mathrm{FT}}(t)}$ represents the true hazard ratio holding all other variables constant. Holding all other variables constant is the same as adjusting for or controlling for all other variables in the model; so e^{β_1} represents the true adjusted hazard ratio associated with previous injury. Consequently, all the β's in the regression model can be transformed and interpreted as adjusted hazard ratios.

Because e^{β_1} the represents a ratio, determining whether the previous-injury variable is associated with the time to return to play is the same as determining whether the hazard ratio $\frac{h_{\mathrm{p}}(t)}{h_{\mathrm{FT}}(t)}$ is significantly different from 1.

RESEARCH HYPOTHESIS: The hazard ratio $\frac{h_{\mathrm{p}}(t)}{h_{\mathrm{FT}}(t)}$ is not 1, after controlling for all other variables in the model.

NULL HYPOTHESIS: The hazard ratio $\frac{h_{\mathrm{p}}(t)}{h_{\mathrm{FT}}(t)}$ is 1, after controlling for all other variables in the model.

Adjusted hazard ratios for dichotomous, nominal, ordinal, and continuous regressors have the same interpretations as the adjusted odds ratios for dichotomous, nominal, ordinal, and continuous variables discussed in Chapter 5. The only difference is that interpretations involve hazards or risks, not odds.

Interpreting the Results of a Proportional-Hazards Regression

A proportional-hazards regression was performed to investigate how factors (previous injury, cause of injury, and pain) are related to time to return to play, while controlling for confounding variables (age and gender).

In this example, the proportional-hazards regression model is

$$\ln[h(t)] = \ln[h_0(t)] + \beta_1(\text{prior}) + \beta_2(\text{ground}) + \beta_3(\text{person})$$
$$+ \beta_4(\text{gender}) + \beta_5(\text{pain}) + \beta_6(\text{age})$$

where $h(t)$ represents the true hazard at time t, and $h_0(t)$ represents the unspecified (but positive) baseline hazard.

Using statistical software, the output in Table 7-12 results from implementing a proportional-hazards regression and indicates that previous injury is associated with the time to return to play. In fact, the estimated risk of returning to play for those with previous injury is approximately half of the estimated risk of student athletes who were injured for the first time ($\widehat{HR}$: 0.491). The p-value ($p = 0.0009$) is quite small. Therefore, there is sufficient evidence to reject the null hypothesis that the hazard ratio is not 1, controlling for all other variables in the model. This conclusion is further supported by the 95% confidence interval for the hazard ratio [0.32, 0.75]. Because the 95% confidence interval provides a set of plausible values of the true hazard ratio, this suggests that the true hazard ratio is, in fact, less than 1.

In addition to previous injury, both pain score and cause of injury are associated with the time to return to play. As the pain score increases by 1 point, the risk of returning to play increases by 5.8% ($p = 0.0011$), controlling for all other variables. Although the risk of returning to play is nearly twice as great for student athletes injured by contact with the ground compared to those injured by repetition, there is no significant difference between contact with a person and repetition. Finally, age and gender do not appear to be related to the time to return to play but are left in the model because they are known confounders.

TABLE 7-12 **PROPORTIONAL-HAZARDS REGRESSION RESULTS**

Type 3 Tests			
Effect	DF	Wald Chi-Square	Pr > ChiSq
prior	1	10.9994	0.0009
gender	1	1.7769	0.1825
age	1	0.4324	0.5108
cause	2	7.6291	0.0220
pain	1	10.5974	0.0011

Analysis of Maximum Likelihood Estimates								
	Level	Parameter Estimate	Standard Error	Chi-Square	Pr > ChiSq	Hazard Ratio	95% Confidence Limits	
prior	1	−0.71055	0.21424	10.9994	0.0009	0.491	0.323	0.748
gender	0	−0.25677	0.19263	1.7769	0.1825	0.774	0.530	1.128
age		−0.04313	0.06559	0.4324	0.5108	0.958	0.842	1.089
cause	ground	0.67013	0.27154	6.0906	0.0136	1.954	1.148	3.328
cause	person	0.15460	0.28877	0.2866	0.5924	1.167	0.663	2.056
pain		0.14216	0.04367	10.5974	0.0011	1.153	1.058	1.256

© Cengage Learning, 2012.

CONCLUSION: Previous injury, cause of injury, and pain are all related to return to play, controlling for age and gender. Specifically, previous injury, contact with ground (versus repetition) and higher pain scores are associated with increased "risks" of returning to play.

Diagnostics

Models provide a way for investigators to understand how the data might have been produced. Therefore, a model is helpful only if it is appropriate for the data. Residuals can be used to help in assessing how well the proportional-hazards regression model fits the data. However, the residuals in a proportional-hazards regression are not simply observed dependent variable minus predicted dependent variable, as in linear regression. In fact, several different types of residuals have been developed for proportional-hazards regression: Martingale, deviance, Schoenfeld, and Score residuals all have different properties and uses. In particular, the deviance residuals can be used to detect possible outliers, and the Schoenfeld residuals can be used to assess whether the proportional hazards assumption has been violated.

The *deviance residuals* perform similarly to those from the linear regression (Chapter 3) because they can be used to detect outliers (see Figure 7-9). In particular, deviance residuals should be distributed around 0.

- Negative residuals indicate longer than expected survival times for a subject.
- Positive residuals indicate shorter than expected survival times for a subject.
- Very large or very small deviance residuals indicate potential outliers.

The *Schoenfeld residuals* provide a way of checking the proportional hazards assumption. The residuals are computed with one observation per categorical regressor. When these residuals are plotted with time or ln(time), the plot provides a curve for each

Figure 7-9 Example of deviance residuals.
© *Cengage Learning, 2012.*

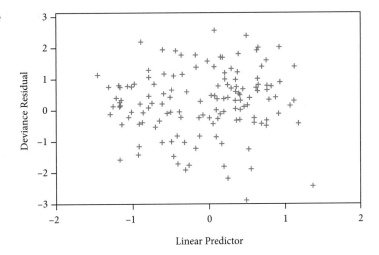

level of the regressor. These curves can be examined to determine whether the pattern indicates proportional hazards or not. If one group has a different time trend compared to another group, then the pattern indicates nonproportional hazards.

An additional strategy for checking the proportional hazards assumption is to include interactions with time in the model. Because the proportional hazards assumption is that the hazards change in the same way over time, a violation indicates that the hazards change differently over time. By definition, group hazards changing differently over time is an interaction. Hence, to test for nonproportional hazards, a regression is performed that includes an interaction of the regressor and time, typically ln(time). Type 3 effects tests can be used to determine whether the interaction is significant (small *p*-value); a significant interaction effect indicates a violation of the assumption of proportional hazards.

The benefit of investigating the proportional hazards assumption with an interaction is that, if the interaction term is significant and indicates a violation, a possible solution is to incorporate the interaction term in the model, which is already done.

Variable Selection

Choosing the variables for a multiple-variable regression can be challenging, and the choice of regressors may depend on the purpose of the study. Hence, variable selection strategies depend on the goals of the regression analysis. There are two primary reasons to perform use regression:

- Forecasting/prediction
- Covariate-adjustment (adjusting for confounders)

Forecasting/Prediction

When forecasting is the primary goal of the regression analysis, the research question focuses on explanatory variables (regressors) and how they impact/predict the outcome. Therefore, choosing an appropriate set of explanatory variables is very important. These regressors need to do a good job of explaining changes in the outcome; so model fit is particularly important. In addition, outliers and influence points must be considered because they may alter the regression estimates. Furthermore, the assumptions of the regression analysis must be rigorously tested because the model is being used to predict outcomes. In fact, other regression models may be more appropriate than the proportional-hazards regression and should be considered.

Covariate-Adjustment

When the research question involves a comparison of groups, while controlling for confounders, the data are generally obtained from an observational study whose groups are defined by something other than random chance. To get a better estimate of the differences between groups, regressors related to group membership and the outcome are included in the regression analysis. Unlike regression analyses whose primary goal is prediction, the selection of regressors in this scenario has much more to do with published literature and an understanding of the groups/outcome than model fit. Although good model fit is important, the primary rationale for selecting a regressor is based more on the context of the problem and less on statistical justification. Accordingly, the first step to variable selection in covariate-adjustment is to consult the literature, and identify variables used in other analyses as potential confounders. A next step can involve data analysis, especially considering descriptive statistics, simple statistical tests, and/or simple regressions. In time-to-event analyses, considering the Kaplan-Meier curves can be very informative as well. Finding unadjusted hazard ratios and conducting simple statistical tests may also be helpful. Generally, candidates for the model are variables that result in small p-values when investigating simple statistical tests. However, the p-value does not at have to be smaller than 0.05 to determine whether variables are potential candidates (e.g., p-values of 0.2–0.3 may be considered). The goal is not to determine statistical significance but to create a subset of variables. If the p-value cutoff for variable selection is too stringent (i.e., $p < 0.05$), important variables may be omitted. When trying to determine whether a variable has an impact, do not focus entirely on the p-value; consider the statistics too.

Strategies for Performing the Regression

A good strategy for performing a regression analysis is to follow the strategies for regression diagnostics.

- Plotting the data is a good first step in identifying variables that may be related to the outcome. Descriptive statistics and bar graphs are helpful. Log-rank tests, Kaplan-Meier plots or proportional-hazards regressions with one regressor may be helpful.
- Once the literature has been consulted, simple tests have been performed, and plots have been created and reviewed, a set of potential variables can be identified.
- Some variables may be measuring the same thing; so potential variables can be further reduced by removing variables that demonstrate multicollinearity.
- With a potential set of regressors, the assumptions of the model can be check and potential outlier/influence points identified. Although outlier and influence points are generally not omitted, an investigation of how removing these points affect estimates may be useful.
- In evaluating the regression output, some variables may not really contribute to the prediction of the outcome. Unnecessary variables can be removed from the model. Be careful in eliminating variables here. If a variable is removed from the model, the estimates are no longer adjusted for that variable.

Using automatic model selection strategies, statistical software can provide a set of variables for the regression model. Although this strategy is reasonable if many potential variables have to be included without guidance for choosing among them, relying solely on automated model selection strategies should be avoided. Many public health problems include variables in the regression for covariate-adjustment and the primary reason for keeping a variable may be based on the literature or on knowledge about the subject, not necessarily on statistical rationale. Hence, relying on automated model selection strategies may have little justification.

SUMMARY

This chapter began with a public health problem: the prevention of injuries in student athletes. Student athletes cannot get the benefits of participating in athletics if they are sidelined by injuries. Moreover, students who return to play too early may be at serious risk for further, more severe injuries. Therefore, understanding factors related to returning to play after an injury is important for coaches, athletic trainers, parents, and policy makers.

The outcome in this study (time to return to play) is a time-to-event outcome and requires special statistical methods for summarizing, comparing, and investigating associations. The concepts of hazard rates and survival probabilities were discussed in the presence of censoring for one, two, and multiple groups. Kaplan-Meier curves and log-rank tests were used for simple comparisons. The chapter concluded by investigating multiple-variable relationships with time to return to play using proportional-hazards regression.

SUMMARY OF CHAPTER CONCEPTS

GOAL	COMMON METHODS	COMMON SUMMARIES	
		Graphical	Numerical
How do I estimate the survival probability?			
Limited number of time intervals	Life-table	Survival curves	Survival probabilities
Many time points	Kaplan-Meier		
How do I compare survival curves (hazard rates)?			
	Log-rank tests	Kaplan-Meier survival curves	Hazard ratios
How do I investigate the association explanatory variables with a time-to-event outcome?			
	Cox proportional-hazards regression	Kaplan-Meier survival curves	Adjusted hazard ratios
How do I compare a hazard rates while controlling for confounding?			
	Cox proportional-hazards regression	Kaplan-Meier survival curves	Adjusted hazard ratios

KEY TERMS

hazard   survival   censoring

PRACTICE WITH DATA

1. COMPARING GROUPS

    a. Provide Kaplan-Meier curves to compare time to return to play for males and females. Perform a log-rank test to compare the curves. What can you conclude?

    b. Create a categorical variable (with at least three levels) for pain. Provide Kaplan-Meier curves to compare time to return to play for different pain levels. Perform a log-rank test to compare the curves. What can you conclude?

2. PROPORTIONAL-HAZARDS REGRESSION

Suppose it is of interest to determine whether cause of injury is related to the time to return to play. Perform a proportional-hazards regression to investigate this relationship while controlling for potential confounders (age, gender, previous injury). Based on the results, provide a conclusion.

PRACTICE WITH CONCEPTS

1. Consider the following research questions/study scenarios. For each study, discuss the most appropriate methods for describing the data (graphically and numerically). What statistical method would be *most* appropriate for addressing the research questions? Be sure to provide a justification of the statistical method. When a statistical test is needed, provide appropriate null and research hypotheses.

    a. Based on the results of a focus group, it is believed that there is a racial disparity in the time it takes physicians to see patients in family practice clinics. A multicenter study is planned to investigate whether there is a difference in the waiting room time for white versus nonwhite patients.

    b. Consider the study in part (a). Suppose the researchers also want to consider the level of injury/sickness, the age of the patient, and the size of the clinic (small, medium, large).

    c. A study was performed to determine whether a new treatment was effective in preventing relapses of Crohn's disease (CD). In the study, 338 patients with irritable bowel syndrome (a possible precursor to CD) were randomly assigned to receive either the new treatment or standard therapy. Data were collected a year after randomization. The primary outcome was time to relapse. Race, blood tests measurements (continuous), and the number of visits to the doctor in the last year were also collected.

    d. A prospective study of subjects undergoing either bariatric surgery or intense diet/exercise regimes is planned. The subjects will be followed for approximately 10 years. The outcome of interest is the time until death. Confounding variables include original weight, comorbid conditions, age, and smoking status.

2. "Older people (aged 65 years and older) are an increasingly important population seen in hospital emergency departments (EDs). Compared with those of younger ages, older people use hospital EDs at higher rates, are more likely to make a return visit, use more resources during a visit, subsequently experience greater

functional decline, and have higher rates of utilization of hospital and community health services. Descriptive studies indicate that early return visits (variously defined) are more often due to the same unresolved problem than later return visits and that many return visits could have been prevented by better management (including treatment and patient and family education)."
(McCusker et al., 2007, pp. 426–427)

a. One of the aims of this study was to investigate the relationship between time to the first return visit (with or without hospitalization) and the relative crowding level, and specialized ED staff to handle elderly patients. Confounding variables included age and gender of the patient, diagnosis at the initial ED visit, and comorbid conditions). Would proportional-hazards regression be appropriate?

b. Below are Kaplan-Meier curves that could result from analyzing data obtained from the study mentioned in part (a). What would you conclude from these curves? Suppose a log-rank test was performed and a chi-square statistic of 4.44 resulted. Provide the hypotheses and conclusions for this log-rank test. (See Figure 7-10.)

c. The authors reported an adjusted hazards ratio estimate of 0.93 (0.87, 0.98) for patients treated in hospitals with geriatric units. Interpret.

Figure 7-10 Kaplan-Meier curves for time-until-first-return visit. © *Cengage Learning, 2012.*

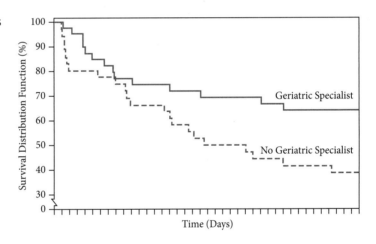

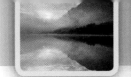
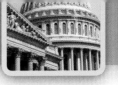
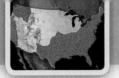
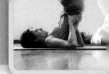

appendix
additional topics

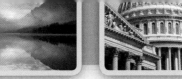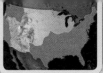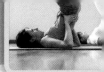

APPENDIX A

correlated data
longitudinal studies

The methods discussed in Chapters 1–7 focus largely on analyses in which each subject contributes one and only measurement, with the goal of comparing groups or looking to see how a variable or a set of variables is related to a single outcome. The methods for analyzing these data assume that the outcomes for the subjects represent a set of independent observations. However, many times in public health, the research requires studying the same subjects over a period of time. *Longitudinal data* occur when the subjects are studied over a period of time and multiple *outcome* measurements are taken on each subject, that is, there are multiple measurements of the dependent variable for each subject. When subjects have an outcome measured multiple times, the observations for each subject are not independent. Measuring subjects at multiple time points allows for research questions that involve comparisons between groups, changes over time, and how groups change over time.

Longitudinal data can be collected on a single group or on multiple groups. Many times the research question involves how some intervention or condition impacts the outcome, and data are collected before the intervention/condition, during the intervention/condition, and for some period after the intervention/condition began. For each subject, there are multiple measurements, usually before, during, and following the intervention/condition. For a particular subject, the measurements before, during, and following the intervention/condition are related or correlated.

If the goal of the study is simply to investigate the change between time points (e.g., the change between before and after the intervention/condition), then a single change outcome is calculated and the methods presented in Chapters 2 and 3 can be used. However, if the goal is to use all time points to investigate a research question, then it is not possible to have a single outcome for each subject. Furthermore, different methods are needed because the outcome is measured a number of times for each subject, and the analyses need to account for the potential correlation that may exist between measurements observed on the same subject.

LEARNING OBJECTIVES

What are longitudinal data?

Understand how and why longitudinal data occur.

Understand how longitudinal data are different from data measured at one point in time.

Why take correlation of observations into account?

Understand the problems with ignoring correlations due to longitudinal data.

What methods are available that account for correlated observations?

Identify potential methods for analyzing longitudinal data.

Understand the advantages of longitudinal data analysis.

Public Health Application

Anemia continues to be a public health problem of global proportions. Severe anemia (hemoglobin <70 g/L) is of particular concern because it poses a significant health and mortality risk. Pregnant women and young children (6–24 mo. of age) are the two groups at highest risk. Severe anemia in pregnant women is associated with an elevated risk of maternal and perinatal mortality (1, 2) and an increased risk of low birth weight and preterm by three-to-five-fold (3). Furthermore, maternal iron status is associated with fetal and infant iron stores and incidence of anemia in infancy (4). Antenatal iron-folic acid supplementation reduces low birth weight and preterm in both developed and developing country settings (5–7).

Few studies have examined the effectiveness of the current treatment recommendations for severe anemia, neither has the efficacy of a different regimen of anthelminthics nor the additional benefit of multivitamin supplementation been tested. Thus, the primary objective of the study was to evaluate the effectiveness of the current standard of care and test the efficacy of an alternative dose of mebendazole and daily multivitamins in the treatment of severe anemia in pregnant women in a periurban, poor population of Karachi, Pakistan.

To test the effectiveness of the standard of care (iron-folic acid and single-dose mebendazole) for treatment of severe anemia, we examined treatment response at the end of the treatment period. To test the enhanced regimens a 2 × 2 factorial, randomized, controlled study design was used. The four treatment groups were as follows: group A received iron-folic acid, mebendazole 500 mg (single dose), and placebo; group B received iron-folic acid, mebendazole 100 mg twice daily for 3 days, and placebo; group C received iron-folic acid, mebendazole 500 mg (single dose), and multivitamins; and group D received iron-folic acid, mebendazole 100 mg twice daily for 3 days, and multivitamins. Group A represents the standard-of-care control.

Characteristics of women at enrollment were compared across the treatment groups. Linear mixed effects regression analyses were done separately for each type of treatment to examine the change in hemoglobin concentration over the duration of treatment (21). This method allows accounting for the within-subject correlation of repeated measurements in estimating the regression variables and their SEs. All analyses were conducted with the use of SAS version 9.1 (SAS Institute, Cary, NC).

[Christian, P., Shahid, F., Rizvi, A., Klemm, R.D.W., Bhutta, Z.A. (2009). Treatment response to standard of care for severe anemia in pregnant women and effect of multivitamins and enhanced anthelminthics. *American Journal of Clinical Nutrition*, 89(3), pp. 853–861.]

In Chapters 2 and 3, a study was described that involved investigating the association of drinking water exposed to herbicides and changes in hemoglobin in pregnant women. Measurements on each of the women in the study were collected throughout the pregnancy—a longitudinal study. However, the analyses presented in Chapters 2 and 3 did not use the longitudinal nature of the data. In fact, the difference between week 9 and week 36 hemoglobins (hemoglobin change) was used as the outcome for each pregnant woman. By taking the difference in the measurements, each woman contributed one and only one outcome, transforming the data from multiple outcomes per subject to one outcome per subject. Although it may be interesting to investigate the change from week 9 to week 36, analyzing the data in this way ignores trends throughout the pregnancy. Analyzing the change allows tests hypotheses about the change between the exposure groups. It does not address research questions regarding how hemoglobin changes throughout pregnancy or whether hemoglobin changes differently throughout pregnancy for different groups.

To investigate how the hemoglobin changes throughout pregnancy for the different groups, multiple measurements of hemoglobin for each participant have to be considered. However, if multiple hemoglobin measures are being observed on each pregnant woman, then the hemoglobin measurements from the same pregnant woman would be related or correlated. For example, if a pregnant woman had a hemoglobin measurement of 10 g/dL at baseline, then a hemoglobin measurement of 14 g/dL would not be expected a few weeks later. In other words, the measurements from time point to time point potentially depend on each other (Figure A-1). When measurements are correlated, then independent observations is no longer a reasonable assumption.

The statistical methods presented in Chapters 2 and 3 assumed that the hemoglobin outcomes were independent. To take into consideration the multiple hemoglobin measures throughout the pregnancy, statistical methods are needed that account for the fact that the measurements are no longer independent.

Like the example presented in Chapters 2 and 3, the public health application study investigates hemoglobin over the course of the pregnancy. In this example, however, severely anemic women were randomly assigned one of four treatments: a standard of care control group (A) and three supplement groups (B, C, and D). In this example, women were assessed at baseline, and a 7, 28, 60, and 90 days post-treatment. Utilizing the longitudinal nature of the data allows for subject-specific and population-level research questions.

RESEARCH QUESTION:
Are there hemoglobin changes over the pregnancy within subjects, and/or are there changes in hemoglobin over the pregnancy between subjects?

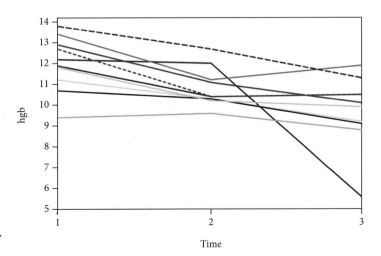

Figure A-1 Hemoglobin profiles.
© *Cengage Learning, 2012.*

The Assumption: Independence

In Chapter 3, the discussion of linear regression (and ANOVA) involved assumptions on the error term. Specifically, the errors for the models are supposed to be independently and identically distributed as normal variables with a mean of 0 and a constant variance. In longitudinal studies, the assumption of independence is violated.

For linear regression (and ANOVA) models, the assumption of independence can be visualized by considering the **variance-covariance** matrix (Table A-1). A variance-covariance matrix has the subjects as rows and columns. The subjects match up along the diagonals, and this diagonal contains the variance. Covariances occur when different subjects are in the row and column combinations.

The common variance assumption implies that each error has the same variance. The independence assumption implies that all errors are uncorrelated or that the correlation for any two errors is 0. Recall from Chapter 3 that the correlation is $r = \dfrac{\text{Covariance } (e_i, e_j)}{\sigma_i \times \sigma_j \times n}$. Therefore, if all of the correlations are 0, then the covariance for any two errors is also 0. In summary, the independence of the errors implies that the variance-covariance table has

- The variances in the diagonal cells
- 0's everywhere else (Table A-2)

The 0's everywhere else represent the independence assumption, and the same variances on the diagonal represent the common variance assumption.

In this example, where hemoglobin is measured throughout the pregnancy, measurements were made at baseline, day 7, day 28, day 60, and day 90. The variance-covariance matrix is now more complicated because each subject has multiple measurements (Table A-3).

There are still 0's wherever the row subject is different from the column subject because the subjects are still assumed to be independent. However, for each subject. there is now a variance matrix, which represents the relationship between the time points for each subject. In this example, each subject has three measurements (Table A-4). In the table, the variances can still be the same, but assuming the covariances are all 0 is not valid. The hemoglobin measured at day 28 is expected to be correlated to the hemoglobin measured at day 60 and day 90 because

TABLE A-1 VARIANCE-COVARIANCE MATRIX

	Subject 1 Error	Subject 2 Error	...	Subject N Error
Subject 1 Error	Variance	Covariance	Covariance	Covariance
Subject 2 Error	Covariance	Variance	Covariance	Covariance
...	Covariance	Covariance	Variance	Covariance
Subject N Error	Covariance	Covariance	Covariance	Variance

© Cengage Learning, 2012.

TABLE A-2 VARIANCE-COVARIANCE MATRIX (COMMON VARIANCE AND INDEPENDENCE)

	Subject 1 Error	Subject 2 Error	...	Subject N Error
Subject 1 Error	Variance (σ^2)	0	0	0
Subject 2 Error	0	Variance (σ^2)	0	0
...	...	...	...	...
Subject N Error	0	0	0	Variance (σ^2)

© Cengage Learning, 2012.

TABLE A-3 **VARIANCE-COVARIANCE MATRIX (MULTIPLE MEASUREMENTS)**

	Subject 1 Time1 Time2 ... Time *t*	Subject 2 Time1 Time2 ... Time *t*	...	Subject N Time1 Time2 ... Time *t*
Subject 1 Time 1 Time 2 ... Time *t*	Variance Matrix	0's	0's	0's
Subject 2 Time 1 Time 2 ... Time *t*	0's	Variance Matrix	0's	0's
. . .	0's	0's	Variance Matrix	0's
Subject N Time 1 Time 2 ... Time *t*	0's	0's	0's	Variance Matrix

© Cengage Learning, 2012.

TABLE A-4 **VARIANCE-COVARIANCE MATRIX FOR A SUBJECT (MULTIPLE MEASUREMENTS)**

	Baseline Error	Day 7 Error	Day 28 Error	Day 60 Error	Day 90 Error
Baseline Error	Variance	Covariance	Covariance	Covariance	Covariance
Day 7 Error	Covariance	Variance	Covariance	Covariance	Covariance
Day 28 Error	Covariance	Covariance	Variance	Covariance	Covariance
Day 60 Error	Covariance	Covariance	Covariance	Variance	Covariance
Day 90 Error	Covariance	Covariance	Covariance	Covariance	Variance

© Cengage Learning, 2012.

the hemoglobin values come from testing the same pregnant woman. Hence, if the measurements are correlated, the errors associated with them are correlated, and the assumption of independent errors is violated.

Impacts of Violating the Assumption

The violation of the independence assumption is more than just an issue of an inappropriate model. The lack of independence in the errors actually has an impact on the inferences. Recall that the *p*-values resulting from statistical tests and confidence intervals all involve the standard error. The standard error is actually obtained from the variance-covariance matrix. When observations are correlated, this affects the standard error. In particular, in longitudinal studies, observations measured on the same subject are generally positively correlated. When they are, the positive correlation causes the variances between groups to be larger. If the correlation is ignored, then the variances (and standard errors) used to compare groups are underestimated. In other words, ignoring the correlation results in a smaller standard error. Small standard errors mean smaller *p*-values and tighter confidence intervals. Therefore, ignoring the correlation could incorrectly result in a significant *p*-value (increases the type 1 error rate). When investigating within-subject effects, ignoring the positive correlation can result in overestimating the variance. In this case, the standard error is too large, and potentially significant associations may be missed. Additionally, ignoring the correlation can lead to biased parameter estimates as well.

Correcting for the Violation: Linear Mixed Models

Luckily, several options are available for addressing the potential correlation within subjects. These options exist for continuous outcomes (as in this example) and for categorical outcomes. Also, the methods (and statistical software procedures) are not very different from the methods for independent observations. For continuous outcomes, the most common (and flexible) method is the linear mixed model.

When there are only two correlated observations and the goal is simply to compare differences in one group, the method that handles correlated continuous outcomes has already been discussed: the one-sample paired *t*-test. This test subtracts the two correlated observations (before and after, for example), providing a statistical test that accounts for the correlation between the two measurements. However, the test does not allow for comparison between groups. When there are only two measurements and comparison between groups is desired, an alternative is to calculate the change score and to compare the groups using an analysis of covariance (ANCOVA). This was done in Chapter 3. When the change score is calculated, it is important to control for the initial measurement; so an ANCOVA is necessary. Often, if there are only two measurements, then the preferred approach is to calculate the change score and to use the initial measurement as a confounder. Also, given only two measurements, the data are not really longitudinal and investigating how subjects or groups change over time is less interesting.

When there are multiple time measurements, however, these simpler methods do not provide sufficient methods for analyzing the data and for investigating the research question. To investigate changes within subjects and/or to determine whether groups change differently over time, a linear mixed model can be used. Linear mixed models, like linear regression models, allow for the investigation of multiple explanatory and confounding variables at the same time.

The most important feature of a linear mixed model is that it can handle correlated outcomes. In particular, it has the flexibility to handle many different types of variance-covariance structures. For example, hemoglobin measurements at the end of the study would be expected to be more correlated than the first and last hemoglobin measurements. A linear mixed model can be implemented to specify this relationship between the measurements. Using the linear mixed model framework, the correlation among the errors can be handled by selecting the variance-covariance structure most appropriate for the longitudinal data. Additional options for linear mixed models account for subjects with different starting values (baseline hemoglobin) and/or situations where the subjects change differently over time.

Another advantage of using linear mixed models for longitudinal data is how missing data are handled. One of the challenges with longitudinal data is missing outcomes. Because data are collected over time, subjects are unlikely to be available for all measurements. Missing data can occur throughout the study. Instead of deleting subjects without a complete set of outcomes, a linear mixed model analyzes all available data for each subject. Therefore, in a linear mixed model, the sample size can differ from time point to time point.

In the linear mixed model, the structure of the data is said to be *long*. There is a variable for time and a variable for the outcome. Subjects occur in multiple rows, making the dataset long. In the example in Table A-5, there would be three values for the time variable; so subjects have up to three rows of data.

So far, only continuous outcomes have been discussed, but it is likely that longitudinal studies in public health will result in multiple measurements of a discrete or categorical outcome. For example, suppose the outcome was anemia at each time point. If that is the case, the outcome would be dichotomous (Table A-6). Linear mixed models are no longer appropriate because the outcome can no longer be described with a mean. However, *generalized* linear mixed models allow for different distributional assumptions and models. For example, a generalized linear mixed model with the binomial distribution and logit(p) can be used to investigate how the probability of anemia changes over time and whether the groups impact the probability of anemia over time. Hence, this generalized linear mixed model would essentially be a longitudinal version of logistic regression.

TABLE A-5 **EXAMPLE OF DATA STRUCTURE FOR LINEAR MIXED MODEL**

Subject ID	Age	Race	Time	Hgb
12221-A	25	W	0	11.1
12221-A	25	W	7	10.9
12221-A	25	W	28	10.1
12227-A	34	B	0	11.2
12227-A	34	B	7	11.1
12227-A	34	B	28	11.0
12227-A	34	B	60	10.2
12227-A	34	B	90	9.3
13445-A	21	O	0	10.2
13445-A	21	O	7	10.1

© Cengage Learning, 2012.

TABLE A-6 **EXAMPLE OF DATA STRUCTURE FOR LINEAR MIXED MODEL**

Subject ID	Age	Race	Time	Severe Anemia
12221-A	25	W	0	0
12221-A	25	W	7	0
12221-A	25	W	28	0
12227-A	34	B	0	0
12227-A	34	B	7	0
12227-A	34	B	28	0
12227-A	34	B	60	1
12227-A	34	B	90	1
13445-A	21	O	0	0
13445-A	21	O	7	0

© Cengage Learning, 2012.

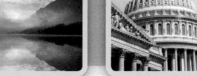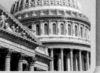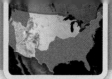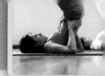

correlated data
clustering and
hierarchies

The methods discussed in Chapters 1–7 focus largely on designs in which each subject is independent and no correlation exists between subjects. However, especially in public health studies, assuming that the subjects are independent is not always appropriate. Often, public health studies involve interventions and policies that impact whole communities or groups, not just the individual. When individual subjects are studied as part of a whole community or group, it is not fair to assume that subjects belonging to the same community or group are not correlated.

For example, suppose a sample of physicians are recruited to help study the impact of a healthy lifestyle intervention. The patients of the physicians are surveyed to obtain data on weight and lifestyle characteristics. A patient chooses to see a particular physician for many reasons (insurance, location, gender, etc.). Furthermore, physician interactions with patients differ from one physician to another. Therefore, patients associated with the same physician are likely to be correlated. Subjects belonging to the same group or community are not a set of independent observations; these subjects form clusters of observations. Studying subjects in clusters is often referred to as *cluster trials*, where the intervention or characteristic being studied is applied to the cluster and measurements are obtained from the subjects in a cluster. When subjects are considered as clusters, special analyses are needed to account for the potential correlation between subjects within the same cluster.

What is a cluster?

Understand how and why clustering of data occurs.

Why take clustering into account?

Understand the problems with ignoring correlations due to clustering.

What methods are available when clusters are suspected?

Identify potential methods for analyzing data that naturally occur in clusters.

Public Health Application

Insecticide-treated bed nets (ITN) provide real hope for the reduction of the malaria burden across Africa. Understanding factors that determine access to ITN is crucial to debates surrounding the optimal delivery systems. The influence of homestead wealth on use of nets purchased from the retail sector is well documented, however, the competing influence of mother's education and physical access to net providers is less well understood.

The study set out to look at predictors of use of nets by children <5 years of age obtained from the retail sector, as these represent the principal sources of nets during the periods leading up to the time of the survey. Therefore, children who used nets purchased from the retail sector were compared to those who did not use nets. Children who used nets from sources other than the retail sector were excluded from the regression analysis. First, a univariate regression analysis was performed to identify which of the predictor variables were significant to the outcome measure, that is, use of nets purchased from retail sector by children. These predictors defined homestead, mother and child characteristics. In the univariate analysis the odds ratio (OR), p-value and 95% confidence interval (CI) for each factor's association with nets purchased from the retail sector were computed. Any factor with a p-value <0.15 was considered to be a potentially important covariate of retail-net use. The

factors examined were homestead wealth assets index; gender of homestead head; homestead demographics; travel time to the nearest market centre; homestead use of insecticide residual spraying (IRS); whether any homestead member attended public malaria awareness meeting (baraza) or owned printed education materials on malaria; whether mother could read; mother's education level (no education, primary incomplete, primary complete and secondary and above); mother's main source of income; mother's marital status; whether mother was pregnant; age of the child; sex of the child; and child's ownership of a health card.

All variables meeting the entrance criteria were used to estimate a multivariable logistic regression model to identify their combined effect on the use of nets purchased from the retail sector among children. The model was fitted using the STATA xtgee command with an exchangeable working correlation matrix. This procedure uses generalized estimating equations (GEE) to account for the potential correlation of use of nets purchased from the retail sector among children seen in the same [area] while accounting for the variability between clusters.

[Noor, A.M., Omumbo, J.A., Amin, A.A., Zurovac, D., Snow, R.W. (2006), Wealth, mother's education and physical access as determinants of retail sector net use in rural Kenya. *Malaria Journal, 5*(5).]

Many times, conducting studies as cluster trials is more economical and practical. For example, if the goal is to investigate the impacts of using insecticides in a region, treating an entire area may be more feasible than treating individual homes. A cluster trial might randomly select sites for implementing (or not implementing) the insecticide treatment. The purpose of using insecticide is to decrease the occurrence of disease, and whether a disease occurs is measured on the individual. For example, it may be of interest to compare the percentage of new malaria cases for those living in insecticide-treated areas versus the percentage of those living in untreated areas. The insecticide-treated area (or cluster) was the unit that was randomized to receive or not receive the treatment, but the individuals were measured for the outcome. In a cluster trial, the unit that is randomized (or assigned a treatment) is not necessarily the unit that is measured. When there are really two levels of subjects—cluster and individual—designing and analyzing the study can get a bit confusing.

Because cluster trials have (at a minimum) two levels, planning a cluster study involves planning at least two levels. It would not be appropriate to perform a cluster trial on only two areas—one that received an insecticide treatment and one that did not—because there is only one cluster per treatment. Thousands of individuals may be living in the cluster, but only one cluster receives each treatment, making it a sample size of 1 at the cluster level. Although there are many individuals, this study would have limited power to compare the differences between the groups. Hence, when planning for cluster trials, having a large number of smaller clusters is better than having a small number of large clusters.

Another example of a cluster trial occurs in studies involving children and schools. Suppose insecticide-treated nets are to be dispersed at schools. An intervention is planned in which some schools receive instruction on the benefits of net use along with insecticide-treated nets, and control schools only receive insecticide-treated nets. This is another example of when randomizing the individual children is not practical. Even if the children were randomized, the children in the same household could be randomized into two different groups Furthermore, even if schools or classrooms were randomized to receive the intervention, parents in the intervention group could communicate to parents in the control group and thus cross-contaminate the study group. For this reason, it may be more practical to randomize school districts. Randomizing school districts would limit the potential for cross-contamination of the intervention. Therefore, a hierarchy develops where schools within a school district may be correlated, grades within a school may be correlated, classrooms within a grade may be correlated, and students within a classroom may be correlated. A hierarchical structure of increasing correlation quickly develops. Cluster studies are sometimes referred to as *hierarchical studies* because there is a hierarchy of relationships. Hierarchical and cluster studies can use the same types of statistical methods as other designs where the subjects are no longer independent. Given the hierarchies that naturally exist in the data, when presenting the results of a cluster/hierarchical study it may be helpful to provide a flowchart describing the clustering/hierarchies (Figure B-1).

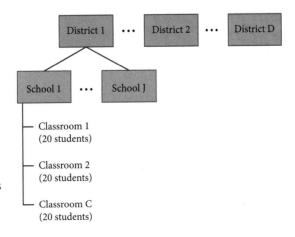

Figure B-1 Example of hierarchies of clusters.
© *Cengage Learning, 2012.*

Point to Ponder

Not all trials where subjects are clustered result in more complicated analyses. The complexity all depends on the unit of analysis. When the unit of analysis is a member of a cluster, then the independence assumption is violated. If, however, the unit of analysis is the cluster, the same methods discussed in Chapters 2–7 can be used. For example, suppose districts were randomized to receive (or not receive) instructions on using mosquito nets. If the research question involves the children in the district, this is another example of a cluster study. However, if the research question involves the rate of absenteeism in each district, this is not a cluster study because the measurement is on the same unit that receives the treatment: the district and the districts (subjects) are not correlated. In this case, a set number of districts are randomized to receive or not receive the assembly, the subject is the district, and the absenteeism rates between the two groups of districts are compared. This comparison of absenteeism rates can be easily made using the methods discussed in Chapter 6 (or even Chapters 2 and 3) because there is no violation of independence between the subjects.

The Assumption: Independence

RESEARCH QUESTION: What factors are related to net utilization for children under the age of 5?

In this example, a comparison of children under 5 years of age using and not using nets was conducted. Specifically, children using nets purchased from a retail sector were compared to children who did not use nets (Figure B-2). Children associated with a particular retail sector might be similar. For example, the households using the same retail sector may be located in the same region, share the same water source, or attend the same schools. Therefore, children associated with the same retail sector form a cluster of children, and children in the same retail sector cluster are not assumed to be independent.

To investigate net utilization in this study, methods that take into consideration the potential correlation of subjects in the same cluster must be used.

In Chapter 5, logistic regression was used to investigate the factors involved with net utilization. However, the assumption was that each household was independent and that the actions of one household had nothing to do with those of another. In this example, the children who used insecticide-treated nets were selected using the retail sector. Because children whose parents use the same retail sector may be correlated, assuming independent subjects is no longer valid.

The correlation between children in the same retail sector is not expected to be very strong. The measure of correlation between subjects in the same cluster is referred to as the *intracluster correlation coefficient*, which is a correlation (discussed in Chapter 3). An intracluster correlation coefficient, however, is a correlation between any two subjects in the same cluster.

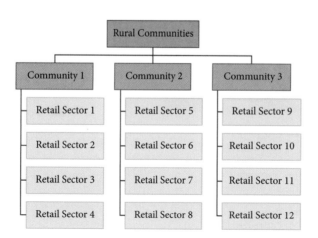

Figure B-2 Clustering of households.
© *Cengage Learning, 2012.*

When observations are independent, the correlations between subjects are all 0, and there are no relationships between subjects. A correlation matrix represents how the subjects are related to each other. When the subjects are independent, the correlation table has the correlations of 1 in the diagonal cells and 0's everywhere else (Table B-1). The 0's everywhere else represent the independence assumption.

In this example, where the retail sectors serve as clusters, children belonging to the same retail sector are considered correlated. The correlation matrix is now more complicated because subjects within a cluster are correlated (Table B-2).

There are still 0's whenever the row cluster is different from the column cluster because subjects in different clusters are still assumed to be independent. However, for each cluster, there is now a correlation matrix, which represents the relationship between the subjects for each cluster. In this example, with M subjects for each cluster, the M subjects within a cluster are not assumed to be independent (Table B-3).

The intracluster correlation coefficient (ρ) is typically positive and small in cluster trials. In fact, values around 0.02 are reasonable. Even though this value is quite small, it can have significant impacts on inferences and sample sizes.

TABLE B-1 **CORRELATION MATRIX (INDEPENDENCE)**

	Subject 1	Subject 2	...	Subject N
Subject 1	1	0	0	0
Subject 2	0	1	0	0
...	...	...	...	...
Subject N	0	0	0	1

© Cengage Learning, 2012.

TABLE B-2 **CORRELATION MATRIX (CLUSTERS)**

	Cluster 1 Subject 1 Subject 2 ... Subject M	Cluster 2 Subject 1 Subject 2 ... Subject M	...	Cluster K Subject 1 Subject 2 ... Subject M
Cluster 1 Subject 1 Subject 2 ... Subject M	Correlation matrix	0	0	0
Cluster 2 Subject 1 Subject 2 ... Subject M	0	Correlation matrix	0	0
. . .	0	0	Correlation matrix	0
Cluster K Subject 1 Subject 2 ... Subject M	0	0	0	Correlation matrix

© Cengage Learning, 2012.

TABLE B-3 **CORRELATION MATRIX FOR A CLUSTER (*M* SUBJECTS)**

	Subject 1	...	Subject M
Subject 1	1	ρ	ρ
...	ρ	1	ρ
Subject M	ρ	ρ	1

© Cengage Learning, 2012.

Impacts of Violating the Assumption

The violation of the independence assumption entails more than just an issue of an inappropriate model. The lack of independence actually has an impact on the inferences. Recall that the *p*-values resulting from statistical tests and confidence intervals all involve the standard error. Correlated observations affect the standard error. In particular, these observations are positively correlated, and the positive correlation causes the variances between groups to be larger. If the correlation is ignored, then the variances (and standard errors) used to compare groups are underestimated. In other words, ignoring the correlation results in a smaller standard error. Small standard errors mean smaller *p*-values and tighter confidence intervals. So ignoring the correlation could quite possibly and incorrectly result in a significant *p*-value (increasing the type 1 error rate).

Furthermore, sample size calculations are based on how large or small the variance is; the larger the variance is, the larger the required sample size will be. The correlation for subjects within the same cluster inflates the variance. Hence, cluster trials often require larger sample sizes.

Correcting for the Violation: GEEs and GLMMs

Luckily several options are available for addressing the potential correlation of subjects belonging to the same cluster. These options exist for dichotomous outcomes (as in this example), categorical outcomes, and continuous outcomes. Also, the methods (and statistical software procedures) are not very different from the methods that do not allow correlated observations.

For categorical outcomes, a common method for accounting for the correlation due to clusters is called *generalized estimating equations (GEEs)*. In this example, a generalized estimating equation is really just a logistic regression that allows for a more flexible correlation matrix. The most important feature of a generalized estimating equation is that it can handle correlated outcomes. In particular, it has the flexibility to handle many different types of correlation structures.

Generalized estimating equations are fairly straightforward to implement because they can be reduced to generalized linear models (logistic regression, log-binomial regression, negative binomial regression, Poisson regression, etc.) when there is only one cluster. Furthermore, the regression estimates obtained from using generalized estimating equations are fairly robust, even with many clusters or an incorrectly specified correlation matrix. Finally, the regression estimates that result from using generalized estimating equations are considered to be population-averaged, or marginal, estimates.

In addition to generalized estimating equations, *generalized linear mixed models (GLMMs)* may also be used. Generalized linear mixed models offer a considerable amount of flexibility in specifying the structure of correlations due to clustering. Furthermore, these models are useful when subject-specific estimates are of interest. These types of models are often utilized when implementing analyses that involve hierarchical models.

Another advantage of using generalized estimating equations and generalized mixed models for clustered data is that both of these models can handle clusters of differing sizes. (Clusters are not likely to be exactly the same size.)

For generalized estimating equations and generalized linear mixed models, the structure of the data is said to be *long*. There is a variable for the cluster and a variable for the outcome. Subjects occur in multiple rows, making the dataset long. In the example in Table B-4, there are three subjects in retail sector A and five subjects in retail sector B.

When cluster or hierarchical studies are implemented, the outcome may be continuous and normally distributed. In this case, linear mixed models can be used in a similar way to account for the potential correlation between subjects belonging to the same cluster.

TABLE B-4 **EXAMPLE OF DATA STRUCTURE**

Subject ID	Age	Wealth Index	Retail Sector	Net Use
12221-A	3	1	A	14.1
12222-A	2	2	A	13.9
12223-A	1	4	A	10.1
12237-B	3	3	B	12.2
12236-B	4	3	B	12.1
12237-B	4	2	B	11.0
13445-B	2	1	B	13.2
13445-B	1	1	B	9.3

© Cengage Learning, 2012.

adjusted mean: The mean that has been estimated while controlling for potential confounding variables.

adjusted odds ratio: An odds ratio that is created while controlling for confounding variables.

age-adjusted rates: Event rates that have been standardized using a reference population; used when comparing event rates to another population that has a different age distribution. A common reference population is the 2000 U.S. population obtained from the U.S. 2000 Census.

association: A measure of how much one variable changes when the other variable changes. When the variables move in the same direction, the association is positive but when the variables move in different directions the association is negative.

balanced design: A design when a study is planned to compare different groups and the groups have the same number of subjects.

biased sample: A sample in which only certain members of the population are chosen so that the sample systematically misrepresents the population.

categorical variables: Variables where the possible responses are limited to a certain set of values or categories.

censoring: Occurs when an event occurs outside the observation window. Events can be *right censored*, *left censored*, or *interval censored*. Right-censored events occur when the event time is greater than the last time the subject was observed. Left-censored events occur when the event time is less than the first time the subject was observed. Interval-censored events occur when the event time is between two observation times.

census: A survey or collection of data on all members of the population.

conditional probabilities: the proportion of subjects with an outcome given they have a particular characteristic.

confounding variables: Variables that are not of primary importance but that are collected and included in the model because they could potentially influence the relationship between the response and explanatory variables.

contingency table: A table in which the categories of one variable make up the rows and the categories of another variable make up the columns. The cells of the contingency table provide the number of subjects that belong to a particular category of the row variable *and* a particular category of the column variable.

continuous variables: Variables where the possible responses are numeric values without natural *gaps* between the values.

count variables: Variables where the possible responses are only positive, whole number values (0, 1, 2, …).

data: Pieces of information that result when measurements are obtained from the subjects of interest in the research question and/or hypothesis.

degrees of freedom: Independent pieces of information needed to estimate parameters and variability; found in several distributions (e.g., *t*-distribution and *F*-distribution).

dichotomous variables: A type of categorical variable that *can have only two levels*.

distribution: A summary of the possible values for a variable and the number of times (either by count or proportion) that the values occur.

dummy variable: A variable that takes on values 0 and 1. Often used in regression analyses so that nominal variables can be included in the model.

effect modifier: A confounding variable that alters the relationship between the explanatory and response variables. An interaction exists when the relationship of two variables depends on the level or category of another variable. Effect modification occurs when there is an interaction between the explanatory and confounding variables. *Also known as* interaction.

explanatory variable: A variable that explains a change in the response or dependent variable.

F-distribution: A common distribution used for statistical inference that is dependent on degrees of freedom for its shape. The F-distribution has two sets of degrees of freedom: one for the numerator ($n_1 - 1$) and one for the denominator ($n_2 - 1$). The F-distribution starts at 0 and is skewed to the right. How skewed it is depends on how large the degrees of freedom are in the numerator and the denominator.

five-number summary: The summary of the median, first and third quartile, and minimum and maximum.

hazard: A hazard function provides a description of the event rate at different time points. The hazard at any particular time is just the risk of the event at that particular interval of time: number of events divided by the time interval. Therefore, the hazard function is simply hazard rates over time.

historical controls: Estimates of the true parameter that were found using data from a different study; for example, from a different time period, a different region, different population, or a different exposure; often used in one-sample studies when the control data are not collected concurrently within the same study.

hypotheses: Statements that describe an expected result and that can be tested using empirical results.

independent groups: Groups of subjects where the measurements obtained from one group have nothing to do with measurements obtained from any other group.

influence point: A point that has extreme explanatory values; generally discussed in the context of a regression analysis.

longitudinal study: A study whose subjects are followed for a period of time and whose outcome is measured multiple times throughout the study.

margin of error: The amount that is added or subtracted to the point estimate to make it an interval estimate.

multicollinearity: When any of the regressors are highly correlated, the regressors are collinear and the regression is said to suffer from multicollinearity. When multicollinearity is a problem then the estimates become unstable and inferences (statistical tests and confidence intervals) become unreliable.

nominal variables: A type of categorical variable that can have multiple levels but the order of the levels does *not* matter.

odds: The ratio of the proportion of successes to failures.

one-sample paired *t*-test: A test in which the mean is obtained from the paired differences of one sample; determines whether there is sufficient evidence against the null hypothesis.

ordinal variables: A type of categorical variable that can have multiple levels and the order of the levels matters.

outlier: A point that lies outside the pattern of the other datapoints; can be an extreme point with respect to the explanatory variable, the response variable, or both; generally discussed in the context of a regression analysis.

overdispersion: In Poisson regression models, it is assumed that the outcome comes from a Poisson distribution, where the mean and variance or equal. When the variance is larger than what would be expected, the model suffers from a problem of overdispersion.

***p*-value:** The proportion of statistics that are even farther from the null parameter than the observed statistic.

paired differences: The difference or between two responses measured on the same subject. Paired differences are often found when considering the change or the difference between pre- and post- measurements taken on the same subject.

parameter: A number that describes the population; the numerical summary of the population that answers a research question.

percentiles: A proportion of all the observations that are less than the value of interest.

person-time: In studies where count is the outcome, subjects may have varying amounts of observation time. The total amount of time each subject contributes is the person-time. It represents the denominator of an event rate and so rates are often reported in units of person-time. *Also known as* subject-years, subject-months, or subject-days depending on the unit of time measured.

point of curvature: The point at which a curve goes from concave down to concave. In the normal distribution, the point of curvature represents one standard deviation.

population: All possible subjects of interest.

power: The probability that a null hypothesis will be rejected when it is false.

prevalence rate: A proportion obtained from a study where the data were collected at one point in time (cross-sectional study).

random sample: A sample from the population in which the subjects in the sample were chosen by random chance.

regressor: A variable that appears on the right-hand side of the model equation; any variable that is associated with a slope in a regression.

reliability: A characteristic of measurements that have little variability. (Variability in measurements occurs when multiple measurements are taken on a subject.)

response variable: The outcome of interest. *Also known as* dependent variable.

risk: A proportion obtained from a study where the data were collected prospectively.

robust: The term used to describe a numerical summary that is not easily affected by extreme points.

sample: A smaller set (or a subset) of the members of the population.

sampling frame: A list of the population.

sampling variability: When different samples of subjects are chosen, the samples will not be exactly the same.

sensitivity: A conditional probability often used to determine how well screening/diagnostic tests perform in identifying unhealthy subjects; the probability that the screening test correctly classifies sick subjects as sick.

sequential random sampling: A sample in which a random number generator is used to select a single number *s*, after which every *s*th subject is selected.

significance level: The probability of making a type 1 error. The significance level is often set at 5%, or 0.05, and is represented as α.

skewed: A distribution having extreme values (large or small) so that a tail of the distribution extends longer in one direction. The distribution is *left skewed* when the histogram has a tail that extends farther to the left or where there exists a set of observations with lower values than the majority of the observed responses. The distribution is *right skewed* when the histogram has a tail that extends farther to the right or where there exists a set of observations with higher values than the majority of the observed responses.

specificity: A conditional probability often used to determine how well screening/diagnostic tests perform in identifying healthy subjects; the probability that the screening test correctly classifies healthy subjects as healthy.

standard deviation: The square root of the variance; always positive.

statistic: A number that describes the sample; the numerical summary of the sample that answers a research question.

stratified odds ratio: The odds ratios for each level of a confounding variable.

stratified random sample: Potential subjects are first divided into subgroups, or strata, and simple random samples are conducted within the strata.

survival function: Provides a description of the non-event rate at different time points. The survival at any particular time is just the probability that the event will occur at a time later. Therefore, the survival function is just a series of proportions of subjects that have event times beyond each time point.

symmetric: A characteristic of a distribution by which the distribution can be folded in half so that each half is close to a mirror image of the other.

systematic random sample: A sample obtained when a number *s* is randomly selected so that every *s*th subject is selected to be in the sample.

***t*-distribution:** A common distribution used for statistical inference, resembling a normal distribution in shape. The mean and the median are in the center at the peak. However, the tails of the *t*-distribution are a little thicker than those of the normal distribution. Thicker tails imply a greater possibility of observing values in the tails. As the sample size increases, the *t*-distribution more closely resembles a normal distribution.

test statistic: A numerical summary from the sample that is standardized or transformed so that common, known sampling distributions can be used to test hypotheses.

total sum of squares: The sum of the squared differences from the mean.

type 1 error: The error occurs when the null parameter is rejected as the true parameter when the null parameter really is the true parameter.

type 2 error: The error that occurs when the null hypothesis is not rejected but is false.

underdispersion: In Poisson regression models, it is assumed that the outcome comes from a Poisson distribution, where the mean and variance or equal. Underdispersion occurs when the variance is smaller than expected.

variance: The average squared distance that each observation is from the mean.

Agresti, A., & Corporation, E. (1990). *Categorical data analysis* (Vol. 5). Wiley Online Library.

Agresti, A., & Finlay, B. (1997). *Statistical methods for the social sciences.* Upper Saddle River, NJ: Prentice Hall.

Aiken, L., West, S., & Reno, R. (1991). *Multiple regression. Testing and interpreting interactions.* Thousand Oaks, CA: Sage Publications, Inc.

Allison, P. (2005). *Fixed effects regression methods for longitudinal data using SAS.* Cary, NC: SAS Publishing.

Allison, P. (2010). *Survival analysis using SAS. A practical guide.* Cary, NC: SAS Publishing.

Brown, H., & Prescott, R. (2006). *Applied mixed models in medicine.* Chichester: J. Wiley and Sons.

Chow, S., Shao, J., & Wang, H. (2007). *Sample size calculations in clinical research.* 2nd ed. Boca Raton, FL: Chapman & Hall/CRC Biostatistics Series: CRC Press.

Cohen, J. (2003). *Applied multiple regression/correlation analysis for the behavioral sciences.* Mahwah, NJ: Lawrence Erlbaum.

Cummings S.R., & Melton L.J. (2002). Epidemiology and outcomes of osteoporotic fractures. *The Lancet, 359*(9319), 1761–1767.

Donner, A., & Klar, N. (2000). *Design and analysis of cluster randomization trials in health research.* Wiley.

Edward, HS (2001). Visualizing multiple regression. *Journal of Statistics Education, 9*(1) http://www.amstat.org/publications/jse/jse_2001/v9n1/ip.html.

Fleiss, J., Levin, B., Paik, M., & Wiley, J. (1981). *Statistical methods for rates and proportions.* 2nd ed., New York: John Wiley.

Francis, L., Weiss, B.D., Senf, J.H., Heist, K., Hargraves, R. (January–February 2007). Does literacy education improve symptoms of depression and self-efficacy in individuals with low literacy and depressive symptoms? A preliminary investigation. *Journal of the American Board of Family Medicine, 20*(1), 23–27.

Hosmer, D., & Lemeshow, S. (2000). *Applied logistic regression.* New York: Wiley-Interscience.

Hosmer, D., Lemeshow, S., & May, S. (2008). *Applied survival analysis: Regression modeling of time to event data.* Hoboken, New Jersey: Wiley-Interscience.

Jewell, N. (2004). *Statistics for epidemiology.* Boca Raton, FL: CRC Press.

Littell, R. (2006). *SAS for mixed models.* Cary, NC: SAS Publishing.

Littell, R., Stroup, W., & Freund, R. (2002). *SAS for linear models.* Cary, NC: SAS Publishing.

Liu, P., Yuen, Y., Hsiao, H.M., Jaykus, L.A., Moe, C. (2010, January). Effectiveness of liquid soap and hand sanitizer against Norwalk virus on contaminated hands. *Applied and Environmental Micorbiology, 76*(2), 394–399. (E-eub: November 20, 2009).

Loong, T-W. (2003, September). Understanding sensitivity and specificity with the right side of the brain. *British Medical Journal, 327*(716).

McCusker, J., Ionescu-Ittu, R., Ciampi, A., Vadeboncoeur, A., Roberge, D., Larouche, D., Verdon, J., Pineault, R. (2007, May). Hospital characteristics and emergency department care of older patients are associated with return visits. *Academic Emergency Medicine, 14*(5), 426–433. (E-pub: Mar 16, 2007).

Milliken, G., & Johnson, D. (2001). *Analysis of messy data, volume III: Analysis of covariance* (1st ed.). Chapman and Hall/CRC.

Rosner, B. (2006). *Fundamentals of biostatistics.* Boston: Duxbury Resource Center.

Scheffé, H. (1999). *The analysis of variance.* New York: Wiley-Interscience.

Snedecor, G. (1938). Statistical methods applied to experiments in agriculture and biology. *The Journal of the American Medical Association (JAMA), 110*(16), 1312.

Stokes, M., Davis, C., & Koch, G. (2000). *Categorical data analysis using the SAS system.* Cary, NC: SAS publishing.

Walker, G. (2002). *Common statistical methods for clinical research with SAS® examples.* Cary, NC: SAS Publishing.

Warner, R. (2008). *Applied statistics: From bivariate through multivariate techniques.* Thousand Oaks, CA: Sage Publications.

West, S.D., Nicoll, D.J., Wallace, T.M., Matthews, D.R., Stadling, J.R. (2007, November). Effect of CPAP on insulin resistance and HbA1c in men with obstructive sleep apnoea and type 2 diabetes. *Thorax, 62*(11), 969–974. (E-pub: June 8, 2007).

Young, G., & Smith, R. (2005). *Essentials of statistical inference,* Cambridge University Press.

Zelterman, D. (2002). *Advanced log-linear models using SAS* Cary, NC: SAS Publishing.

sample range, for continuous data, 38–39
samples, 4–5
    sample size, 29–30
    random, strategies for obtaining, 5–6
    statistics for, 10
    variability between, 20–21
sample size, 29–30
    categorical variables, 164–166, 191, 286
    continuous variables, 51–55, 69–72, 82, 117, 149
    for correlation, 117
    for multiple regression, 149
    for multiple samples, 82
    for one-sample, 51–55, 164–166
    for two-sample, 69–72, 191, 286
    time to event variables, 286
sampling distributions
    central limit theorem and, 21–23
sampling frame, 5, 6
sampling variability, 20
scatterplots, 92–93, 96
Scheffe adjustment, 81–82
Schoenfeld residuals, 294–295
sensitivity, in numerical summaries, 200–201
sequential sum of squares, 127
signed rank tests, 56–57
significance levels, 28
    Bonferroni adjustment to, 81–82
simple linear regression. *See* linear regression
simple random sample, 5
skewed data
    continuous data, 37
    distributions, 36–37
    numerical summary, 103
    outliers as, 113
skewed distributions, 17–18
slope
    confidence levels for, 109–110
    for count dependent variables with multiple
      regressors, 250
    equation for, 102
    hypothesis tests for, 107–109, 130–132, 252–253
    for logistic regression, 210–211
    in logistic regression, hypothesis tests
      for, 213–214
    in models, 100
    for multiple linear regression, 121
    for proportional hazards regression, 288–289
    in simple linear regression, 99
Spearman rank correlation coefficient, 95
specificity, in numerical summaries, 200–201
spread, measures of, for continuous data, 36–39
SSM (sum of squares model), 126, 128
standard deviations, 10
standard errors
    for Kaplan-Meier method, 276
    for one-sample proportions, 163–164

    for one-sample *t*-tests, 47
    for proportion differences, 183
    for proportions ratios, 185–186
    for rate ratios, 247
    for unequal variances, 66
statistical inference, 1, 23–29
statistics
    definition of and notations for, 10–11
    test statistics, 23
stratified contingency tables, 203–205
stratified odds ratio estimates, 203
stratified random samples, 5
study designs, 6–7
    balanced designs, 69
    cross-sectional, 7, 160
    hypothesis testing in, 25–29
    longitudinal, 35
    planning, 29–30
    prospective, 6, 159
    retrospective, 6
    See also planning studies
subjects of study, 4
    determining number of, in planning
      studies, 29–30
    graphical summaries of, 11–23
    numerical summaries of, 9–11
    study designs for, 6–7
    variable types, 7–9
    See also populations
Sum of Squares Total (SST), 76
survival analysis, 267
survival functions, 271–272
survival probabilities, 272, 274
symmetric distributions, 16
systematic random samples, 5

T

t-distribution (*t*-test)
    nonzero correlation *t*-test, 97–98
    one-sample *t*-tests, 46–47
    for two-group comparisons, 80–81
    two-sample *t*-test with equal variances,
      60–61
    two-sample *t*-test with unequal variances, 67
telephone sampling, 6
testing studies, 30
test statistics, 23
time-to-event data, 267, 270
    censoring in, 272–279
    group comparisons for, 279–286
    Kaplan-Meier method for, 274–277
    life-table method for, 277–279
    numerical and graphical summaries of,
      270–272
    planning two-sample studies using, 286
    proportional hazard regression for, 287–296

Tukey adjustment, 81–82
two-sample studies
    with continuous outcomes, 57–73
    with continuous outcomes, with equal
        variances, 59–63
    with continuous outcomes, nonparametric
        tests for, 72–73
    with continuous outcomes, planning, 69–71
    with continuous outcomes, with unequal
        variances, 63–69
    with count data, 244
    with count data, rate ratios for, 244–248
    with dichotomous outcomes, 191–192
    effect size, 54
two-sample *t*-test with equal
    variances, 60–61
type 1 errors, 27–28
    in multiple-sample studies, 81–82
    statistical power and, 28–29
type 2 errors, 28
    statistical power and, 28–29
type 3 effects, 212–213
    in logistic regression, 212–213, 218
    in Poisson regression, 251
    in proportional hazards regression, 291

U

unadjusted means, 140
unimodal distributions, 16

V

variability
    between samples, 20–21
    within and between subjects, 20
    total variability, 104

variables, 1
    associations between, 92
    confounding variables, 138–139, 202–203
    continuous variables, 33, 89
    count variables, 8–9
    explanatory and response (independent and
        dependent) variables, 98
    noncontinuous regressor variables, 133–136
    regressor variables, 118
    time to event variables, 267. *See also* specific
        types of variables
    types of, 7–9
variable selection
    in logistic regression, 226–227
    in multiple linear regression, 147–148
    in Poisson regression, 260–262
    for proportional hazards regression, 295–296
variance
    Analysis of Variance, 76–77
    of binomial distributions, 14
    for continuous data, 36–37
    in Poisson distribution, 18–19
    in two-sample studies, with equal
        variances, 59–63
    in two-sample studies, with unequal
        variances, 63–69

W

Wilcoxon (Mann-Whitney) U test, 73
within subject controls, 48–50
within (residual) sum of squares (SSE), 77

Z

z-scores, 19
z-tests, one-sample, 161–162